*Stories of Illness and Healing*

જી

*Literature and Medicine*
MARTIN KOHN AND CAROL DONLEY, EDITORS

# Stories of Illness and Healing

ૐ

## Women Write Their Bodies

ૐ

Edited by Sayantani DasGupta

& Marsha Hurst

ૐ

The Kent State

University Press

KENT, OHIO

ૐ

For Kirin, Sunaya, Caleb, and Oliver

૪ð

© 2007 by The Kent State University Press, Kent, Ohio 44242
ALL RIGHTS RESERVED
Library of Congress Catalog Card Number 2007005266
ISBN 978-0-87338-916-7
Manufactured in the United States of America


11  10  09  08  07     5  4  3  2  1


LIBRARY OF CONGRESS CATALOGING-IN-PUBLICATION DATA
Stories of illness and healing : women write their bodies / edited by Sayantani DasGupta
and Marsha Hurst.
p.   cm.—(Literature and medicine ; no. 10)
Includes index.
ISBN 978-0-87338-916-7 (pbk.: alk. paper) ∞
1. Women—Diseases—Psychological aspects.  2. Patients' writings—History and criticism.
3. Body image in women.  I. DasGupta, Sayantani.  II. Hurst, Marsha.
R726.5.S764 2007
616.0082—dc22
2007005266


British Library Cataloging-in-Publication data are available.

# Contents

ഉ

# *Preface*

୫ବ

THIS COLLECTION of women's narratives was compiled in order to examine
the powerful variety of women's experiences regarding illness and healing.
In doing so, it gives voice to alternate experiences of illness that go beyond
prescriptive medical categories of disease. In addition, by presenting personal
stories alongside more academic analysis, this collection aims to place women's
subjective experience on an equal ground to more traditional scholarly writing
in the construction of knowledge. This collection is intended for both scholars
and students of narrative, illness, and women's experience, as well as men and
women interested in, affected by, and working with illness.

The authors in this collection are a group of women diverse in age, ethnicity, education, socioeconomic background, sexual orientation, nationality,
profession, and writing experience. The work of three authors is published
posthumously. Although the majority of authors are from the United States and
Canada, we have contributors from India, Australia, the United Kingdom, the
Netherlands, and former Yugoslavia. While some contributions were solicited
from known scholars and authors, the majority of authors in this collection
found us—having seen our call for submissions, or, more frequently, having
been encouraged to submit by friends and family who had seen our call. This
collection represents a variety of women's illness narratives—poetry, essays,
short fiction, short drama, analyses, and even transcribed oral testimonies.

The editors of this collection are two health care educators; one of us is a
political scientist and the other a physician by training. We have both done additional advanced work in community and public health and have been involved
in developing curricula and teaching health care professionals to appreciate the
experience of sickness and suffering through narratives of illness. Our common
work involves the teaching of health advocacy to master's degree students who
come to our program from health care disciplines, including nursing, medicine, speech therapy, and social work, and from other professions and careers,
including law and business, and, in a few cases, directly from undergraduate
training. In addition, one of us (SD) is also involved in training medical students
and pediatric residents through the reading and writing of narrative texts, as

well as teaching at a writing seminar for health care professionals, ill individuals, and their families. We approach our work with this anthology not only as educators and professionals, but as a white woman and a woman of color, of middle and younger adult years, as daughters, mothers, and spouses who have experienced illness personally and in our familial circles. We aim, in our own analyses and in our teaching, to acknowledge the variety and richness of illness experiences and to value the impact of gender, culture, ethnicity, nationality, class, and sexuality. We wish to hear not only individual voices and stories, but how those voices are interconnected.

This book draws on the important distinction between illness and disease. While disease, a malfunctioning of biological processes in a patient, is usually the focus of traditional medical practices, illness represents that individual's personal reaction to the disease or discomfort. Illness is shaped by subjective perceptions, symbolic meanings, and value judgments that arise from an individual's culture, identity, and environment.[1] Although the work in this collection will encompass individuals with diseases that fall into traditional categories, including cancer, mental illness, eating disorders, and chronic diseases, the impact of these diseases on women's lives lies beyond these potentially limiting categories. Therefore, this book is organized with an organic framework that emerges from the narratives themselves rather than groupings based on disease alone. In doing so, we acknowledge that women's illness experiences are more than their diseases; they encompass their entire lives as workers, teachers, writers, and family and community members.

The writing in this book is divided into seven sections: Narratives of Body and Self: The Experience of Illness; Narratives of Diagnosis and Treatment: Relationships to the Medical Community; Narratives of Womanhood: Social Constructions of Body, Sexuality, and Reproduction; Narratives of Family Life and Caregiving; Narratives of Professional Life and Illness; Narratives of Advocacy: From the Personal to the Political; and Narratives of Advocacy: Activism, Education, and Political Change. Of course, these categories are fluid; there are essays about the experience of illness that have activist themes, stories about family life that have to do with diagnosis and treatment, and so on.

We would like to acknowledge, first and foremost, our students, without whom this anthology would never have been written. Not only was this book born of a desire to find such a collection that we could use in our classroom teaching, but it was inspired by the innovative and revealing writing of our students regarding their own illness experiences. We are indebted to them for teaching us to appreciate the nuance, richness, and power of expressions of illness. We would like to also thank our colleagues who supported and encouraged us in the writing of this book, including Rita Charon, Cortney Davis, Arthur Frank, David Watts,

Penny Wolfson, and Carol Levine. The faculty in our respective departments at Sarah Lawrence College, Columbia University, and Montefiore Hospital, as well as the Narrative Medicine Program at Columbia University and the Writing the Medical Experience Seminars at Sarah Lawrence College, provided professional and moral support. This book could never have been completed without the work and support of the staff of the Health Advocacy Program at Sarah Lawrence College, especially Crystal Greene and graduate assistants Alexandra Roberti, Emily Macel, and Diana Alvarez. We must profusely thank, for tireless hours given in support and childcare, Sujan DasGupta, Shamita Das Dasgupta, and Boris Mueller. Finally, we gratefully acknowledge Elsie Hurst for her invaluable organizational assistance and Richard J. Hiller for generous and loving pro bono legal counsel.

NOTES

1. Arthur Kleinman, *The Illness Narratives: Suffering, Healing, and the Human Condition* (New York: Basic Books, 1988).

# The Gendered Nature of Illness

SAYANTANI DASGUPTA AND MARSHA HURST

THIS BOOK IS AN INVITATION into the suffering body. What lies within this text concerns the experience of illness, a territory that was once the sole purview of the medical practitioner, hidden from even the sufferer. This book is a collection of voices speaking what was once unspoken, making public what was once private. This book is a collection of illness narratives, each one "a story that the patient tells, and significant others retell, to give coherence to the distinctive events and long-term course of suffering."[1] The illness narrative does not merely reflect the experience of illness; it contributes to that experience by giving coherence, symbolism, and meaning to what might otherwise have been a chaotic experience. Telling stories about illness puts the experience in personal and social contexts, reflecting the individual's symbolic cultural interpretation of events.

"Telling stories about illness is to give voice to the body," writes sociologist Arthur Frank. Bodies are not just the topics of stories, but "the body sets in motion the need for new stories when its disease disrupts the old stories."[2] Particularly in Western cultures, where mind and body are often constructed as dualities, illness carries with it the potential for not only physical but psychic devastation—whereby the ill person may be forced to confront a previously unconsidered physical self. The illness narrative has the potential to bridge this fractionated personhood. Self-stories allow individuals to construct meaning from otherwise devastating life events, repair the disruption caused by illness to their healthy life narrative, and reclaim power from other narratives of the experience, including the medical narrative.

This book is, in addition, an invitation into the experience of the female sufferer and, ultimately, the relationship between gender and illness. This relationship is nuanced and complex, impacted by the gendered constructions of medicine, health, voice, and vulnerability. It is ultimately also impacted by the construction of gender itself. Although this book does not include the voices of transgendered individuals, we do acknowledge that the notion of two fixed, distinct genders is an inherently social construction. Within the traditional

male-female framework, we know that certain diseases do seem to discriminate by gender: prostate and certain sex-specific cancers including testicular
for men, and cervical, uterine, ovarian, and, usually, breast cancer for women,
not to mention rheumatologic diseases, which predominantly seem to affect
women and girls, or sex-linked diseases like Duchenne muscular dystrophy,
which predominantly affect men and boys. But what this book addresses is not
just the *what* of illness (as in, what disease?) but the *how* of it—as in, how does
illness affect our lives? How does it fit into our life stories or culturally based
explanatory models of health? How does it affect our self-image, family relationships, professional identity, sexuality, and spirituality? How does it impact
the care we receive and the interactions with our health care providers? How
does it inspire activism or draw us into new communities of fellow sufferers?
This *how* of illness is fundamentally tied, of course, to who we are and our
many complex identities—gender being but one of them. Women's stories, like
the stories of other marginalized communities, have the potential of revealing
alternate truths that expand traditional medical narratives since the way that
women experience illness and medical treatment is very much dependent on
broader social constructions of gender in society. In addition, both men's and
women's stories are impacted by the gendered construction of health and illness
in medicine itself.

Pediatrician-writer Perri Klass has a story about her medical school experiences called "Macho" that illustrates as well as any theoretical essay the impact
of gendered constructions upon the medical profession:

> Macho in medicine can mean a number of things. . . . You can hear echoes of
> it in the strongest praise one can receive in the hospital, "Strong work," which
> may be said to an intern who got a very sick patient through the night or to
> a medical student who successfully fielded some obscure question on rounds.
> And the all-purpose term of disparagement is "Weak." They're being really
> weak down in the emergency room tonight, admitting people who could just
> as well be sent home. Dr. So-and-so is being weak with that patient—why
> doesn't he just tell him he *has* to have the surgery? . . . Macho can refer to your
> willingness to get tough with your patients. . . . It can refer to your eagerness to
> do invasive procedures—"The hell with radiology, I wanna go for the biopsy"
> . . . . Macho can mean territoriality: "These are *our* patients and *we* make all
> the decisions." . . . The essence of macho, any kind of macho . . . is that life is a
> perpetual contest.[3]

If doctors, potentially of both genders, are supposed to be "macho," then
patients are constructed as the opposite—weak, passive, feminine. Indeed, in

the Western tradition of Cartesian dualism, the intellect has been primarily associated with the masculine, while the body, with its frailties, illnesses, and disabilities, has been associated with the feminine. The Western origins of this dichotomy regarding illness can be traced to the late nineteenth century. The frail woman patient of that time was set in stark contrast to the capable male physician. Medical practices created this dichotomy by promoting a cult of female invalidism and notions of hysterical women.[4] A classic example of this notion is in Charlotte Perkins Gilman's "The Yellow Wallpaper," in which a woman suffering from neurasthenia—and who is quite pointedly the wife of a physician—is robbed of paper, pen, and essentially all adult intellectual activity while she is treated with the "rest cure."[5] And even though today the "macho" physician may be a woman and the "weak" patient may happen to be a man, these gendered constructions of health and illness remain.

Both male and female writers of illness narratives must grapple with this gendered stereotyping of health as masculine and illness as feminine. It is in the work of some male writers of illness narratives that the feminization of illness can be seen clearly. Illness and disability may be the first time that these men have been forced to contend with the social construction of their bodies. In an essay titled "Occasional Notes: Compounding the Ordeal of ALS: Isolation from My Fellow Physicians," Dr. David Rabin writes that when he initially passed off his disabilities as resulting from essentially masculine activities such as sports injuries, he was still socially accepted among his peers. However, when his ALS (amyotrophic lateral sclerosis) diagnosis became known, it made him professionally invisible—with one colleague literally pretending he did not see him as he lay in the middle of a hospital courtyard after a fall. Although Rabin does not explicitly call his disease emasculating, he does articulate the requirements for belonging to the profession of medicine. He writes, "The dichotomy of being both a doctor and a patient threatens the integrity of the club. To this fraternity of healers, being ill is tantamount to treachery."[6]

Similarly, writer and journalist John Hockenberry writes in his memoir *Moving Violations: War Zones, Wheelchairs, and Declarations of Independence*[7] about his experiences as a disabled man in America. In a section where he struggles to do as simple a task as hailing a cab in New York from a wheelchair, Hockenberry is explicit about the different treatment he received while on assignment in the Middle East: in his narrative, it is New York that is the war zone. While Hockenberry resists the label of what he calls the "supercrip"—the disabled person able to overcome all odds through personal willpower—his narrative is in many ways an aggressive reassertion of his masculinity. He tells of the dangers of reporting from war-torn countries, of his sexual exploits, and of his reaction to NYC cabbies resistant to picking him up—puncturing their tires with a Swiss Army knife or in one case punching in the driver's side glass of the car. Hockenberry's narrative is both an analysis of and reaction to the sociocultural construction of male disability.

Conversely, women have historically been circumscribed, judged, and silenced through their bodies, irrespective of their illness status. Lucy Grealy's *Autobiography of a Face* chronicles her life with Ewing's Sarcoma of the jaw and multiple reconstructive surgeries. "My face, my self,"[8] she writes, risking reinforcing the notion that women's realities are determined solely through their bodies. However, hers is a narrative continuously aware of not only her physical disability, but the social disability of a woman whose appearance and therefore beauty, femininity, and sexual attractiveness deviate from a socially determined normalcy. Although male writers like Hockenberry also contend with the impact of illness and disability upon sexuality, Grealy's experience is uniquely feminine. Rather than being ignored by taxi cab drivers, Grealy is actively ridiculed for deviating from the accepted feminine norm.

"Children stared at me," she writes, "and I learned to cross the street to avoid them. This bothered me but not as much as insults I got from men. They weren't thrown at me because I was disfigured, they were thrown at me because I was a disfigured woman . . . Had I been a man, would I have had to walk down the street while a group of young women followed and denigrated my sexual worth?"[9]

In her essay "Carnal Acts," Nancy Mairs writes about the double shame of not only openly discussing the details of disability, but female disability. "By speaking about it, and about the whole experience of being a body, specifically a female body, out loud . . . drowns out the frantic whispers . . . 'Ssh! Ssh! Nice girls don't talk like that. . . Don't mention sweat . . . Don't mention menstrual blood . . . Don't tell.'" Like Lucy Grealy's disfigured face, Mair's leg brace is an additional burden to a woman already struggling with sexual and social acceptability. Writes Mairs, "The idea of going around with my bare brace hanging out seemed almost as indecent as exposing my breasts."[10] Like ethnicity, sexuality, or class, illness adds yet another layer to the identities of these women writers.

Illness narratives are, then, perhaps particularly important for women, who have historically had their bodily experiences defined, categorized, and encapsulated through narratives structured by the patriarchal medical system. The medicalization of women's health has sought to narrowly define experiences such as puberty, childbirth, or menopause, attributing them to biological "truths" and ignoring the impact of culture, ethnicity, nationality, class, or sexuality. To listen to women's individual voices is to acknowledge the variety of women's experiences and move beyond narrow, medically defined categories. Prior to the professionalization of medicine, illness was a private experience located within families and traditionally under the dominion of women. With the rise of the medical profession, the illness experience became primarily removed from private suffering to a public experience mediated by physicians. Therefore, listening to the stories of women allows for a new understanding of the relationship of those individuals to themselves, but also to their medical caregivers, their families, and their communities. The story of women's illness narratives is the story of the personal made public, or, if you will, made political. In the words of medical educator Delese Wear, this sort of storytelling recognizes that "when we write ourselves through our bodies . . . [we] affirm the fluidity of women's corporeality; generate ways of knowing that may take us beyond ourselves—certainly beyond prescriptive medical narratives; and serve as fertile ground for the construction of collective, always shifting realities."[11]

The invitation into this text is not without risk. In the words of physician and writer Richard Selzer, "I feel some hesitation to invite you to come with me into the body. It seems a reckless, defiant act."[12] By inviting you into these stories of suffering, this book risks participating in and facilitating a kind of voyeurism, whereby suffering is "construed at a safe distance, without the social responsibility of real engagement."[13] At the very least, these narratives run the risk shared by both medicine and literature, a risk emerging from their nature as representational, a risk of becoming totalizing enterprises. In the words of Levinas scholar Craig Irvine, "A work of literature is not the naked face of a patient's suffering. Rather it is the representation, the identification of this face."[14]

Recent published illness narratives of otherwise public figures, including, among others, athlete Lance Armstrong, reporter John Hockenberry, and television film critic Joel Siegel,[15] reflect a very literal desire to "identify the face" of illness. This is totalizing to an extreme, whereby there exists a story that is *the* cancer narrative, *the* Alzheimer's narrative, *the* woman's narrative, and so on. It is important to remind ourselves that illness narratives, and particularly published illness narratives, represent a distinct minority of those who suffer from disability and illness. For each individual who has the skill, facility, and time to translate her story into writing, let alone the ability to publish that writing, there are countless others whose stories remain unheard. These stories are often those that are difficult to hear—angry stories of medical mistreatment, stories of socially marginalized individuals such as prisoners, and stories that are unresolved and still in the midst of chaos.[16] The practice of eliciting, witnessing, and recording oral stories is one methodology by which to bring to public attention these stories that might otherwise have remained private suffering.

Whether written or oral, illness narratives are not only important to those who do the telling but to those whom they are told. Indeed, illness stories are inherently social and usually presuppose an audience. This audience can be the physician or the friends and family who listen to the ill person's verbal tale, the support group who reacts to the shared journal entry, the community of sufferers who reads a personal story in a newsletter, health care scholars and students who study a published poem about sickness, or the wider public who reads a variety of published work about illness and health. How, then, is the reader of this volume to position him or herself? It can perhaps be posited that not only listeners, but readers of illness narratives can engage in what Arthur Kleinman calls "empathetic witnessing." Empathetic witnessing involves "the existential commitment to be with the sick person and to facilitate his or her building of an illness narrative that will make sense of and give value to the experience."[17] And so, in answering this call of the suffering body—these narratives of women's illness experiences—the reader becomes engaged in a very critical and special position: the reader becomes witness.

What, then, is the responsibility of the reader in the face of this volume's invitation? Whether man or woman, student or teacher, health care provider or patient, policy maker or family caregiver, you, the reader of this volume, are invited to engage with these narratives and allow them to engage with you—impacting not just your personal understanding of illness but the public ways in which you apply that understanding. Be it activism, education, policy making, advocacy, family caregiving, or personal transformation, this book is ultimately an invitation to translate the witnessing of suffering into empathy, care, and action.

## Notes

1. Arthur Kleinman, *The Illness Narratives: Suffering, Healing, and the Human Condition* (New York: Basic Books, 1988) 49.

2. Arthur Frank, *The Wounded Storyteller: Body, Illness, and Ethics* (Chicago, IL: U of Chicago P, 1995) 2.

3. Perri Klass, "Macho," *A Not Entirely Benign Procedure: Four Years as a Medical Student* (New York: Plume, 1994) 80.

4. Barbara Ehrenreich and Dierdre English, *Complaints and Disorders: The Sexual Politics of Sickness* (Old Westbury, NY: Feminist Press, 1973).

5. Charlotte Perkins Gilman, *The Yellow Wallpaper* (New York: Feminist Press, 1973).

6. David Rabin et al., "Occasional Notes: Compounding the Ordeal of ALS—Isolation from My Fellow Physicians," *New England Journal of Medicine* 307 (1982): 508.

7. John Hockenberry, *Moving Violations: War Zones, Wheelchairs, and Declarations of Independence* (New York: Hyperion, 1995).

8. Lucy Grealy, *Autobiography of a Face* (New York: Harper Collins, 1995) 170.

9. Grealy 67.

10. Nancy Mairs, "Carnal Arts," *Minding the Body: Women Writers on Body and Soul*, ed. Patricia Foster (New York: Anchor Books, 1994) 267–82.

11. Delese Wear and Lois LaCivita Nixon, *Literary Anatomies: Women's Bodies and Health in Literature* (Albany, NY: SUNY Press, 1994) 2.

12. Richard Selzer, "The Surgeon as Priest," *Mortal Lessons: Notes on the Art of Surgery* (New York: Simon and Schuster, 1996) 25.

13. Arthur Kleinman and Joan Kleinman, "The Appeal of Experience; The Dismay of Images; Cultural Appropriations of Suffering in Our Times," *Social Suffering*, ed. Arthur Kleinman, Veena Das, and Margaret Lock (Berkeley: U of California P, 1997) 10.

14. Craig Irvine, "The Other Side of Silence," *Literature and Medicine* 24 (2005): 10.

15. Lance Armstrong with Sally Jenkins, *It's Not About the Bike: My Journey Back to Life* (New York: Putnam Adult, 2000); Hockenberry, *Moving Violations;* Joel Siegel, *Lessons for Dylan: From Father to Son* (New York: Public Affairs Books, 2003).

16. Frank.

17. Kleinman, *Illness Narratives* 54.

# The History of Women's Illness Narratives: Private Relationships, Public Voices

## Marsha Hurst and Sayantani DasGupta

MODERN AMERICAN women's illness narratives are a product of a long history of women's illness stories. The history of women's illness narratives reveals a tension between private experience and public voice. In addition, the history of women's illness narratives is a history of women's relationships—their caregiving and caring connections.

Very few, if any, historic records remain of women's oral illness narratives. However, women's diaries and letters give a glimpse into their experiences of illness and caregiving. For instance, the diaries of Martha Ballard, a turn-of-the-nineteenth-century New England midwife, reveal much about the social connections surrounding women's illness and reproduction. Ballard earned a material living attending births and caring for the sick while she mothered her own children, attended to her husband, and struggled with the ardors of rural life.[1] Similarly, diarist Martha Farnsworth from late nineteenth-century midwestern America cared for first one, then another husband, an infant daughter and a niece, and lived a life so exhausting that the deaths of those she loved felt liberating. The diary that Farnsworth leaves sets her personal experience within a changing context of health care: during her first husband's illness, she was supported by the caring of friends and neighbors; during her second husband's illness, caring had become an isolated and lonely endeavor—friends called on the newly adopted telephone instead of coming to help.[2] These women's diaries very much set personal experience in the context of social and cultural life at those historic times. As diaries, however, the question of intended audience is a looming one: Is the gaze of the modern reader an intrusion into an experience that had no access to public expression?

Women's narrative voices have historically also been expressed in letters, particularly important as women used these written accounts of their lives to maintain the social and familial connections so important to the structure of their worlds. One of the most famous surviving breast cancer narratives is English novelist and diarist Fanny Burney's chilling account of her 1811 mastectomy—without anesthesia. Burney tells this story in a letter to her sister, Esther.

My dearest Esther, not for days, not for Weeks, but for Months I could not speak
of this terrible business without nearly again going through it! I could not think
of it with impunity! I was sick, I was disordered by a single question—even now,
9 months after it is over, I have a headache from going on with the account! &
this miserable account, which I began 3 Months ago, at least, I dare not revise,
nor read, the recollection is still so painful.[3]

Burney tells us that she found even the recollection painful, and we feel her pain
not only in the operation but in the telling of her story. She tells this story not only
to Esther, her sister, but to "all my dears" to whom Esther retells the story. Hers
was very much a narrative meant to be shared. Although the particular medical
details of Burney's experience may not be shared by modern women with grave
illness, the legacy of Burney's letters to this collection's modern narratives is this
impetus to tell one's story and give voice to what feels unspeakable.

Similarly, Deborah Vinal Fiske, a mid-nineteenth-century New Englander,
used letters written, as she grew increasingly sick from consumption, to express
her remaining sense of agency as a mother, wife, and friend. Fiske's was a narrative of "chronic illness and social obligation."[4] She wrote two sets of letters, one in
a public voice—letters of morals and manners for her daughters, lessons meant
to continue Fiske's caring motherly duties beyond her own death—and one in
a private and personal voice, connecting her suffering with ties of friendship
and family, and, as her illness progressed, expressing intense bonds with other
female "invalids." These letters tell of an experience of illness that undercuts
women's duties as wives, mothers, and community members.

Diary and letter writing, albeit in electronic forms, continue to be a common
way in which women express their illness stories. Like the private voice of the
diary, the limited intended audience of Fiske's personal letters perhaps makes
them more problematic. Does making public a private documentation of suffering amount to a type of voyeurism? In the case of letters, which are one step
removed from the personal intimacy of the diary, the reader is perhaps still an
interloper, albeit one whose gaze is aligned with an external, intended recipient.
The modern technology of e-mail is for this reason interesting; e-mail combines
the intimacy and informality of a diary with the connectedness of a letter. Modern
women often use both diary excerpts and e-mail correspondence to share their
experiences of sickness, particularly when they choose to have their narratives
reflect the rawness of the immediate experience of illness and healing.

Most modern women's illness narratives are, however, not written in diary
or e-mail form. Rather, they are essays and stories written for a wider audience.
Historically, too, we see women writing stories with illness themes. In 1892,

Charlotte Perkins Gilman wrote the famous short story "The Yellow Wallpaper."[5] Although Gilman had written this classic narrative of illness constructed by and through women's societal role, she refused to let the narrative of her own life be one of illness. When she was diagnosed with incurable breast cancer in 1932, Gilman "chose chloroform over cancer." She left her readers only the epilogue to her autobiography, a narrative testament to the importance of choice in dying, not to the experience of living with illness.

By the time Gilman died of cancer in the 1930s, however, women were writing about their illness experiences in popular magazines. In particular, narratives of breast cancer, because it is primarily a woman's disease, can provide a historical thread of women's illness narratives more than any other disease. In this way, the historic thread of one disease acts as a frame for the way women experiencing illness see themselves as women, and see their role in society.[6] Unlike the previous historic narratives that were written in order to share a painful experience with friends and loved ones, these published articles were often narratives of advocacy written for a public audience to "remove the terror" from the experience of illness in the hope that women would come forward sooner for medical help—to "put themselves in the hands of their doctors."[7]

In the writing of women of the New Deal era we hear the experiences of women who were outspoken, activist, and socially involved, and who turned their illness experience into advocacy. The women of the 1950s were more focused on their post–World War II role as wives, mothers, and homemakers, and their physical image of hourglass perfection was part of the picture. Terese Lasser had a radical mastectomy for breast cancer in 1952.

> There is, indeed, a Valley of Despair, desolate, solitary, swept by anguish, darkened by confusion. I, too, have been there. . . . [W]hen told that my right breast had been removed, I wanted to shrivel up and die. How could I face life, a scarred woman? . . . How could such a life be worth living? . . . And—most tormenting thought of all—what about my husband? . . . Suppose, in spite of his love and his devotion, he should be repelled by me? . . . Was it possible for a man to desire a woman who wasn't whole? Suppose all my husband could feel for me now, all he would ever be able to feel, was pity?—so that never again would he need me, or reach for me as a man reaches for a woman? If that were to be so, better not to be alive at all. [8]

Lasser's private experience became a public crusade. Her program, Reach to Recovery, survives today because Lasser marched into women's hospital rooms and told her story to women who thought they were completely alone. Historic and modern readers of her writing are an audience being invited to action. Here, we see the early history of women's personal storytelling being translated into public, political advocacy. Lasser's is a narrative of sharing, a woman-to-woman telling of the story, caring, and acting.

Women's illness narratives of the 1970s have been called "memoirs with a mission,"[9] a mission that focused on women's agency and the patriarchal medical practice that dominated cancer treatment. Women's narrative voice found expression once again in women's magazines. In a 1971 *McCall's* article, Rosamund Campion, fiction editor of *Seventeen* magazine, recounted her refusal to sign a consent form for a one-step biopsy/radical mastectomy procedure. She tells us her surgeon's response:

> "You are being a very silly and stubborn woman. You ask too many questions. I could have performed the mastectomy while you were under, and you would not have to go through this trauma twice and everything would have been fine. . . . Now with a radical mastectomy you'd have a nice clean area." Urban renewal I thought. Or a pleasant place to picnic. A nice, clean, empty, useless area.[10]

Rose Kushner's now classic 1977 advocacy narrative *Why Me? What Every Woman Should Know to Save Her Life* recounts days of calling and visiting doctors in search of one who would separate biopsy from treatment, and a breast surgeon who would perform a modified rather than a radical Halstead mastectomy. "No patient is going to tell me how to do my surgery," Kushner recounts one physician growling when she asked for a two-stage operation—biopsy now, mastectomy later. "You're absolutely ridiculous!" another exploded. Her narrative linked her own personal experience with a clear advocacy message:

> Separating biopsy from mastectomy gives women a voice in controlling their own destinies. . . . The point of this book is to show that we women should be free, knowledgeable, and completely conscious when the time comes for a decision, so that we can make it for ourselves. Our lives are at stake, not a surgeon's.[11]

These narratives of the 1970s were part of the context of women finding their own voice and becoming empowered in their lives. Individual women's narratives and the collective voice that constructed knowledge from this experience formed the basis for the groundbreaking *Our Bodies, Ourselves,*[12] first written as a pamphlet to be used by groups of women to educate each other about their bodies and their health and now being published in its fifth book edition. Here again we see women's illness narratives as texts of inclusion, written with an eye to a reader who will utilize her reading to become empowered herself, educate others, or take wider public action.

Many of the breast cancer narratives of the 1980s and 1990s were more inward looking, giving voice to individual suffering and personal battles. This trend perhaps reflects late twentieth-century American society's focus on self-help, individual responsibility, and, for many, the role of personal faith. Yet at the same time, these personal stories gave rise to probably one of the most effective disease-specific advocacy movements in the United States since the March of Dimes.

There is, throughout the history of women's illness narratives, the prevalent theme of connection, whereby the story of the individual experience is connected to a caring relationship, to family, and to community. In addition, all through the history of women's illness narratives there has also been the connection of one woman to public womanhood, an advocacy connection that sought to change the experience of many through the voice of one.

## READING WOMEN'S NARRATIVES AS RELATIONAL

From the diaries of Ballard and Farnsworth on, women's illness narratives throughout history have narrated more than their individual, personal experiences. These are stories that engage in what oral historian Alessandro Portelli calls the multiple narrative modes of history telling—the personal, communal, and institutional.[13] Women's narratives not only reveal realities about familial and social groups but larger sociopolitical forces. Therefore, listening to women's voices does not only help readers "hear" the uniqueness of individuals, but learn to "hear" in entirely different ways.

We see in modern narratives as much as in historic ones a rich literature of women caregivers writing about the illness experiences of those for whom they care. Indeed, women and caring relationships are deeply connected historically and across cultures. Hilary Rose argues that women's work involves the production and reproduction of people, which is emotionally demanding labor.[14] Whether women care for others as paid or as unpaid laborers, the caring is "grounded in the real and material practice of taking care of both our own and the bodies of others." For this reason, women learn to "read the body," to empathize with and care *about* as well as *for* others. Women's construction of knowledge, including scientific knowledge, includes emotional caring about others.[15]

Whether the culture of caring is rooted in any "essential" nature of woman or is, however ubiquitous, fundamentally a social construction, it need not affect our argument for the importance of women's narrative voice in understanding the experience of illness. That voice is most often a voice of caring and connectedness. Empirically, woman's caring voice is rooted in her caring roles. In her discussion of feminist ethical models, Susan Sherwin argues that "because women are usually charged with the responsibility of caring for children, the elderly, and the ill as well as the responsibility of physically and emotionally nurturing men both at work and at home, most women experience the world as a complex web of interdependent relationships, where responsible caring for others is implicit in their moral lives"[16] This is clearly reflected in both professional and relational caregivers' narratives, as well as in narratives of women experiencing illness.

As Ann Smitow writes in her classic essay, "A Gender Diary," "Culture offers a variety of rewards to women for always giving attention to others first. . . . Some feminists," she says, "see this female giving as fulfilling and morally powerful." For others, "any job relegated to the powerless is one undervalued by the society as a whole."[17] Historians explicitly explore these interconnections in the "undervalued" and "powerless" profession of nursing. In the pointedly titled *Ordered to Care: The Dilemma of American Nursing, 1850–1945,* Susan Reverby explores the duality of caring as an emotional and a material activity in nursing, a "form of labor shaped by the obligation to care."[18]

In contemporary narratives too, caregivers and women experiencing illness find their voices through relationships. Penny Wolfson, the author of an essay in this collection, finds "language" in the external experiences and landscapes of her life, but her "voice" is "set free" only as she hears the diagnosis of her son's Duchenne muscular dystrophy:

> I wrote about Ansel immediately, the day after his diagnosis, at the counter of a coffee shop a block away from his special ed nursery school. I wrote about him furiously, in a way I never had written about anything. I wrote about him to create art from his small existence, which I was told would be short. I wrote about him because I thought I would drown in the identity of disabled-child's mother, in the endless cycles of doctor's appointments, and the ugliness of clinic corridors and the devastating prospect of my child in a wheelchair. I wrote about him because I knew my own life would be limited by this disease, by this increasingly dependent child, and writing was something I could do, at home, where he needed me. I wrote about him to savor his life, to save his life; I wrote about him to save mine. And suddenly I had a voice, a much louder and clearer voice than I'd ever had.[19]

Kathlyn Conway's cancer narrative, *Ordinary Life: A Memoir of Illness,* is a modern narrative about her cancer experience, but it is also a narrative of connections. She refuses to write the "transformative" narrative that portrays the cancer experience as one of "lessons learned," of patient growth and survivor enrichment.[20] Conway's voice is angry, but it is also relational. Conway and her husband had gone through her Hodgkin's disease together as graduate students, and now she would experience breast cancer within her family of parents and children and grandparents. She experiences her illness through its impact on each family member, through shifting relationships with friends and the reaction of neighbors, through changes in the way she cares for and about others and they care for her. And because she experiences illness in terms of relationships, she needs to connect with her own caregivers through that relational understanding. At the office of the breast surgeon before her biopsy, Conway envisions her doctor:

> On his wall is a painting of a man who I imagine is his father, perhaps the other doctor named Cody whom we found in the phone book. I'm glad he has a father. Does he have children? I want him to know that what matters most about possibly having breast cancer is that I am part of a family. I have parents, a husband, and children.[21]

We know as readers that Conway's illness is inseparable from her caring relationships. We also know that for Conway, empathy on the part of the health professional would require familial consciousness.

Women's narrative voices challenge professionals to confront the social structures as well as the personal experiences of caring by translating the illness experience into political action. Carol Levine, a personal caregiver for her severely disabled husband and a public advocate for long-term caregivers, calls family caregivers "invisible, as individuals and as a labor force."[22] Levine, who also writes an essay in this collection, found her narrative voice as she ceased being a wife and became a family caregiver: "No one advocates on my husband's behalf except me; no one advocates on my behalf, not even me." She cares for her husband out of "love and devotion," but also out of obligation. And her caregiving structures an increasingly public voice. Why, she asks, should caregiving be a personal and family responsibility? Why not a community and social responsibility?

Narratives of women experiencing illness also inspire activism by making explicit relational identities based on community and cultural groups. Few modern illness narratives are as openly political as Audre Lorde's *The Cancer Journals.* Lorde writes about going beyond the isolating personal experience and uses her voice to summon other women to raise theirs in activist protest:

> Each woman responds to the crisis that breast cancer brings to her life out of a whole pattern, which is the design of who she is and how her life has been lived . . . . Breast cancer and mastectomy are not unique experiences, but ones

shared by thousands of American women. Each of these women has a particular voice to be raised in what must become a female outcry against all preventable cancers . . . may these words serve as encouragement for other women to speak out and act out of our experiences with cancer and with other threats of death, for silence has never brought us anything of worth.[23]

Although she recognizes that the process of writing about her pain, fear, and transfiguration is "work (she must) do alone," her strength emerges from her group identities: "a black lesbian feminist mother lover poet all I am."[24] In her narrative, she gives importance to the circles of women around her: her daughter, lover, friends. "From the time I woke up to the slow growing warmth of Adrienne's and Bernice's and Deanna's and Michelle's and Frances' coats on the bed, I felt Beth Israel hospital wrapped in a web of woman love and strong wishes of faith and hope for the whole time I was there, and it made self-healing more possible, knowing I was not alone."[25]

Nancy Mairs similarly discusses how giving voice to her body's illness, multiple sclerosis, allows her to gather other women to her. Expressions of illness are inherently political, she writes, since speaking about the female body, particularly a disabled female body, is breaking sociocultural taboos of silence and secrecy around the feminine experience. In writing, she reverses the silencing power of shame imposed upon women:

I can subvert its power, I've found, by acknowledging who I am, shame and all, and, in doing so, raising what was hidden, dark, secret about my life into the plain light of shared human experience. What we aren't permitted to utter holds us, each isolated from each other, in a kind of solipsistic thrall . . . one of the strangest consequences of publishing a collection of personal essays . . . has been a steady trickle of letters and telephone calls saying . . . 'Oh, me too! Me too!' It's as though the part I thought solo turned out to be a chorus. But none of us was singing loud enough for the others to hear.[26]

NOTES

1. Laurel Thatcher Ulrich, *A Midwife's Tale: The Life of Martha Ballard, Based on Her Diary, 1785–1812* (New York: Vintage Books, 1990).

2. Emily Abel, "A 'Terrible and Exhausting' Struggle: Family Caregiving during the Transformation of Medicine," *Women and Health in America*, ed. Judith Walzer Leavitt, 2nd ed. (Madison: U of Wisconsin P, 1999) 573.

3. Fanny Burney, "A Mastectomy, 30 September 1811," 25 Aug. 2004 <http://wesclark.com/jw/mastectomy.html.>

4. Sheila M. Rothman, *Living in the Shadow of Death* (New York: BasicBooks, 1994) 79.

5. Charlotte Perkins Gilman, *The Yellow Wallpaper* (New York: Feminist Press, 1973).

6. Charles Rosenberg, "Introduction—Framing Disease: Illness, Society, and History," *Framing Disease: Studies in Cultural History*, ed. Charles E. Rosenberg and Janet Golden (New Brunswick, NJ: Rutgers UP, 1992) xiii–xxvi.

7. Ellen Leopold, *A Darker Ribbon: Breast Cancer, Women, and Their Doctors in the Twentieth Century* (Boston: Beacon Press, 1999) 233.

8. Terese Lasser and William Kendall Clarke, *Reach to Recovery* (New York: Simon and Schuster, 1972) 21.

9. Leopold 251.

10. Rosemund Campion as quoted in Leopold 224.

11. Rose Kushner, *Why Me? What Every Woman Should Know to Save Her Life* (Philadelphia, PA: Sounders Press, 1982) 23.

12. See www.ourbodiesourselves.org for a history of their publications.

13. Alessandro Portelli, "There's Gonna Always Be a Line: History-Telling as a Multi-vocal Art," *The Battle of Valle Giulia: Oral History and the Art of Dialogue* (Madison: U of Wisconsin P, 1997) 27.

14. Hilary Rose, "Thinking from Caring: Feminist Construction of a Responsible Rationality," *Love, Power, and Knowledge: Towards a Feminist Transformation of the Sciences* (Bloomington: Indiana UP, 1994) 28–50.

15. Rose 49–50.

16. Susan Sherwin, *No Longer Patient: Feminist Ethics and Health Care* (Philadelphia, PA: Temple UP, 1992) 47. Sherwin (1992) offers a longer review of the debate regarding women's moral thinking, and in particular the debate surrounding Carol Gilligan's proposed dualism and the argument by Sara Ruddick and others that all women share the moral perspective of maternal thinking. This is a discussion germane to our paper but beyond its limited scope.

17. Ann Smitow, "A Gender Diary," *Conflicts in Feminism*, ed. Marianne Hirsch and Evelyn Fox Keller (New York: Routledge, 1990) 23.

18. Susan M. Reverby, *Ordered to Care: The Dilemma of American Nursing, 1850–1945* (Cambridge: Cambridge UP, 1987) 1.

19. Penny Wolfson, "Voice Lessons," *Sarah Lawrence Magazine* (Spring 2003): 14.

20. Kathlyn Conway, *Ordinary Life: A Memoir of Illness* (New York: W. H. Freeman, 1997), distinguishes between the "writing that transformed the experience of cancer" and the cancer as a transformative experience. Writing made her feel alive, "not deadened by the cancer or the chemicals" (254).

21. Conway 15.

22. Carol Levine, "Loneliness of the Long-Term Care Giver," *New England Journal of Medicine* 340.20 (1999), 15 June 2003 <http:content.nejm.com>.

23. Audre Lorde, *The Cancer Journals* (San Francisco: Aunt Lute Books, 1980) 9–10.

24. Lorde 25.

25. Lorde 29.

26. Nacy Mairs, "Carnal Acts," *Minding the Body: Women Writers on Body and Soul*, ed. Patricia Foster (New York: Anchor Books, 1994) 279.

# Narratives of Body and Self: The Experience of Illness

ৰ্কੈ

PATRICIA STANLEY'S ESSAY "The Patient's Voice" examines isolation caused by illness, including isolation from the healthy, isolation from loved ones, and isolation from the body and self. Stanley draws from published narratives in order to reflect upon such isolation in the wider community of women; yet it is through the act of writing narratives that are then read, of telling stories that are then witnessed, that the isolation of illness can be minimized. Her challenge to not only health care professionals who can elicit and witness the suffering of a patient but to us as readers of illness narratives is to engage in an ethical practice of reading whereby the act of witnessing becomes an impetus for action and advocacy. This essay frames our task as readers of the collection.

The remaining work in this section explores what it is like to have such diverse diseases as food allergies, cancer, cystic fibrosis, manic depression, and a cerebral artery dissection. These narratives describe aspects of the illness experience while at the same time struggling with the indescribability of illness, the incommunicability of suffering. This emerges, in part, from the inadequacy of written language, which is bereft of the engagement, dynamism, and facial and body language that accompany oral narrative. Indeed, many of the written works in this section are transcriptions of oral narratives—a theme that recurs again in the last section of this collection. Not only was Laura Rothenberg's radio diary recorded for and played on NPR, but Victoria Maxwell's contribution to this volume is the script of her one-woman theatrical show about manic depression, "Crazy for Life." And although written as an essay, Robyn Ringler's "Dissection," with its ominous, text-disrupting "WHOOSH WHOOSH WHOOSH," reads as if it were meant to be performed, perhaps because of the author's experience recording personal essays for radio. Similarly, Angelee Deodhar's *haibun*, describing the experience of having a pulmonary artery embolus, relies upon aural description of nature and the body: "cough outshouts thunder, ribs rattle like the windows after each thunderbolt. Wheezing whistling laboured breath like the wind outside. Each thunderclap like the rasp of the cough."

This section teaches us that not just the written word but language itself may be inadequate to describe the experiences of illness. As quoted by Stanley, "physical pain does not simply resist language but actively destroys it, bringing about an immediate reversion to a state anterior to language."[1] In the words of Lara Birk in "The Listening Room," "Pain cannot be told. . . . The story that can be told, the story that can be taken in, is never the whole story." The origins of this idea of incommunicability lie in the asymmetry of access to the experiential knowledge of pain, whereby only the sufferer is sure about it—she, being asked to respond to another's pain, is necessarily in doubt about its existence. Yet in his volume *Social Suffering*, Arthur Kleinman posits that from a perspective of social suffering, a preoccupation with individual certainty is less important than how "acknowledgement of pain as a cultural process is given or withheld."[2] Therefore, the moral act is not to imagine another's pain but to acknowledge it. The incommunicability of pain lies not with the solitary writer grappling with language but with the narrator in relation to her empathetic or nonempathetic listener.

## NOTES

1. Elaine Scarry, *The Body in Pain: The Making and Unmaking of the World* (New York: Oxford UP, 1985) 4.

2. Arthur Kleinman, Veena Das, and Margaret Lock, "Introduction," *Social Suffering*, ed. Arthur Kleinman, Veena Das, and Margaret Lock (Berkeley: U of California P, 1997) xiii.

# *Faith**

## Laurie Stroblas

Don't tell me this is living.
It's late in the summer
and the bees are circling.
The tree bones are dry rot.

It's late in the summer
and my legs aren't moving.
The tree bones are dry rot
but I don't believe.

And my legs aren't moving
through the marrow-heavy grass
but I don't believe
it is happening to me.

Through the marrow-heavy grass
and the bees are circling,
it is happening to me.
Don't tell me this is living.

* Pantoum: a form of poetry in which the second and fourth lines of each stanza are repeated as
the first and third lines of the next; additional rules apply to the final stanza. The meaning of
repeated lines may shift, although the words remain the same.

# The Female Voice in Illness:
## An Antidote to Alienation, a Call for Connection

### PATRICIA B. STANLEY

It was Monday, after a lonely Thanksgiving weekend, the fifth weekend of our two-month stay in the bone marrow transplant unit. I had risen at dawn to drive to the city to be at my husband's side for the doctors' rounds. He had seemingly declined during the holiday weekend and I was frantic to get information. We had spent long days with no one to talk to and little information on his condition. Feeling isolated is part of any illness, but it is an essential part of the atmosphere in the bone marrow transplant unit. By necessity. God forbid anyone get near those bodies lying vulnerable and exposed, waiting for their immune systems to kick in. The holiday only sharpened the contrast between the real world participating in the Thanksgiving feast and our living behind that hermetically sealed door in a sterile box with antibacterial soap, latex gloves, plastic wrapped food, and limited human contact.

This experience in the bone marrow transplant unit only heightened what I had learned about isolation and illness as my husband's caregiver during his ten-year siege with cancer. Isolation is inherent in many aspects of biomedical treatment, and it is rooted in Western cultural barriers, which separate the ill and their caregivers from healthy society. It is also true that the very nature of pain from illness disconnects the patient from traditional channels of communication. Writer Elaine Scarry maintains that "physical pain does not simply resist language but actively destroys it, bringing about an immediate reversion to a state anterior to language, to the sounds and cries a human being makes before language is learned."[1] The question that must be asked is whether this inarticulateness is inherent to pain and illness or to its socially constructed experience or to both.

Ironically, this experience of isolation is one that has no voice in traditional spaces. The code of medical science informs us about facts in a language incomprehensible to lay individuals and incapable of expressing their personal stories. By reading illness memoirs, however, we gain a phenomenological explanation of illness that addresses this void left by medicine. In particular, the memoirs of women will be explored here for their power to project beyond the patriarchal attributes of science and the "male-biased model of human nature and social reality."[2] As Audre Lorde writes in the introduction to her powerful memoir, *The*

*Cancer Journals,* "Our feelings need voice in order to be recognized, respected, and of use."[3] And Nancy Mairs tells us, "Speaking about the whole experience of being a body, specifically a female body, is an antidote to shame, shame for who I am . . . What we aren't permitted to utter holds us, each isolated from every other, in a kind of solipsistic thrall."[4]

A focus on isolation in illness narratives reveals several kinds of isolation—isolation from the healthy, isolation from loved ones, and isolation from the body and the self. In the following pages, I offer selected narratives based on personal experience as a way to share the vision of women who deal with these categories of isolation and to show how their collective realities might inspire the listener to create communities of caring.

## ISOLATION FROM THE HEALTHY

The segregation of the ill from the healthy is perhaps a uniquely modern phenomenon in Western cultures. Historically, illness was often experienced as a normal part of life and did not generate feelings of isolation. Particularly for women, the treatment of illness was rooted in their expected roles as mother and housewife. In mid-nineteenth-century New England, tuberculosis was widespread and the treatment gendered: women with illness stayed home and remained part of the family while the men were sent away on long curative sea voyages.[5] In America before industrialization, people lived in rural and small communities and dealt with most illness within the family and local community,[6] where it was often women who were expected to be the caregivers of the ill. In the twentieth century, the advances in biomedicine changed the location of the illness experience from within family and community to physical separation from the healthy. As cities grew, the treatment for the ill shifted to commercial institutions and professional experts, including hospitals and licensed fee-for-service doctors.

Much of illness's isolation is also a result of the social and cultural intolerance of illness, which leads to a construction of the ill person as "other." Nancy Mairs, afflicted with multiple sclerosis, writes, "We've never been too fond of the other. We prefer the same. I feel shame for my body . . . : it is a crippled body."[7] Medicalization, or the categorization and consequent treatment of life experiences as pathologies or illnesses, has alienated women from their own bodies; women's life changes and events, from menarche through menopause, become "medical conditions," separating them from "normal" life. The more medicalized we become, the less accepting we are of differences, the greater our need for labels and categories, the more walls we put up between the diagnosed person and the "normal" person, the more marginalized people we create. Activist Audre Lorde writes in her breast cancer memoir about a woman from the advocacy organization Reach to Recovery who tried to convince her to wear a prosthesis so that she could return to "normal" life: "I ached to talk to women about the experience I had just been through . . . But I needed to talk with women who shared at least some of my major concerns and beliefs and visions . . . And this lady, admirable though she might be, did not."[8] The draw of the prosthesis, critiques Lorde, is a reaction to the isolation of illness, "The terror and silent loneliness of women attempting to replace the ghost of a breast leads to yet another victimization."[9]

The high hurdles created by the insurance system in our country and the increasing millions of people without health insurance lead to systemic isolation that intensifies personal isolation. In her unsentimental account of living with stage-four breast cancer, *Seeing the Crab*, Christina Middlebrook writes,

> So many of my fellow metastatic cancer patient friends who soldiered through a world that did not want to know what was going on with them are dead now. The others who are living cannot afford to be bunnies. They have had to develop hard and burdensome shells. They are tortoises, now, stumbling and slow. . . . Money, expenses, bills, debts, credit, disability payments—I have them all. And though I move money around like peas under walnut shells, I have the peas. I have the walnut shells. . . . I have been very lucky.[10]

Isolation does not end with recovery. Isolation, alienation, and separation continue to be experienced by those who have recovered but fear relapse, those who are chronically impaired from either the effects of the primary illness or its medical cure, those who are disabled, and all those who were once ill and now struggle daily to stay well—in short, those who are members of what sociologist Arthur W. Frank calls "the remission society."[11] Sandra Steingraber, a cancer survivor, environmental activist, and author of *Living Downstream: An Ecologist Looks at Cancer and the Environment,* expresses her fears in the last two stanzas of the poem "Post-Diagnosis":

> Look that meant nothing,
> I am restored, put back.
> I am not like those others,
> full of metastases, who are returned
> to their lives as guests,
> who have only a journey,
> who are packing their bags,

who are leaving now.
A week ago my surgeon rose
from his instruments and laughed.
"Sandra, let's grow old together."
The tests were negative. He is a young man
and I told him this was a good place,
a good place to live.

But sometimes late at night
I still see the lights of the hospital—
the white hushed comings and goings,
the gray partitioning curtains,
the slow dripping in tubes.
Outside this window the last
summer flowers hemorrhage
in the garden and winter lies
like a tumor beneath the earth.[12]

## Isolation from Loved Ones

The construction of illness as failure or weakness impacts ill individuals' social acceptability. The pervasive American attitude that control is always possible on both the individual and social levels influences both the patient's illness experience and others' perception of her. Failure—including illness—is the result of not enough will, determination, or character. The American way is to believe that even someone with a chronic illness should have control and the ability to determine outcomes through sheer will and strength. The culture repudiates acceptance of the limits set by the disease, as Barbara Webster observes:

> My disease reflects the imperfection of my nature. . . . I am continually faced by the judgment that my disability is a moral outcome, not an objective reality. If I were to deny the implications of my disease, were to struggle and fight against the reality of my disability, were to rely on hope as a response and a way out, I would be more in tune with my culture and would be viewed in a more favorable light by most people.[13]

Although it is a common belief that illness brings families together, often, in response to inherent and culturally induced stress, illness separates patients and caregivers from those they love. In her memoir, *Moonrise: One Family, Genetic Identity, and Muscular Dystrophy,* Penny Wolfson writes about her reaction to her son's diagnosis of Duchenne muscular dystrophy that propels the family into chaos:

> I live for a time in a blurred dark universe, one in which real feelings fuel my dreams but the day-world is meaningless . . . I am in the middle of a whirlwind, and all I can do is hang on. . . . I am aware of Joe [her husband] as compatriot, but we lie separately, emotionally apart, because we have to preserve our strength and our own resources."[14]

Later she refers to an afternoon spent skiing with her husband, during which they suddenly realize they are on top of a frozen lake and the ice is cracking. This becomes a metaphor for how the chaos of chronic illness divides them as parents: "We are out in the center of a large, dangerous place, a place no one can reach us. But we cannot be close. To survive we've got to separate, at least a few steps, at least for a while."[15]

The American culture of denial can pervade the most intimate relationships. Christina Middlebrook writes, "I want interest and curiosity. I want the same concern I'd get if I said that I had been laid off from a job or had a broken leg. I want someone to say 'God, how awful. How're you doing?' I want someone to ask, 'What's it like?'"[16] She goes on to describe in grim detail phone conversations with her mother and sister who have remained estranged from her during her bone marrow transplant. They refuse to believe that she is dying.

> There is nothing in my family's godlessness, no clue, no yearning, no instinct, nothing that enables them to share with me the inevitability of my early death. . . . We are not meant to talk about the odds. We are not meant to speak the unspeakable, that my odds are not good. . . . My brother also calls. . . . I tell [him] . . . that our mother has told me that I did not have a recurrence. "Maybe you'll have only *one* recurrence." I sigh the deep sigh of the lonely. One recurrence is all it takes. I cannot breathe for the loneliness.[17]

Illness can separate friends, peers, and colleagues as well as family members. Kathlyn Conway, in her memoir *Ordinary Life: A Memoir of Illness,* quotes a woman with cancer who, when running into a friend on the street, found that the friend immediately ran away from her shouting, "I haven't called you because I just can't handle it."[18] The final isolation occurs when patients acutely, inevitably face death. For some cultures, particularly those with a spiritual belief in an afterlife, fear, isolation, and suffering may not even exist. But in-dividuals without that belief may well experience horrible fear. Middlebrook quotes Barbara Rosenblum who, ten months before she died, wrote of the fear of leaving loved ones behind and of traveling alone on the journey to death: "If you think standing by yourself waiting for someone to talk to is lonely, if you think holidays alone are lonely, if you think that not having a relationship for a long time is lonely, if you think that the long, frightening nights after a divorce are lonely—you cannot know the aloneness of one who faces death looking it squarely in the eye."[19]

## ISOLATION FROM THE BODY AND THE SELF

Illness threatens not only the individual's physical integrity but also the individual's identity and sense of self in the world. The separation of *me* from my *self* is terrifying. As Barbara Webster explains in her book *All of a Piece: A Life with Multiple Sclerosis*, "Disturbance of body image is very shattering. It disturbs the very experience and root of self. I think one has no real awareness of the centrality to self of that body image or, indeed, no awareness that one holds that image, until it is disturbed."[20]

Illness evokes change with the hallmark of difference—it isolates patients from their previous lives. Isolation comes both from others and how they regard the sick person and also from how the patient regards herself. Conway writes, "For me, hearing the diagnosis of cancer meant entering a closed circle inside of which I was separated from my ordinary life, my ordinary self, from the very people I loved . . . I felt like a creature from a different species. . . . I looked the same, . . . but my spirit had been taken away."[21]

The procedures designed to treat and cure the patient—iron lungs, oxygen tanks, IV poles, external artificial hearts, dialysis machines—can add a cyborg isolation to the patient's suffering that separates her from the healthy self. The bone-marrow transplant is a particularly dramatic example of forced isolation necessitated by a procedure. Chronicling what she underwent for her bone-marrow transplant, Christina Middlebrook describes herself as a "zoo creature" trapped in the room she lay in for twenty-five days in isolation. She has become not only not herself but not human at all:

> The zoo creature is very dopey. Its left eyelid sags. Its back is covered by a hid-eous rash that itches. The body has no hair, not on its head, its face, arms, legs,

underarms, or now-sexless crotch. There is no buffer between it and the world, no hiding. Mammals hide inside their hair. The zoo creature does not know if it is a mammal anymore. Its warm blood is cooled by chemotherapy. It is hairless and no longer able to nurse its young. . . . Worst of all, the zoo creature cannot think or remember. It says things in a language that makes no sense. . . . It cannot respond to solicitous messages left on the answering machine. . . . It does not know what day it is or whether it is day or night. All it knows is to look to the chair at the side of the bed in hopes that a visitor is there, keeping watch.[22]

## CONNECTING WITH PATIENTS: GIVING VOICE

Narrative approaches to illness and health advocacy propose that giving voice to patients can help minimize the isolation of illness. Through storytelling, the patient can begin to heal and the listener, through witnessing, can facilitate in that healing. Kathlyn Conway talks about her writing as a way to save her life: "The writing is like a magnet that draws together all the stray parts of myself."[23] Nancy Mairs, too, uses her voice to counter ostracism:

> I speak as a crippled woman. At the same time, in the utterance I redeem both "cripple" and "woman" from the shameful silences by which I have often felt surrounded, contained, set apart; I give myself permission to live openly among others, to reach out to them, stroke them with fingers and sighs.[24]

There may be therapeutically useful ways that health care professionals can encourage patients to give voice to their illness experiences. The health care provider has the opportunity to witness the suffering of the patient fully by hearing, understanding, and compassionately helping patients break through isolation. Without this true listening, the provider is defeated and the patient is left alone with no one to hear his or her fears and suffering. Rita Charon, a general internist and director of Columbia University's Program in Narrative Medicine, explains:

> Once we allow ourselves to listen with compassion and to let the full implica-tions of their suffering register on us, we are in a position to change the state of affairs. It will not always lead to cure, and it will not always lead to a change in the medical treatment, but it can lead to a radical change for the patient. It can confer recognition and communion, ending the isolation and strangerli-ness of sickness.[25]

Through stories, connections are created and combined into communities of caring. I am reminded of the powerful narrative in Andrew Solomon's book on depression, *The Noonday Demon: An Atlas of Depression*, about Phaly Nuon and her method of treating fellow female survivors of the atrocities inflicted by the Khmer Rouge. Initially, she would get the women to tell her their stories. Then she would teach them to forget, then to work, and then to love by uniting them in a community of caring for each other. Eventually they build enough trust and support to tell each other their stories: "They have learned how to make friends, so that they will never have to be so lonely and so alone again."[26] The last step is the integration of the forgetting, working, and loving, and once they have understood the practice of these three things together, they are ready to reenter the world. Audre Lorde reminds us of the power of the call for connection:

> Each of these women has a particular voice to be raised in what must become a female outcry against all preventable cancers . . . May these words serve as encouragement for other women to speak and to act out of our experiences . . . for silence has never brought us anything of worth. Most of all may these words underline the possibilities of self-healing and the richness of living for all women.[27]

These voices represent the familiar call from women who care, but they are for all people to hear. If we choose not to listen, they are voices crying in solitude. But if we are moved by their song, we can—through conscious reading, writing, and witnessing—build communities of caring that connect us to those suffering voices and thereby reduce the anguished isolation of illness.

## Notes

1. Elaine Scarry, *The Body in Pain: The Making and Unmaking of the World* (New York: Oxford UP, 1985) 4.

2. Emily Martin, *The Woman in the Body: A Cultural Analysis of Reproduction* (Boston: Beacon Press, 2001) 21.

3. Audre Lorde, *The Cancer Journals* (San Francisco: Aunt Lute Books, 1997) 9.

4. Nancy Mairs, "Carnal Acts," *Minding the Body: Women Writers on the Body and Soul*, ed. Patricia Foster (New York: Anchor Books, 1994) 279.

5. Sheila M. Rothman, *Living in the Shadow of Death: Tuberculosis and the Social Experience of Illness in American History* (Baltimore, MD. Johns Hopkins UP, 1995) 18–20.

6. Paul Starr, *The Social Transformation of American Medicine* (New York: Basic Books, 1982) 22.

7. Mairs 272.

8. Lorde 42.

9. Lorde 67.

10. Christina Middlebrook, *Seeing the Crab* (New York: Basic Books, 1996) 189.

11. Arthur W. Frank, *At the Will of the Body* (Boston: Houghton Mifflin, 2002) 138.

12. Sandra Steingraber, *Post-Diagnosis* (Ithaca, NY: Firebrand Books, 1995) 32, lines 42–63.

13. Barbara D. Webster, *All of a Piece: A Life with Multiple Sclerosis* (Baltimore, MD: Johns Hopkins UP, 1989) 83–4.

14. Penny Wolfson, *Moonrise: One Family, Genetic Identity, and Muscular Dystrophy* (New York: St. Martin's Press, 2003) 41.

15. Wolfson 56–7.

16. Middlebrook 135.

17. Middlebrook 115–6

18. Kathlyn Conway, *Ordinary Life: A Memoir of Illness* (New York: W. H. Freeman Press, 1997) 120.

19. Middlebrook 205.

20. Webster 124.

21. Conway 255–6.

22. Middlebrook 55–6.

23. Conway 240.

24. Mairs 281–82.

25. Rita Charon, "Let Me Take a Listen to Your Heart," *Caregiving: Readings in Knowledge, Practice, Ethics, and Politics,* ed. Suzanne Gordon, Patricia Benner, and Nel Noddings (Philadelphia: U of Pennsylvania P, 1996) 304.

26. Andrew Solomon, *The Noonday Demon: An Atlas of Depression* (New York: Scribner, 2001) 37.

27. Lorde 10.

# Dissection

ROBYN DESANTIS RINGLER

In the dark of night, at the age of forty-one, I should have been nestled in my husband's arms, listening for my daughter's even breathing in the next room. Instead, I lay on my bed, very still, eyes tight, my face pressed to the sheet, thoughts focused on just continuing to breathe. I had never felt such pain. I could hardly lift my head off the mattress. A repetitive, rushing sound echoed through my ears with every heartbeat.

*Whoosh. Whoosh. Whoosh.*

Sliding to the floor and crawling to the bathroom, I urinated then threw up. Breathing shallow and rapid, hands and lips tingling, head in agony, the room spun. My husband, Bob, in his underwear on the cold tile floor, cradled my shivering body with his arms as I leaned heavily against his chest between bouts of sickness.

My moment has come, I thought. Funny how difficult it is to imagine a medical emergency before it happens. I always thought mine would involve crushing chest pain or a hard lump in the breast. I never imagined it would be my head.

Back in bed, I held my afflicted head in my hands, trying to block out the pain, noise, and fear and fighting to think only of my nine-year-old daughter, Lily.

*I can't be sick. I will not be sick. I refuse to be sick.*

Wanting desperately to go anywhere but the hospital, I was terrified that I would never come home.

*Please don't take me to the hospital.*

In the emergency room, the doctor's expression changed from an unconcerned smile as we explained I had an excruciating headache, to a look of gravity when I added there was a whooshing noise in my head. A day of tests—brain MRI, carotid ultrasound, blood tests, and X-rays produced no answers. Then, the neurologist came in.

"I'm afraid the noise in your head indicates that you probably have a venous malformation in your brain. If so, it will require surgery." A venous malformation is a congenital problem that can cause bleeding.

I know I should have felt relieved to have an answer, but instead, I felt angry. I did not want to hear his words. Until this moment, everyone had been smiling and hopeful. All of the tests had been negative. This doctor was serious and unwavering and was telling me I needed brain surgery.

Brain surgery—something most of us never think we will need. Brains are taken for granted. I could not imagine having brain surgery.

I needed one last test—an arteriogram—in which the artery in my groin would be punctured, a catheter inserted and threaded up through my aorta and into my brain arteries, where dye would be squirted while we all watched it on television.

The test had risks—bleeding, paralysis, death. The neuroradiologist came in with a consent form, assuring me that none of his patients had ever suffered any of these problems. Signing the form, I wondered whether the statistical probabilities were against me.

On the way to radiology, the breeze in the hallway blew through my hospital gown and the thin blanket covering me as I lay on a stretcher, the pain and noise in my head constant. Two male technicians wheeled me into a cold operating room where everything was stainless steel. They moved trays of utensils onto tables laid with white sheets. The table was hard, lights bright.

I tried to joke so they would like me and fight hard for my life. We talked about line dancing, Girl Scouts, local restaurants. They allowed me to sit up even though I was supposed to lie down. One said the neuroradiologist did not think this test would show anything. What did that mean? Should I even have this test?

The doctor injected my groin six times with a local anesthetic. Then he prepared to pierce the artery with a catheter. Having my groin punctured was just like it sounds—someone stabs you hard with a sharp instrument. I endured several stabbings before it was successful.

Once the catheter made its journey from groin to brain, dye was intermittently injected. Each time, I felt a rush of hot, prickling nerve endings dancing on a section of my face. Finally, the rush came to an area in the back of my head.

"You are touching exactly where the pain comes from," I said.

"You mean I'm making it hurt more?" asked the doctor.

"No, you are touching the very spot exactly."

The neuroradiologist took pictures from every possible angle in that area of my brain and found what we were all looking for—the vertebral artery was dissected or torn. The noise in my head was caused by swelling in the artery, which was so bad that the blood almost couldn't get through. Every time the blood tried to force its way through the almost occluded artery, it made a whooshing sound.

Vertebral artery dissection was a better diagnosis because the treatment did not include brain surgery. Given time, the artery should heal itself. However, because blood was having such a hard time getting through the swollen artery, I was in danger of having a stroke.

Being in danger is a frightening thing. My head overflowed with images of the worst-case scenario—paralysis, blindness, my family living on without me. Yet being obsessed with the unthinkable showed that my brain was still functioning.

The doctors discharged me after one night in the hospital with few instructions: pain medication and bed rest as needed, activity around the house as tolerated, call the office for an appointment.

For weeks, the pain and noise were unrelenting. Nights were worse, as the pain inexplicably intensified, at times making me frantic. Bob fixed cool washcloths for my head, rubbed my back, distracted me, and enfolded me in his arms.

Over three months, the noise in my head gradually disappeared, but I was left with frequent intense headaches. Headaches interfered with my activity and commitments. I kept trying but, at times, had a feeling of suspension, of holding my breath and waiting for my life to get back to normal.

Sometimes, not knowing the extent of your limitations is a good thing. But, eventually, a time comes when it is better to acknowledge the truth—that you are, in fact, altered. At the end of two years, I finally understood that I had suffered a permanent loss. Although my body looked the same, pieces were missing.

# Storm Warning*

## Angelee Deodhar

Drenched in rain, catch cold, run fever, cough outshouts thunder, ribs rattle like the windows after each thunderbolt. Wheezing whistling labored breath like the wind outside, each thunderclap like the rasp of the cough. Storm peaks, trees crash, electricity poles spark, lights go off, a great black cloud blankets the house from the aerial attack. As suddenly as it came the storm abates, inside me the storm goes on, three weeks of sleepless tormented nights, a turn in bed and the pulse races, breath comes in spasms, chest hurts, head aches, cough like distant thunder rumbles, grumbles on, threatening to deluge me.

He suggests cognac and we drink it with hot water and honey. Over cheese and crackers we laugh ourselves silly till the bronchospasm stops me in my tracks. Nothing helps, X-ray chest reveals white clouds on black, the cardiologist's sinister whisper over the abnormal whoosh of the echo, so unlike any sea except the troubled one inside me. Worst of fears confirmed need hospitalization, can't wait, the thrombus in the pulmonary artery might turn killer. The tide's racing in, the angry sea rising, breathlessly, I beg for eighteen hours grace before admission till my son's examinations are over.

An IV heparin line, a tributary to the turbulent sea and oxygen, the foam on that surf helps me breathe. Laughing through the mask, I fight the great black clouds of fear. Soon the clots start breaking up and moving freely in the lungs. Cough worsens, "showers" they call them, outside a light refreshing drizzle, longing to be out there, barefoot in the rain, removing the mask I laugh and talk again, black clouds forgotten in the fragrance of wet earth.

> now calm outside
> still the cough
> —an angry sea

* Haibun: A combination of brief prose and embedded haiku, usually recording a scene or a special moment

# The Listening Room

## Lara Birk

It has been almost thirteen years since I left a high school soccer game on a stretcher, alarmed and bewildered by a sudden onset of unfathomable pain, and entered into a world no sentences could ever wrap their words around no matter how I cast or stretched them. It has been years, and yet I still don't know how to tell the story—the short story—though I've heard myself try a thousand times. Every time I see a person catch a glimpse of the lump or the scars that mark both my legs, I silently start rehearsing the words.

None of these strangers wants the long story, although a lot of them think they do. What they want is an explanation. A promise. *Tell me what you went through won't happen to me. Tell me I'm safe.*

The onset of the pain was sudden. I had an acute muscular disease no one knew I had. It had masked itself at first as "shin splints," the pain of which I had stubbornly run through all summer. My "no pain, no gain" philosophy seemed to pay off. I made the varsity soccer team and played as stopper in our first preseason game. I remember running, watching the ball as it moved from player to player on the other side of the field, ready at any moment to defend our goal.

Suddenly, I could not pick up my foot. I no longer had control over my ankle. And then the pain came. I raised my hand to be taken out, but my coach motioned to me that we had no subs. I nodded and tried to continue. My teammates tell me I "crumpled" to the ground, seemingly without warning, and had to be carried to the bench. Me, who at age two did not cry when both of my eardrums ruptured and was only taken to the doctor when my mother found the fluid on my pillow, me who ran no matter what I felt like—*me* on the bench. I was writhing, squirming, whimpering.

My vision was blurred with the pain. I only remember being carried to a car, bumped around on the interminably long ride home, my mother's face, the alarming speed with which she drove us to the ER, the green-capped faces rolling me to X-ray, and the white-coated man who called me a "sixteen year-old crybaby" when no breaks were found in the bone. Then, the struggle to get me in the car, the trip home, the long night waiting for relief, the cries my mother could no longer stand, the early morning trip back, the palpations by different hands, and finally blackness. Emergency surgery and admission to the hospital.

For some reason, still a mystery, I had developed acute compartment syndrome simply from playing soccer. Later, in an article documenting my case, the doctors called it acute *exertional* compartment syndrome. Now people know about it, but at the time, no one knew. The pressure escalated within the fascial sheaths encasing the muscles of my leg. The compartments became so tight, the tissues within could no longer receive the oxygen-enriched blood which keeps them alive. As the muscles began to die, the pain raged and the necrosis spread. It could have killed me had it reached my kidneys. I did not know that. I did not know that this was only the beginning.

When they slit the skin, the internal pressure pushed the flesh apart, cleaving a purple river from knee to ankle. I awoke to find five inches between one edge of my skin and the other. The nurses were on intensive watch for signs of a potentially lethal infection. I could not move. The staff hummed busily around me, hovering dangerously close to my leg, which was heavily draped with ice and propped up above my heart on an unsteady pile of pillows. An errant elbow could knock my leg from its precarious perch, plunging it, me, into wrenching pain.

After the principal of my small private school made an announcement about my hospitalization, I soon had a stream of visitors toting balloons and flowers. But my classmates hovered by the door when they came bearing chocolates; they left notes for me saying, "I would have stayed but you were asleep," even though I could see them scurry past the double doors of my room as I waited. When worried nurses poked through IV wires and struggled with stubborn, sticking bandages to undress my wound, "just to take a peek," the smell of necrotic flesh drove my frightened visitors from the room. They said things like, "You're through the worst of it!" or "Chin up!" before excusing themselves and sounding their footsteps down the hall in quick departure.

Marty Joseph and Sam Robeson were different. We'd been friends for about a year—not close, but I thought they were "cool," cooler than me certainly, which is why I was especially surprised when they decided to visit. The first time they came, Marty and Sam didn't seem fazed like the others. They looked around and then told me with wry grins that they'd parked in the space marked "clergy" in front of the maternity ward so that they wouldn't have to pay for parking or worry about the time.

"You guys are terrible!" I said, shamefully elated at the image of Mrs. Robeson's "grocery-getter" taking up an enormous, illegal space just for me.

When I laughed, their faces lit up.

After this, they started to visit me every day—even befriending the fourth-floor nurses. No one asked them to leave when they stayed past visiting hours. Whenever the nurses' desk was unattended, they stole wheelchairs. They would race each other up and down the hall. The ambulant kids on the ward giggled shyly from their doorways and then screamed and clapped when Sam beat Marty to my door, adding "wheelies" for everyone's amusement. I looked forward to their visits.

One afternoon, sometime during my third or fourth week in the hospital, Marty came by himself. When he walked in, I was still a little groggy, recovering from another emergency surgery. My surgeon walked in just then on his post-op afternoon rounds and clapped his clipboard on the side rail of my bed, creating a clanging reverberation throughout my body.

"Well, you almost lost that leg of yours," he said, looking at his notes. "We considered amputating due to all the necrosis you've still got in there, but we decided that a real good excision of all that stuff will hopefully do the trick. You'll keep seeping, of course, but we've got you on for three-times-a-day dressing changes."

The surgeon looked at me then. "You're a lucky girl, you know," and he turned and left the room.

In the wake of the silence left by my doctor, I heard the words, several times, in random order, as they banged around inside my head. I forgot Marty was there. I forgot everything. Then, after a while, I could feel Marty's presence again.

He stared at me. His mouth hung open and his eyes were wide. "Oh my God. I had no idea it was *that* serious. You don't deserve this." Marty was tall, a football player with deep brown skin, but he looked small and pale now.

"Marty, it's okay. Things are chaotic, random, you know. Things just happen to people . . ."

"No. Not like this. You *must* have done something—something bad, something really bad—to deserve all this." He stared at me, looking bigger again. "What did you do?"

I looked at him, thinking that if I waited long enough he would change the subject and tell me a joke or something. But then Marty drew himself away from me, his chair screeching on the floor. I was suddenly cold. I heard my voice groping at words but I just laughed.

"I'm not kidding," Marty continued, looking at me with a ferocity in his eyes I had not seen before. "Think about it. Go into your past—you must have done *something* for all this horrible stuff to happen to you. Things don't just happen for no good reason."

I did not answer. I didn't realize how much he needed an answer. A nurse came in then for the first of the post-op dressing changes.

"Marty, sweetie," she said, "I need you to wait in the hall until this is over. It's pretty painful for our little trooper and we'll need to dose her up. You might hear her crying out a bit, but I'll tell you when we're through and you can go back in again. I know she'll need your company after this one."

I could see her wink at Marty, and then I watched him walk out, his image fleetingly casting a shadow back into my room as Nancy began the slow, interminable process of undressing and redressing my wound. The pain was deafening. Marty was not there when the nurse called for him.

Marty did not visit again. The abruptness and totality of his abandonment embodied a violence that left me painfully aware of his absence. Sam visited me a couple more times, but he didn't park illegally or steal a wheelchair to make me laugh. The steady stream of friends who'd visited in the first couple of weeks had turned into an anemic trickle.

Even months later, after I was out of the hospital and had returned to school, Marty avoided all contact with me. I replayed our last conversation in my head over and over. Maybe Marty—and probably the others too—had conceived of me as a *nice girl,* someone pretty much like him. And then suddenly I was in a white bed in a white room facing surgeries, doctors, disability, and pain. It was dangerous for him to continue to think of me as like himself. There had to be something to differentiate us, something that could explain all the suffering I'd had to endure and he hadn't. There had to be something to assure him he would never have to endure the kind of horror that had befallen me. By severing all connections with me, Marty eliminated the possibility that I might further challenge or threaten him.

We want to have faith that we are the authors of our own lives. When people see me on my cane today or witness a spell of my awkward and intrusive pain, they ask me questions. "But you're so young—what twenty-eight, twenty-nine years old?—why the cane?" "What's wrong with you?" And the question that still stings the most: "What'd you do to yourself?" They want the tragic story, they crave it, but only when it leaves enough space for them to feel that things could have been different, better. That space is their listening room, where they can sit in a comfortable chair and project themselves into the scene and imagine all the ways *they* would have done things differently, all the signs they would have heeded that would have delivered them safely back home. Without that space, true listening is unbearable. But the listening room cannot encompass all the stories that add up to the truth that is my life. Pain cannot be told. Yet, in isolation, it grows. It longs to be wrapped in words, just as these strangers long for my gory narrative, but only if told in threads loose enough for them to weave themselves a happy ending. But the listening room does not and cannot protect us. The story that can be told, the story that can be taken in, is never the whole story.

# My So-Called Lungs

### LAURA ROTHENBERG

*Produced by Joe Richman/Radio Diaries, Inc., All Things Considered (NPR) 8/5/02\**

*NPR Host:* Laura Rothenberg is 21 years old, but, as she likes to say, she already had her midlife crisis a couple of years ago, and even then it was a few years late. Laura has cystic fibrosis, a genetic disorder that affects the lungs and other organs. People with CF live an average of 30 years. Two years ago, we gave Laura a tape recorder. Since that time, Laura has been keeping an audio diary of her battle with the disease and her attempts to lead a normal life with lungs that often betray her. This is Laura's story.

[*hospital sounds, beeping*]

*Laura:* Hi this is Laura. It's about 11:02 P.M. I'm here in the hospital. I've been here for five days now. I'm in room 1004 this time. [*coughing*] That's me coughing.

[*hospital sounds, nurse comes in*]

*Laura:* Hello. This is Carina. She's one of my favorite nurses. Yeah, we can put that . . .

[*nurse sounds*]

*Laura:* I have a sort of status in the hospital. They don't even say my last name. It's like "Laura's coming in." You know, I've seen patients come and go, and I've seen nurses come and go. I've seen medical students become interns become attendings. It's like my hotel.

[*talking to nurse*]

*Laura:* Okay, Carina is going to stick me. Twenty-two and three-quarter needle. In we go. I don't feel a thing. Ooh that hurts.

*Laura:* I don't have to be on death's door to go into the hospital.

*Laura:* We got a nice blood return. Now we're flushing.

*Laura:* They call them tune-ups. It's almost like you charge the battery on your cell phone.

* To listen to the audio story visit www.radiodiaries.org.

*Laura:* And now we're going to hook me up to my antibiotics. [*hums Jeopardy theme*]

*Nurse:* I'll be back.

*Laura:* Thanks.

*Laura:* Get back into bed here. My nice comfy electric bed.

*Laura:* I was diagnosed with cystic fibrosis when I was three days old. It was 1981, and uh, I guess at that time, my parents really didn't know how long I would end up living. The average life span of a person with CF was much younger than it is now. When I was twelve and thirteen, I met a lot of kids in the hospital with CF. There was sort of like a whole gang. You know there was a lot of CF kids. And we'd just play cards, and talk dirt about the nurses, and watch TV shows at night. Ride down the hall on IV poles. There was just this sort of bond you know?

*Laura:* Jeana died when we were thirteen. Damien died that year he was seventeen. Nikki Cooli died. Tamisha died. Elizabeth Florin died winter of twelfth grade. My friend Sophie died when I was in eleventh grade. She was one of my best friends with CF. And, my friend Marcy died this past summer.

*Laura:* Do you hear how quiet it is? This is the sort of after hours calm. Everyone's asleep. I like nights in the hospital. Goodnight.

[*hospital sound fades*]

[*car sound*]

*Laura:* This is Laura back again. Dad and I are on the Bruckner. We're driving up to Providence. I agreed to let him drive. I just spent about four or five days in the hospital again for a partial bowel obstruction, so that was thrilling as ever. And luckily it was only a partial obstruction, so they were really excited about that. But of course at the moment I wasn't as excited about it because I had a tube in my butt, and it's a little bit hard to be excited when you have a tube in your butt. Wouldn't you say, Dad? Why are you crying?

*Dad:* Well, I mean, it's hard to talk about this, not knowing, what's going to happen next. And you go ahead with your life the best you can. [*sniffle*] Pause it for a second.

[*guitar, fade under*]

*Laura:* So, now for a little lesson. Here is the deal with CF: Basically your body produces abnormally thick, sticky mucus that resides in the lungs. And the lungs are sort of the deadly part of the disease, in that after years of infection the lungs sort of get worn away and deteriorate. Most people who see me on the street wouldn't realize how much harder I work to breathe. Or even people who know me don't really realize it, because over the years I've got better and better at hiding the fact that I have trouble breathing.

[*coughing*]

*Laura:* It's funny sometimes, sometimes I cough so hard that I can see stars.

[*school, dorm sound*]

*Laura:* So, I'm back here at Brown. Classes started on Wednesday. I think that people who know me, who really know me, who are my friends, don't see me as someone who is sick. They see me as Laura, who's a sophomore at Brown. It's hard for them to imagine, you know, oh, she might not be here in a few years. They know I have CF. They know that it means you get very sick and that you die, but they see me and it's hard for them to make it real, because they don't want to, because no one wants to, because, you know, they want me to live forever, because I'm their friend.

[*people singing in the background*]

*Laura:* The truth is that even though I'm always thinking about health-related stuff, I don't want to come off as someone who is purely thinking about health-related stuff. I think that's kind of boring.

[*singing fades out*]

[*oxygen tank sound*]

*Laura:* Hi. Um, I'm actually wearing my oxygen, because it's easier to breathe with this on. So that's why I'm wearing oxygen. I'm not feeling very well. The past week I get into really bad coughing fits, and I just have trouble, you know walking. Feeling kind of tired. You know? It's frustrating. And even though people say that it's supposed to get so much worse, I don't quite understand how, like how, I'm expected to just watch it get worse. Like this is not okay: the fact that I'm in on a Friday night. I mean, I'm in college. I'm nineteen. I should have gone to this play I was supposed to go to. I should have gone to these two parties that I was invited to, but instead I'm here. It's just frustrating. I want to be like my peers. But I don't know how. [long pause] Anyway, I think I'm going to go to bed.

[*tape recorder clicks off*]

[*guitar music*]

*Laura:* [*clears throat*] Hi. It's a couple days after my birthday, so I'm twenty. It just sort of all hit me today. I was lying on the couch in the living room, and the sun was setting, and I just, I just knew it. It was at that moment that I really felt that I wouldn't be alive at New Years. The last few weeks, I definitely felt that I was starting the dying process, and it's just a matter of when. How fast. How much at a time. It didn't make sense to push the limit, try to see how long I could last with these old lungs. So, I decided, I'm going to try the lung transplant. You know, there are risks with it. The obvious one of course being, if it doesn't go well, and I die. But I don't want to just go down hill without trying to stop it first.

[*commotion, loud whispers*]

*Friend1:* Where is she right now? Wait, so we're waiting until she takes the blinds off and then we're saying . . . ?

*Friend2:* Yes

*All:* Shhhhhh! [*laughter. door opens*] Surprise!

[*screams and laughter, fades under*]

*Laura:* All my friends came to this lung retirement party.

*Friend3:* We are gathered here, this evening, just to send Laura off with a hurrah, as she leaves Brown temporarily as a student. [*sound fades under*]

*Laura:* Well, I've decided to leave college, and go up to Boston—that's where the hospital is, and wait there for my transplant. I have the poster that my friend designed that says "Thank you to the lungs of Laura for twenty years of exemplary service." So that's kind of neat.

*Laura:* [*to friends*] Well. That's a wrap.

[*clapping and laughter, fades*]

[*phone ringing*]

*Laura:* Hello. Julie? Hi. Yeah I haven't talked to you in a long time. Oh, it's okay, you know. I'm just sort of just sitting here waiting for lungs. Hehe. Yeah, but they've had what they are calling a lung drought. You know, there is nothing I can do to make it happen, short of going out and hitting someone with a car. Hehe. Yeah, I do. Okay, I'll talk to you soon. Love you. Bye. [*Hangs up phone*]

*Laura:* Mom? Mom? [*coughing*]

*Laura:* My dad and my mom are very worried; they wish they could do something. But we don't spend a lot of time talking about it.

*Mom:* I remember even when you were younger, before even the question of the transplant came up, I watched you, you know, go through this. I watched you get very ill. Still, I have never really been able to experience what you've been experiencing, and at times, um, had no idea what you were going through.

*Dad:* I remember that we were always wondering about how to talk to you about what the disease meant. And it never seemed to be the right moment. There was no reason to throw this at you. And then there was this particular time, in the news there was something about cystic fibrosis. And you were ah . . .

*Laura:* I was eleven.

*Dad:* You were eleven, and you told me, "Dad, this'll probably be in the paper tomorrow, and why don't you cut it out for me, and I'll read it on the school bus." So I went to the paper, and exactly what I'd feared had happened. In the last sentence it said, "cystic fibrosis the most common genetic disease, and the average life expectancy is, eighteen years, or twenty one years," or whatever it was. So I thought, I can't have you, I can't have my daughter read this on the school bus, go on the school bus and read this that she is going to die at an early age like this, because by now you would understand what it meant. And so I thought to myself, I've got ten minutes to tell my daughter that she's going to die. And I went in the kitchen.

*Laura:* . . . and I was sitting there eating . . .

*Dad:* You were having your Cheerios. And ah, I said to you, Laura, you know this illness you have, this cystic fibrosis, it's a serious illness. And such was the tone in my voice that you kind of got it immediately. And you became very tremulous, and you said, "You mean, I'm going to die?" and when you said it in that tone of voice, I completely broke down, and I was crying, and I said to you, and it's true, that it's my dream that you should outlive me. And at this point, it was really remarkable, you were ah, put an arm around me. And began to comfort me. [*pause, sniff*] I got a phone call that afternoon that said, "Dad, that article, the point of that article, was that there's hope, isn't it. Isn't that the point of it?" and I said "Yes, Laura. That's the point of it."

*Laura:* I remember that conversation.

[*scene fades*]

[*phone ringing*]

*Dad* [*on answering machine*]: You've reached Laura. The news this fifteenth of July is that Laura is today getting her lung transplant. [*beep*]

[*hospital beeping*]

*Laura:* Well, it's about ten to eight in the morning. I'm here in the hospital. The sun has just come up. And the animal curtains are pulled across my window. But there's just a little bit of light showing through into my room. And it's shining on my toes.

*Nurse:* Hi there. I need to get you upstairs.

[*beeping*]

*Laura:* This surgery is going to happen, and it's weird. When I go in the OR, I always like to look at all the monitors when I'm lying on the table, and all the faces and the lights. The lights are really bright. There's sort of this feeling of, once the anesthetic is in, everything sort of hazing out, forcing you to close your eyes. And I always try to keep my eyes open as long as I possibly can, to remember the last moment that I was awake. And it's so hard to do that. It always wins out. [*beeping, fade out*]

*Answering Machine* [*female voice*]: You have one message. [*beep*]

*Lauren, friend* [*on answering machine*]: Hi. My name is Lauren. I am a friend of Laura Rothenberg. She came out of the surgery well last night. She has beautiful new lungs, and more updates will come. Alright, bye-bye. [*beep*]

[*Laura breathing slowly*]

*Laura:* That sound.

[*Laura breathing slowly*]

*Laura:* Those are my new lungs. And this is a picture, it's in the OR, and they're taking the lungs out of the ice, and it's a close-up, and it's in like a metal basin-type thing. That's my lungs! Up close it just looks like a turkey, basically.

[*leaving hospital sounds*]

*Laura:* [*to hospital staff*] Bye. Thank you. Good luck with everything. Thanks.

*Laura:* I'm leaving the hospital after nineteen days, and it's very exciting.

[*commotion, guitar music fades in*]

*Laura:* Most people ask, how does it feel? Like how does it feel different to breathe? And it's funny because it feels like a completely different body. Sort of everything about it seems new. I don't know it like I knew my body before. It's like a whole new ballgame.

[*music fades out*]

[*blowing into the microphone*]

*Laura:* This is Laura. And I'm sitting here with my cat Gus who is asleep. I haven't talked in a while. On Monday it will be a year since my lung transplant. So, I'm happy I made it a year, but it is not the year that I'd dreamed of: complication, after complication, after surgery, after surgery, and rejection and lymphoma. I've had to get a feeding tube put back in because I lost so much weight. You know I think to get to the transplant, I really had to pretend that the transplant would do more than it realistically could do for me. My whole life, I've been searching for something to fix me. And it hasn't.

I definitely think about after I'm gone. I've always been scared that people will forget about me, but I'm also here right now. So it's about trying to come to a place where I can just accept that things have gone the way they've gone, and accept that it's never going to be perfect. You know I'm well enough to go back to school. I'll be a junior. You know, I want to walk from my door to the Main Green, maybe even play soccer which I haven't done for like eight years. But I don't really count on anything anymore. I just go with the flow. I think that's okay.

[*music*]

# Nuts

XAN L. ROBERTI

The device in hand I stride into
the restroom with Margaux in trail.

It's not every night I loosen
my will, say yes to the
double yes whiskey offered.

On Essex St. at 2am I have been
a dartboard for kisses,
I have flung back plenty.

The bartender follows us
into the restroom: *Do you
have a pen in there? I don't want
any graffiti . . .*

Yes I do. Have an
epinephrine pen.

I've translated dinner ingredients
by dictionary in Paris. I restrict
my restaurants even here; cutting
boards carry residue.

Nuts, all nuts, no nuts—

I forgot to check in her mouth
the last time we kissed. She had
cashews, bar-nuts, I licked on her
tongue.

So far, it's been perfect: a night I
would drive, yes drive, through Manhattan
watching people, and a slanted sky
to see the moon descend.

But I sit, pants down, on a lidded
toilet, allergic, with a needle
resolution in my thigh.

# Crazy for Life:
# A True Story about Living with Mental Illness

VICTORIA MAXWELL

I'm at a meditation retreat, desperate to find enlightenment. But my desperation has very little to do with the genuine desire to know God. It has way more to do with wanting to be free from the pain of human experience—my human experience—what I find out later is actually severe clinical depression. I want to transcend this crap we call life into what I pray is something more restful and tranquil.

The meditation starts with a mantra, a silent question I repeat in my head: "Who am I?"

"Who am I?"

I feel something. Sort of like the warm "fuzzies" I feel when I look at my boyfriend. A wave of patience washes over me.

Again: "Who am I?"

Nothing. Literally. Perfect silence.

"Who am I?"

More stillness. My mind doesn't wrestle or cough. It's just quiet. And actually I can feel my mind. Sort of lying there.

A hot syrupy feeling opens from the center of my chest and burns outwards. It bulldozes through my arteries, my arms, into my hands, down my spine, until the feeling of my body completely disappears. But the burning sensation doesn't. I have no idea what's happening. I'm not freaking out though. Having a body doesn't seem very important. A lot of things begin to seem overrated.

My breath mysteriously shifts into imperceptible bubbles of air. Then: nothing. I stop breathing. And am gliding like a plane after liftoff. Consciousness, thick with comfort and an unusual sense of ... curiosity. Emotions aren't fluttering, no jagged edges or anxious bits bouncing back and forth.

This is peace. And I'm watching it all. Then it hits me that "I" am not here ... my usual sense of "me" ... of "I," of Victoria is ... well ... not here ... "Who am I?" suddenly makes sense. This "I" I think I am is not me ..., it's a construct of the mind ... an effective title helping me navigate through this concrete world ... "I" DOESN'T EXIST ... and I am larger than I could ever imagine ... moving into realms of rapture ... pure beautiful nothing ... bliss ...! My breath returns, body remorphs. I open my eyes, experiencing everything as if for the very first time: hearing, seeing, feeling. Don't exactly know what's happened, just that something has.

I'm now sitting in my bedroom, alone, burning up with this cosmic energy. I'm ecstatic. Voracious for liberation. "Who am I" orbits through my mind . . . triggering surges of energy barreling through my body . . . love pours from my heart . . . the room spins: one, two, three . . . then stop. One, two, three . . . stop. And time stands still. And never starts.

I lie on my bed. Heat scorches the underside of my skin. Chills roll over my body. I begin to shake. I'm nervous, but not panicked. The blue walls of my room rumble with both terror and bliss. I walk between sweeping waves of ecstasy, tornadoes of grief . . . gales of laughter erupt from my belly . . . tears stream from my eyes . . . I am blown open! I don't sleep or eat and barely need to drink. I've been awake for over five days.

I talk nonstop, weaving cosmic revelations with opinions about drapery fabric. I see my skin melt, light shine from the top of my head. My dad asks me to get into his new Mazda 626. I think we're going for a nice Sunday drive. Trust me, the hospital is his only option.

We pull into a parking stall. I heave open the door and leap out. I want to tell everyone about what I've discovered. And I do, running around the psych hospital parkade, screaming at the top of my lungs, with my sixty-one-year-old dad chasing me:

"I got it. This is an illusion. There's no separation. I'm everything. Everyone. The Alpha, the Omega. No separation. I'm Meryl Streep! I'm Dolly Parton! I'm David Hasslehoff!"

"Vicki! Vicki! Come back here!"

"THIS is all an illusion! How could I have been so stupid? I'm free. I'm no longer in the illusion!"

The psych nurses, however, are. Next thing I know I'm in emergency, lying in a hospital bed with a pink curtain closed around me. My dad is somewhere on the other side of the curtain, cursing a nurse. I no longer feel the joyous expansion of being my favorite movie star or TV's oldest lifeguard. Now all I feel is terrifying emptiness and death-knell isolation.

The guru's voice echoes in my head: "There is only room for one. You must do this alone. Alone." Looking back, I think he was referring to simple meditation. But back then, I figured he must mean something much more drastic: I needed to eliminate my ego. Kill my ego. That would complete the process.

I rummage through my bed. Rifling through the soft blue blankets. I don't know what I expect to find. Something sharp, anything sharp. I mean business.

My father is still berating the nurse. This is my chance to liberate myself once and for all. I lunge at the row of cotton swabs and bandages I see on a nearby table.

The nurse turns and shouts—and I'm not kidding—"Hey! Stop the crazy woman!"

They chase me down, wrestle scissors out of my hands, but I run for it. I head for the nearest bathroom. Lock the door. Click. Lean against it and breathe. A lot. And wait for salvation. All I hear is their impervious knocking. Do they think I'm stupid? I'm not going to open it. Then: door handle jiggles. Click. Crack! Bang! Door swings open. Nurse tumbles in. But I'm quick and I'm off. I push through the crowd of orderlies and . . . I can't remember exactly how . . . I end up lying face down on a gurney.

Steel "safety" bars up. Both sides. Left wrist—strapped: leather cuff. Right wrist—locked: leather cuff. And my butt, cold as arctic ice, hanging out of what must be the most humiliating piece of clothing ever made. The minty green hospital gown. All I can feel is air. Frickin' air.

To my left—a security guard, gray as silly putty, arms crossed, stone faced, eye line frozen above my feet. I lift my head, trying to catch his eye: "I'm not getting out of here, am I?" He resentfully moves his gaze down, shakes his head, molasseslike, and pins his stare back to the same spot on the wall.

White stockings scuttle past me on the speckled lino. A mauve skirt swinging, orthopedic shoes chirping. I crane my neck. A nurse is tapping a needle: a needle the size of a frickin' 7-Eleven straw! Then, wet cool cotton and jab—a rush of images. Regrets and dreams kaleidoscope. In that moment I realize: I've gone crazy. What everybody calls crazy. God. My heads falls into the pillow. Everything goes black.

After they unchain me from the gurney and the heavy sedatives wear off, I'm told what I went through was "little" more than a brief reactive psychosis. Then after brain scans and assessments the doctor says, "No, no, it's rapid cycling, mixed state bipolar disorder with mild temporal-lobe epilepsy, and generalized anxiety disorder." But I don't buy that. What I'm going through is an illness. I don't doubt there's a chemical imbalance, but a mental illness?

Regardless, I spend a lovely three weeks at the all-inclusive "Club Medication," AKA the psych ward. The hospital does help me "come back," "come down." What doctors like to call "normal," I call "neutral." But getting to neutral isn't the problem. Staying there is. It's like asking a roller coaster to forget about all its dips and peaks. And I'm not so keen on being in "neutral." I mean, who would be? A car can't even move in neutral. So how good can it be?

When I leave "Club Med" I'm handed a prescription. Zoloft and Epival. Antidepressant and mood stabilizer, respectively. Drugs for mental illness. But see, getting those kind of drugs is different than getting ones for, say, blood pressure, high cholesterol, or even a ... yeast infection. It feels like someone's saying, "Your personality isn't okay." Like you're the new kid in school and nobody likes you. You know that "you're too sensitive. You take things too personally. You're too moody, too much. Here, take a pill. It'll make it easier for the rest of us." Well, I don't let people off the hook that easy. I don't take any. I decide to go au naturel. OH MY GOD! No medication. No psychiatrist. No telling what would happen.

Depression. That's what happens. What I fear and respect most. It seeps deep into my bloodstream. I recognize it immediately. I anxiously tread above its current. But eventually I relent, surrender to its undertow, exhausted. No reason for the beast's presence. No lost love. No lost job or dwindled savings. Just a hovering blackbird circling my movements, permeating my entire existence.

Depression. Not the blues, not in the dumps, not down, not self-pity. A physical sensation. Wet laundry soaked in my chest. Pain in my joints. A haze of fatigue. And absolute hopelessness. Infinite and immovable. Relentless. Relentless. I hate myself I'm worthless I'm nothing I'm useless I'm crap I'm dead I hate myself I'm worthless I'm nothing you're useless you're crap you're dead.

My father, my mom, and my boyfriend all listen tenderly to me at first. Then over time and fatigue, they stiffen as I talk. No one wants to admit it, but there is only so much listening, so much support a person can give. Depression has a cutthroat way of dismantling empathy. And I am painfully aware of this.

Over the next few days, I talk to no one. Not to friends. Not to my parents. I'm dangerously silent. Dangerously despondent. And worse? I don't care. I lie in bed for days on end, getting up only to go pee or order pizza. The effort to shower's too much. Answering the phone, too painful. I flip through my address book trying to get the courage to call someone. My hair's stringy, clothes stale. Half empty coffee cups decorate the windowsill and Kit Kat wrappers litter the carpet. Darker and darker thoughts pour into my mind. Days bleed into weeks, passing into one endless suicidal dream. But natural fierceness prompts me to take one last shot at hope.

"I'll talk to somebody, just to say good-bye." I get the name of this counsellor. I don't even know where I got her name. Flipped through the phone book or looked in the classifieds or something. I don't remember where I was when I called her. In fact, I don't even remember calling her. But I must have.

The entrance to her suite is at the back of a dentist office. I always did hate going to the dentist. I'm sitting, swallowed up by an overwhelming salmon pink armchair. Across from me, this woman: a psychotherapist with a triangular forehead and a smile disproportionate for her face. She leans forward. I push back. Silence.

"Did you know," I pipe up, "that therapist is actually 'THE-RAPIST' if you break it up?" There, that'll get her going. Piss and vinegar I am. But nothing, shit.

"How are you?" She looks directly at me, her hands neatly interlocked on her lap. "How are you?"

My eyes well with hot tears. "Fine," I lie. And look away as she leans closer.

"Really? I want to make this worth your while." She shifts her weight, crosses her plump legs. I can see knee-high nylons under her bias-cut skirt. "Do you still want to kill yourself?" She doesn't beat around the bush this one, does she? I'm secretly impressed.

I must have mentioned in our phone conversation that I might take a ticket outta here, do the "big adios," that I didn't know if I want to take it anymore. Perhaps that I *wouldn't*. Funny how offhanded you get when death becomes an option.

"Have you thought of a way?" She's taking me seriously. I appreciate this. It's not like I chose this suicide thing on a whim.

"Pills." I spit out. And choke back more hot tears. "It's not that bad—really." I lie—again.

Do you know there's a whole manual in the library dedicated to suicide? I mean, obviously someone thinks there's a right way and a wrong way to do it. Success or failure. That's a lot to live up to. Sort of. The last thing I want to be is a failure at suicide. I mean that's a killer on the self-esteem.

Well, first there's the jumping off the bridge event: way too much media exposure. And to be honest, I'm a fairly strong swimmer, so what if my natural instincts kick in? And I don't want to go even near the whole gun thing: too expensive, too illegal, too masculine for starters. And razors? That's a whole other ball of wax. Way too scary. I'm way too much of a wuss for that. There is, of course, the classic: pills and booze. Dramatic, very Hollywood, Entertainment Tonight–like, but not necessarily surefire. I'm always afraid I'll just puke and pass out. Not die. Very messy, not to mention embarrassing. Nonetheless, as I mention to her, my method of choice is a pills-and-vodka-with-OJ combo. I did considered apple cider but . . . well, how effective can alcoholized apple juice be?

She eyeballs me: "Where would you get the pills from?"

"Me. And my parents. I haven't taken a whole mess of my own meds for months, but I got the prescriptions filled anyway. I'm always thinking ahead." I lean closer and whisper, "I'm a planner, you know." I hope she recoils or shudders or something, but this one, cool as a cucumber. Nuttin'. "My mom and dad have something for everything. So I'm sure I could find some stuff there too, without them even noticing anything's gone. And vodka. Lots of vodka."

The early evening light streams through the venetian blinds. I stare at my feet. Pick at my cuticles. I think of all the reasons why I won't go through with it and all the reasons why I will. She just waits.

"Ever since I started studying this enlightenment crap," I burp out, "trying to find Utopia, I feel screwed. I bet this suicide thing isn't really any answer at all. You probably become some etheric blob of energy floating around, wanting to kill yourself. Which is even more frustrating because then you don't even have a body to get rid of." We both laugh.

We never really come to any solid conclusions about whether I will or not. Kill myself, that is. But at least someone knows. At least I tried. I look her straight in the eyes when I hand her my money. "I dare you," I'm thinking, "take money from a dying woman." I'm top-notch. Martyr skills down to an art. But nothing.

There's no cure for life. But there are vacations from it. Suicidal thoughts were the cheapest ones for me. Ironically, it's thoughts of death and suicide that kept me alive.

. . .

I'm running . . . running . . . like an exploding jack-in-the-box . . . up West Tenth . . . past Safeway . . . past the Starbuck's . . . turn to my left . . . running . . . 12th and Trimble . . . running . . . west of a fire hall . . . running . . . running . . . I'm running: NAKED. I'M NAKED!

I'm not taking any meds . . . obviously . . . but I am now seeing a shrink. I've moved off the couch of "bingeing-on-Cheetos-and-Pop-Tarts kind of suicidal depression" and am now, once again, in a state of euphoric manic psychosis, riffing on this enlightenment thing. I've discovered not taking medication is a sure-fire way to catapult into the up-and-down chaos of bipolar disorder. I am DEFINITELY on an upswing.

What I'm going through is strictly a spiritual transformation. I'm not gonna take some pills that'll blot out my spiritual awakening. Granted . . . my life is in complete shambles. But shit! Pills to stop the most profound experiences of my life? Who else would I turn to?! . . . God. He'll understand where I'm coming from. Or at least his son will. Christ! Exactly: Christ.

I run past the fire hall. If there isn't an emergency, there sure as hell should be. I guess you could say I'm the best siren there. See, I think taking off my dress is a good way to meet the Beloved (God). You know that purity of body kind of thing? I don't get that naked doesn't always mean purity.

The fire guys must be on their afternoon naps. Because nothing. Nada. Not one firefighter/calendar pinup boy to the rescue. They're sleeping. That's what I tell myself. Otherwise, my rather fragile positive body image will categorically collapse.

I think God purposely put me in a snobby postal code to, you know, shake up the neighborhood. I'm definitely doing something demographically unac-ceptable. Not really a clothing-optional street, if you know what I mean.

So I'm bouncing my way down the street. Well, parts of me are, hoping to meet the Divine. I'm more or less playing hide-and-seek with God. I'm alive, euphoric, like I haven't been in months and all this, the world around me, means nothing. Not like apathetic nothing, but "it's-all-a-dream" nothing.

Colors blur by, green leaves, bright sun, hard concrete. Cars slow down . . . then speed up. Then: something. There—in the bushes. For me to find. So simple, so divine . . . I'm here. It's me. I think I see the Beloved peeking around the stop sign, beckoning me forward, then vanishing into the laurel bush. I run toward the corner. But . . . I stop . . . turn . . . a girl, say, oh, about seven, peers out from behind a porch post. Staring at me, sort of like how a chimpanzee looks into a camera lens. I stand, aware of two worlds at once: ordinary reality, and the heavenly realm, both trying to sting me awake.

The little girl . . . her pointed chin . . . ruddy summer cheeks . . . two white legs jutting out from underneath a pink sundress. The door opens behind her. A tall, liquid woman. Her mother, I guess. She shoos her daughter into the house (no doubt nervous about the naked lady staring at her child). The woman gingerly moves toward me. Warm with a smile. I stand there, frozen—literally shivering. It's cold when you're naked. Especially when everyone else isn't. She asks, "Would you . . . like something to wear?"

A road map to God might have done just as nicely for me, but she offers me clothes. A bathing suit to be exact. Size 4. *Girl's* size 4! Within minutes, the police show up. Then the ambulance. The gig is definitely up. Yup. No escapin' this one.

I'm now wearing the yellow bathing suit, not my birthday suit, sitting in the ambulance, hunched over, poking at all the gadgets. Two paramedics look at me with actually very compassionate eyes. "What's your name? Do you know where you live? How old are you?"

I answer. Ten out of ten. Gold star. I'm pumped. I feel young, very young and quite cute. Why not use it to my advantage? I check out one of the ambulance guys, the one with the hip sideburns and the copper necklace. I wink. Zero. I pout instead. They're taking notes, these two. Very serious. "Can I ride up front? I've never been in an ambulance before."

"Okay," the cute one says, "but no siren." He smiles and wags his finger. I don't get to flick the siren switch, but I do get a front row seat and a wheel chair welcome to my good ol' alma mater, the psych ward.

After they stabilize me—I think that means I stop flirting with the paramedics—I get a very nice south-facing "apartment" for my alumni visit to A 2. Lights out. I'm under my covers. Blue blanket. Soft but sad. "Ill . . . mentally unstable . . . fragile state of mind . . . on med-i-ca-tion . . . PSYCHOTIC EPISODES. Shit." I cry myself to sleep.

. . .

I went bonkers. Did it with flair, if I say so myself. Full on with fireworks and everything, emotional pyrotechnics galore. It's like a thousand watts of electricity went through a 40-watt bulb. I had some amazing insights in meditation, which also blew my circuits in some very vulnerable spots. Diabetes doesn't run in our family; bipolar disorder, clinical depression, and anxiety do.

I'm sitting now. Spread out. On the beach, against a log. Sunset. Birds. Seagulls. A heron. Smell of sweet cherry blossoms. A little girl plays at the water's edge. Huh. Funny. A yellow suit. Two piece though. She laughs and shrieks. Spins. Splitting water with her fingers. Her back to the ocean, she faces her family. Waving. All smiles. "Look at me! Look at me!"

Behind her, a swell, a giant wave. Rolling, gaining speed behind her . . . rolling, gaining speed behind her . . . totally oblivious . . . I call out, try to get her attention, but . . .

She turns. Faces the breaker. Hit! Arms up. Body back. She shakes her head . . . and hugs the water right back. Squeals of giggles mark the sky. Then she starts the whole shebang again: Spin. Waves. Turns. Hit! And embrace . . . all over again.

# Casing the Joints:
# A Story of Arthritis

## Mary Felstiner

### Heat Inversion

Long before morning I wake with a stinging in my shoulders so acute I lie in bed for hours thinking how to drain the acid off; or I get up in the dark—tired, baffled, stiff, and slow. All morning I keep dropping off and waking in a burn. What if I worked on an assembly line where, falling asleep, I'd get maimed?

It's noon and I'm waiting for the ache to go away. Inside the joints there's high influenza—it must be 102 degrees. Anywhere I sit stays hot after I get up. If I reach for a magazine, it slips off my thumbs. If I take a shower, I can't squeeze the tube of shampoo. I try reading but the sense of words simmers away.

And then my heat inversion lifts. By late afternoon I lose sight of how it was. I see friends. They say I look good. Just before sleep, I wave away what will come a few hours later.

A joint disease like mine gives daily meaning to the wicked words "double life."

### Chronic

This joint disease of mine, rheumatoid arthritis, is intractable, incurable, inflammatory, and degenerative, bodywide and long as life. It starts and persists by autoimmune reaction, which means my joints are attacked by an immune system that thinks it's kept me safe.

Rheumatoid arthritis afflicts two million Americans, and over twenty-two million more have somewhat milder joint diseases such as osteoarthritis. So tens of millions of Americans wake most mornings with a jolt: awareness of day is awareness of pain. Imagine the ecological challenge if this populace—larger than whole countries—demanded resources to address its suffering.

As anyone who lives a double life knows, the resources of those close to us are what wear thin. Relatives can only give so much, friends always ask but mostly hear nothing good, kids listen to the same gripes every day. Finally even the sufferers find it hard to keep caring afresh. And it is caring—public pressure, medical focus, and personal storytelling—that raises the social standing of any disease.

The social profile of arthritis has settled way too near the ground for our most common chronic condition to stay in sight. Is this mass illness so threatening to our health practices it has to be overlooked? Is its slow repetitive course always muffled by more glamorous frailties or more clamorous crises of health? Is it pushed back by a medical system favoring acute and infectious patients over those who are ill all their lives? Is arthritis underrated because two-thirds of all Americans who suffer the disease belong to the female sex?

## Female Joints

These days most women are scared of suffering any disease that discriminates by gender. Ovarian cancer. Cervical cancer. Breast cancer. In the name of equality, women now demand public action on illnesses like these.

By contrast, our stiff knees, stinging hands, slow gait, hot skin, lousy days, lifelong complaint, all seem things we have to bear. No one thinks of arthritis as a disease of women in the main or as women's main disease—even though one-third of American women between ages forty-five and sixty-four already have some form of arthritis, and after age sixty-five this rises to 56 percent. Plainly put, more than half of U.S. women will sometime suffer this ailment. What we ought to fear we hardly have in mind.

About its most severe form, rheumatoid arthritis, the public learns scraps from time to time but not the most unsettling fact: the disease collides with women in their childbearing years. One thing Americans rely on to keep them fed and mended (for less than a living wage) is women who won't say, "Take care of me. I'm all crippled up." Who would fill in for these women of childbearing age—lifting babies, mashing potatoes, cleaning cafeterias, grading papers, doing all the jobs where nobody picks up after *them*?

"An unrecognized major women's health problem" is the Arthritis Foundation's label for arthritis. The most common and disabling chronic condition women report, says a 1995 study from the Centers for Disease Control and Prevention (the CDC), is arthritis, far more than any other disease—more than cancer, heart disease, diabetes, hypertension. The CDC estimates that twenty-three million women over age fifteen now suffer from arthritis or rheumatic disease, and in twenty-five years the number will jump to thirty-six million women.

Of course breast cancer is epidemic too, and all we can say so far is that women have more breast tissue than men. Arthritis makes much less sense—our human immune system and our common aging process mostly turn against female joints. If we want to know what to fear, it's that no one thinks it urgent yet to find out why.

## Hidden Disability

An ailment of mostly female joints, when it's devoid of drama and lived with year after year, hardly ranks as a "disability" in American eyes. Over time, this misperception seems cause for concealment. Someone taking a job doesn't let an employer know she has a degenerative disease like mine. "They hired me mainly for my energy," one woman tells me recently, yet she's scared that after a few years she'll falter.

This is the hidden dilemma inside hidden disabilities. It's a buyer's market in the job world today: employers are looking for anyone they can exploit. I've been on committees that studied candidates for their battery power, hiring the ones that looked like they'd work all night. So anyone would conceal a disability if it's not observed. Certainly I sashayed into my first teaching job without giving a hint what I'd been diagnosed with. But a secret fear shadowed my early years of work. What if I couldn't carry on? What if they didn't like why?

A few years into my job I let on I had rheumatoid arthritis, and though no one was sure what it meant, the fact was laid down. Much later, when I got so ill my output reversed to intake, I stumbled into the chairperson's office and announced, "I'll finish this semester, then I've got to go on leave. I know you've set the new schedule but if it's possible . . ." He said, "The rearrangements are my job, just let me know how to help." Of course such leaders come from a kinder planet, but I'd prepared him for something like this years before; he knew his teachers were a susceptible tribe.

Revealing a disability can jump-start a helping reaction right away. I've noticed how my colleagues accommodate an outspoken disabled professor, how I grab a seat beside him at gatherings to feed him the best stuff: A little more pâté? I ask (with my own grip shaky on the cracker). He strengthens me.

By saying out loud what we're struggling with when we have to go home early or need help stapling two papers together, we ease the fear that our coworkers will think we're drunk or lazy or drugged. It's better to pop pills in sight of all than worry someone will discover them and wonder what's up. And if we lead with the worst news first, then people figure we'll handle the next-to-worst bulletin without missing a beat. We actually get credit for being steady-eyed when we describe our distress. Because it's our own voice saying, "Here's the trouble," others open up right back. Time and again, I'm told a humbling secret once someone realizes my hands are useless and my feet are killing me.

Every handicap made visible becomes an example to another person—in my case to students who have covert worries about themselves. They want to know an honest job can be done with a disability. They even want to know an honest job can't be done the same way everyone else does it. They now think that if disability strikes them, they won't wash up, they'll tack along like me.

So whatever disclosures we make (and this depends on our condition) we ought to be able to make without risk, without shame. That's more likely to happen if I confess and then you confess and then someone else, until it's clear we're no cowering minority in the family of humankind.

## SCALP

I confess: I'm the woman with stiff ankles and snapping knees, arms like T-squares and hands curled up. I'm the woman who can't open the car door or the toothpaste tube or the salt shaker or the window blind. I'm the one with pouches under the eyes and a scratchy voice, a dry mouth, bumpy knuckles. Without dyed hair—without much hair at all. The one with no eye makeup, my eyes being dry and sore. This is the way some of us women look, and I'd like to think for this condition I look just right.

I've been the one without much hair since I started taking a drug called methotrexate, an immunosuppressant used against rheumatoid arthritis (RA for short) and also as chemotherapy against cancer. One difference is, if you have RA, you don't stop taking methotrexate. It helps suppress symptoms but your disease persists and so do the side effects of the drug. Methotrexate left scattered strands of hair all over my tub. In the mirror I stared at scalp.

That's when last century's paintings of women began to offend my taste. Painting where females glow in their hair (a cover-up of any good hard head) prepared the way for modern ads that nobody can resist. Today hair has become the logo women can't present themselves without.

It's a primary code, a way each woman calls out, "This is me over here." If your hair is worn rowed, it might mean you're proud of African descent. If it's reset every day, maybe you're ready to replace a boss. If it's flying around unwashed, you're not going to be what your parents want. Cut to a brush, it says, look me in the eye.

So what does it mean to lose your hair against your will? You lose access to your code. You're kept from a female way of directing someone else's gaze. You stay mortified, like a mummy, preserved without the one feature you'd arrange.

A friend of mine, after undergoing chemotherapy, forfeiting her breasts, facing the chance of death, said her greatest sense of loss was just her hair. She rejoiced—smack in the middle of cancer—when the first fuzz reappeared. Another friend whose chemotherapy made her bald was at the movies one hot night where she took off her scarf till the last credits rolled and then she had a choice: get that scarf on or show scalp. The lights came up. She walked out of the movies and into her office the next day, and every day, just as she was. Someone took a snapshot—a grinning woman with ears—which later she liked to show around.

Maybe if she thought her inalienable female trait couldn't grow back, her daring might have failed. Women lose their hair forever from man-made toxins, menopause, drug therapies, genetic legacies, autoimmune diseases. So my own body's complex response to rheumatoid arthritis and to its treatment was collapsing into one humiliating loss.

In 1995 I stopped the methotrexate injections and suffered a kickback reaction—when unrestrained immune cells torch the joints—that knocked me flat for months until I started a less invasive (and less effective) drug. Then the disease process between my bones sped up, while the light-brown marsh grass on my head got stringier but not so fast. I asked myself: how should I choose between my need for joints and my need for hair?

Shift Key

The disease process sped up. But my ideas about it seemed slower to form. That's what it felt like when I first shifted from written to oral expression, around 1995. Like slipping sideways into a district where hands-on machines just don't exist. No fax, let alone e-mail; no computer, let alone typewriter; no ballpoint even. The voice is all that's around for transporting thought. You have to make this shift with damaged tendons or joints, with disease or repetitive stress (the epidemic of our keyboard age). First you can't live without fingertip communication. Then you live as if it had never been invented.

After closing up pen and keyboard (at the insistence of my finger joints), I got to speak my business out loud like a herald to scribes: their hands produced each private message of mine, each financial form and medical disclosure and, of course, this paragraph. Since I couldn't rewrite by hand, I dictated every change over and over. Since I couldn't dash off postcards to friends, I got on the phone each evening. After I stopped penciling students' papers, I had to make comments face to face. It was labor-intensive, voice-activated, what social exchange used to be. And I liked it. I liked talking. To everyone who has to give up writing machines, I'd say: oral culture has its uses. It's good to hear your voice again.

Then in 1996 I sneaked back to the written word under the guise of high technology—a speech-recognition computer program petitioned from State Disability so I could work with less expense and effort. The first time I looked into speech recognition I should have been forewarned. A disabled colleague told me he preferred writing flat on the floor with a keyboard and an oxygen tank to using that software. But I plunged ahead.

As someone used to typing quick paragraphs, this speaking to a computer reduced me to precognition, before knowing what word I was trying to form. Four sentences could take forty exhausting minutes of repetition and correction to translate from digital sounds into accurate type. To change one phrase in a document required ten verbal commands, some of which failed to be speech-recognized themselves. From the simplest spoken words the program created arcane utterances that I corrected on the spot because otherwise it proudly committed its mistakes to deep memory. I retrained it with every word until I couldn't stand its backwardness, or mine.

But the most pernicious effect was this: just when I'd grudgingly shifted from using my hands to using my words, this voice-intensive program took away my voice. It wasn't laryngitis. It was my vocal cords acting like my arms and hands: swollen with arthritis, inflamed, and locked. So far as I knew, I'd blown out the essential joint, with no more hope for its return than for straight elbows or bending wrists.

I became the proverbial silent woman. For weeks on end I sat at my kitchen table just moving my mouth in pantomime while those around me guessed. I couldn't write notes because my hands didn't work; and for the same reason I knew I'd never learn sign language. Thoughts welled up in my throat then had to be drained back down. Facial muscles wore out miming delight or dismay at anyone's news. For weeks nothing rose toward my teenage son Alek except "Have a great day," mouthed in the morning, and "How was your day?" after high school.

At the kitchen table one night, Alek started on the harm of hate words versus the insult of censorship—a subject so close to my cortex I could feel thoughts bulging behind my eyes. I said nothing, of course, but understood that for me the end of free speaking was the end of living. In a matter of weeks I'd learned more of human nature than in all my years before, but I couldn't pass a word of it to anyone.

Then things came forward I never watched arrive before. From all over the country my friends made one-way phone calls and wrote notes I couldn't answer, though these friends came in the first place from all the words between us. Though I lost my smoothest hours (the drowsy bedtime talks with John, a habit of thirty years), I found him staying awake to look my way. From a friend came a textile that I decked the computer with, demoting my machinery to drapery. And from my doctor: a sharp dose of cortisone that located my vocal cords, while a speech pathologist slowly taught them ways to make soft sounds.

A shift key took my language from manual to vocal and from vocal to facial, then shifted again to a place where I have to quit talking (or forfeit my voice) whenever a radio's on or a dishwasher's running or a van's going by, where I wait for a noiseless house (no water on) before I talk long distance with my daughter

Sarah, where I mike my own phone and my tape recorder and any conversation that isn't one-on-one, where I dictate only an hour's worth of words to keep my vocal joints from damage. This is a fragile place, just short of speechlessness, where most people think it's too quiet to live. I live there morning to night, casing the joints.

## NOTE

I would like to thank Ruth Rosen, John Felstiner, Gerda Lerner, Joan Weimer, Nina Jo Smith, and Stanford's Institute for Research on Women and Gender for invaluable assistance.

*Narratives of Diagnosis and Treatment: Relationships to the Medical Community*

℘

THIS SECTION BEGINS with an essay by the only male author in the collection. Sociologist Arthur Frank gives us an insightful gendered analysis of women's anger toward the medical community. The narratives in this section, Frank explains, are jarring because they impeach the unimpeachable. He contextualizes women's reaction to the medical gaze and medical technology within a framework of larger social victimization. In his words, "What these stories brought me, as a male reader, to see with renewed clarity is how women arrive at medical treatment with an embodied wariness that is the end product of a lifetime of vulnerability to male objectification."

The medical gaze in this section is isolating, enraging, frightening, and victimizing. In her brief haiku written in the hours before an orthopedic operation, Fran Bartkowski writes of holding her own hand "to calm the pulse of fear." In "Stereotactic Biopsy," Amy Haddad writes about being "Trapped / Waiting" after a biopsy, wondering, "Where did they go?" and then "Thinking I am alone / I start to cry quietly / then sob." Medical diagnostics and technology are here framed as consuming: they devour women's body parts and divide them into fragments. This fragmentation is mirrored in the physical structure of Veneta Masson's poem, "Pathology Report," in which "the specimens" of her body are parceled into "containers" and labeled with numbers. In "What If They Said," Amy Haddad writes, "We have your breasts and lymph nodes. Now we want / your hair, all of it, brows, lashes, pubic hair, / the down that covers your arms and legs." But this consumption requires more than body parts—it threatens the ill woman's intellect, the very self that lives to tell the tale of her suffering. Jan Feldman, who eventually died of her seizure disorder, wrote of her treatment, "I no longer owned my sleep or appetites. Moods and pains could always signify something else. I felt my wit dull and my perceptions slow. Conversations seemed labored." Similarly Haddad's poem "What If They Said" ends, "Your wit, the ability to choose words, / play with ideas—give us all of that as well. / After all, / we're trying to save your life."

The violence of medicine is technologically precise, militaristic. Veneta Masson describes "dispassionate hands," which dissect and ultimately "submit" her body. As Frank notes, medical violence is deemed necessary and therefore unimpeachable. "War licenses extreme and aggressive and often hasty action," writes Rebecca Pope in her essay "White Coat." "In times of war we are less critical of leaders and generals, more willing to go along with what they say must be done . . . We are more likely, in our fear, to mistake propaganda for sound and credible argument, the horrific for the reasonable . . . We tell ourselves that we can't really concern ourselves about collateral damage." This military metaphor finds embodiment in the context of real political conflict, a history of displacement, ethnic violence, and state terror in Jasmina Tešanović's diary-based "All Patients are Political Women." Here, the institutional inhumanity of a hospital ward reflects the larger state violence and vice versa. The patient becomes powerless refugee, without nationality, home, or context.

# The Negative Privilege of Women's Illness Narratives

### Arthur Frank

Any introduction to these women's writing risks taking a stance of authority that would impose another layer of professional pretension on narratives that are written to show how pretentious professionals can be. Commentary is made more dangerous because I as a man impose another male gaze on women whose illnesses have rendered them vulnerable to male gazes. The problem of commenting on narratives is to show ways that individual voices connect but to avoid reducing any one voice to its terms of connection with others. In the ideal commentary, individual stories are empowered by their association with other narratives, but they are not subsumed within that association. The objective is not to analyze—in the sense of claiming to discover some truth that individual writers could not be aware of—but rather to enlarge, giving each story a greater scope through its chaining to other stories.

The stories in this section each depict some facet of what can be called the mundane horror of medical treatment and diagnosis. Alan Radley understands horror in illness narratives as "the appearance of the unthinkable in the guise of the innocuous."[1] In the waiting rooms of the cancer center where I was treated, I was always vaguely disturbed by volunteers serving tea, from a cart, in china teacups and saucers. The utterly pleasant civility of that gesture—so well intentioned on the volunteers' part—was horrible to me, for reasons that Radley explains. The tea service rendered innocuous what was really going on: the systematic chemical destruction of bodies. The service called on us to act as if we were there for a tea party; what we were actually there for what was unthinkable: planning having parts of our bodies cut out; pumping poisonous substances into our central circulatory systems. These stories are each a refusal to conventional gestures to make it all right. They each scream that it is not all right. That is their testimony and truth.

Of course medicine would reply with the great paradoxical rationale that bodies are being violated so that they can be restored. The quality of horror, Radley argues—and the narratives in this section confirm—lies in presenting death, pain, and brutality "in the context of the ordinary, or the unimpeachable."[2] Medical goals are, by definition, unimpeachable. "After all," Amy Haddad's poem ends, after detailing all the horrific effects of her cancer treatment, "we're trying to save your life." That justification is supposed to render all the horrors part of an acceptable trade-off. Many of the narratives in this section question that trade-off; they impeach the unimpeachable, and that is their jarring, dissonant quality.

Rebecca Pope perhaps most explicitly questions the competence of medicine. After making a case that medical treatment has killed her mother, she quotes an influential medical textbook that advises "doing all that is possible," even when "no effective treatment is available." The medical justification for useless intervention would probably cite the need to sustain hope and not let the patient feel abandoned. Pope cites the devastating iatrogenic effects of treating when treatment can be predicted to be ineffective. Other writers—Amy Haddad, Veneta Masson, and Diane Driedger—leave open the question of whether medicine will help or not. They also leave open the equally consequential question posed by Jasmina Tešanović: will they ever be willing or able to forgive medicine, especially if they are cured and have time to think about what happened to them? Tešanović refers specifically to children forgiving their parents for surrendering them to medical treatments, but these stories extend the issue of forgiveness to all patients and their physicians.

What stands in need of forgiveness is the arrogance of medical staff treating people's bodies as the everyday stuff of their tasks. "I relinquish my right breast," Haddad writes; "the tech pulls on it." The biopsy that follows is more a torture than a treatment, and again the violence is rendered innocuous by the physician's departing comment: "Okay . . . / Let's see what we've got." What he has "got" are sixteen tissue samples, extracted from Haddad's breast by repeated mechanical piercing with a wide-bore needle; what he has got is the product of pain and dehumanization. In Diane Driedger's poem the invasion is visual, but her body no less than Haddad's is reduced to what the philosopher Martin Heidegger, in his essay on modern technology, called "stock."[3]

Heidegger's argument, for all its complexities, is grounded on a fundamental observation that these narratives confirm: the nature of technology is to make things as-they-are disappear, so that they can reappear as the raw material that some technology needs to do its job. In Heidegger's examples, the forest ceases to be a natural, living ecosystem and becomes a source of lumber and pulp; the river ceases and becomes hydroelectric power. Technology, Heidegger argues, enframes the world, causing us to see life as stock for technology. Haddad's breast is enframed by medical technology: all that it meant in her life and relationships disappears, and it reappears as an object that exists for the biopsy machine, to which all priority is granted. Haddad—her body, herself—becomes material for the machines and finally for the gaze of the physician. "Let's see what we've got," the doctor says, with detached curiosity. Perhaps, at the end of the poem, as he sees her sobbing, his throat clearing may be a recognition of what she has been subjected to: not only the pain, but the indignity of transformation into medical material, stock, the everyday stuff of people's mundane work. Or perhaps he will proceed to speak to her as if her sobbing were an embarrassment to both of them, best ignored.

Again the question: should medicine be forgiven? Jan Feldman expresses the ambivalence that runs throughout these stories. At the end of her story, it seems that the doctor has "taken care of it," as grating as that phrase has become as a repeated promise. In the course of treatment, Feldman loses her old self by degree. "I started rooting around in old diaries and picture albums," she writes. "I wanted to identify the real me from these snippets of the past and successfully rappel to the present, identity in hand." Yet she remains "compliant," and at the end this seems rewarded: "the doctor had taken care of it as he said he would." In the context of the other writings in this section, Feldman's closing line can be heard as ironic, but it may be utterly sincere—both senses of her phrase compete with each other, and that is many patients' experience of medical horrors. For what Feldman's doctor gives her (freedom from seizures that might be increasingly damaging; not a trivial matter), he demands nothing less than her self—"the real me" she is left to search for. It is unclear how extensive the remaining "side effects" will be. In Feldman's story we see the gap between the physician's version of his patient's problems being taken care of and that patient's experience of how treatment affects her life.

Feldman's story, forcefully but no more clearly than any of the others, raises the final question that I will consider: the effect of gender in how these people are treated. The question nags throughout her story as throughout all these narratives: would that physician have talked to a man as he does to this woman? How many of these stories could be written by men, with adjustments of pronouns and body parts? Having had testicular cancer myself, I know that male bodies are vulnerable to gender-specific cancers; that vulnerability seems an inevitable part of being human. But there is nothing inevitable in how men and women are treated by medicine and nothing inevitable about how a person's history of living as a man or woman predisposes the way that person experiences medical treatment.

What these stories brought me, as a male reader, to see with renewed clarity is how women arrive at medical treatment with an embodied wariness that is the end product of a lifetime of vulnerability to male objectification. At one end of the continuum are sexually oriented glances that may be more innocent curiosity than malicious intent; at the other end are overt violences of molestation and rape. Men are vulnerable to sexual assault, but in no sense do most men spend their lives having to be oriented to that risk. Returning again to Amy Haddad's poem about her breast biopsy, her experience can be compared to descriptions I have heard from men about prostate biopsies. In a formal, procedural sense, the experiences can be compared. But for most men (not all, certainly, but most), the prostate biopsy is not experienced as part of a life spent protecting oneself from being the victim of sexual assault. Haddad's poem has, without any dramatic flourishes being added, the qualities of a scene in sadomasochistic pornography.

Haddad's tears are distinctly women's tears. They are the tears of someone who has been forced to submit to her nightmare *and* treat that nightmarish submission as innocuous. Because the procedure is defined as unimpeachable in its goals, its practice claims similar unimpeachability.

Women have good reasons not to forgive, and women have a better eye for what is unforgivable. Pierre Bourdieu describes what he calls symbolic violence as "instituted through the adherence that the dominated cannot fail to grant to the dominant . . . when the schemes she applies in order to perceive and appreciate herself, or to perceive and appreciate the dominant . . . are the product of the em-bodiment of the—thereby naturalized—classifications of which her social being is the product."[4] In other words, women, as one group of dominated persons, have spent their lives learning to be the patients in these stories. The terms of percep-tion and appreciation that society has offered them, as means through which to know themselves and to know their physicians, render natural (unimpeachable) the domination these women experience. The male/medical alibi is built in from the beginning. As Bourdieu explains, "The particularity of the dominant is that they are in a position to ensure that their particular way of being is recognized as universal. The definition of excellence is in any case charged with masculine implications that have the particularity of not appearing as such."[5]

Bourdieu's *Masculine Domination* also makes the point that women see through this symbolic violence. Here is the gap between perceptions that is expressed by many social theorists: the dominant are most readily convinced that their par-ticular way of being *is* universal; the dominated have the clearest vision of the games that the dominant are playing. "On their side," Bourdieu writes, "women have the *entirely negative* privilege of not being taken in by the games in which privileges are fought for and, for the most part, not being caught up in them, at least directly, in the first person. They can even see the vanity of them [and] look with amused indulgence on the desperate efforts of the 'child-man' to play the man and the childish despair into which his failures cast him" (emphasis in original).[6] The women in these stories are subject to too much pain, and the assault on their bodies is too pressing, for them to look with amusement, at least at the time they write these stories and poems. But these writings are expressions of the "entirely negative privilege" that Bourdieu notes.

The complexity of masculine games of domination, in the idiom of medicine, are most subtle in Muriel Murch's story of Dr. Patel, who is, in so many ways, the doctor many of us would like to have for ourselves and our loved ones. Dr. Patel actually reads his colleague's referral letter and acts on it, immediately. He makes a house call. He speaks to his patient gently and with respect. Yet there is an ominous note from the beginning when he strides into his office without looking at Jane, his secretary, or returning her greeting. Murch describes Dr. Patel as "like an archaeologist." That metaphor is apt in that he views what he discovers as not alive, no longer fully connected to the living; or at least some connections are beyond what Dr. Patel is prepared to acknowledge. When Dr. Patel calls Susan King, the daughter of the woman who will become his patient, he speaks "quickly as he always did when he had already decided what would work for him."

Murch calls our attention to Dr. Patel's repeated use of "of course" when he tells Susan King his diagnosis and prognosis for her mother. "She cannot stay here of course," he says, cutting off any questioning of what he claims. Some of the implications of his diagnosis and prognosis he knows; other implications he cannot fully know, nor are they within his purview. Again, we see the gap between professional reality and lived reality. "Susan's own heart sank at the words. Fifteen years of slow erosion. How could her mother bear it, and there would never be enough money for that." The story ends with an outcome that promises to work, as well as anything might work, for all concerned; yet, inevitably, "There was no longer any safety."

I have difficulty imagining how Dr. Patel could have acted more sympathetically or professionally. Is he nothing more than the messenger whom we should not shoot, or is he somehow enacting the scene? The story is subtle on this question. The horror of the story is expressed in the irony of its title. Dr. Patel comes to tea, but not for tea. He comes to bring news that rends the apparent tranquility of the afternoon scene, even as he acts in ways that preserve that tranquility. Bourdieu observers that "men are also prisoners, and insidiously victims, of the dominant representation."[7] Dr. Patel is caught in a web of classification and options in which he enjoys certain privileges but to which he is as subjected as Susan King and her mother. His privilege is to be the one capable of speaking "of course." His deficiency of vision is to believe that his *of course* assumption applies to how others experience the world. Is that deficiency also a culpability? Should Susan King forgive Dr. Patel?

These stories are the testimony of those who remain uncertain what requires forgiveness and what to forgive. Their voices disrupt healthy people's imaginations of how we would like to imagine ourselves being treated when we become ill. That disruption becomes tangible in the stories' sensuous details. To read them is a deeply disturbing, frightening encounter.

I had cancer too long ago to be able to read these stories and poems with any ease. Today, it takes concerted effort to let myself be reminded.

Once during the years while I was still having regular follow-up examinations with their frightening false positives and just after my mother-in-law had died of cancer, I would have read these stories as telling the truth; not *a* truth but *the* big truth. I would have found in these stories and poems an antidote to the incessant demands of healthy society to have a "positive attitude" toward illness and always to be grateful to medical staff—all the demands to treat the unspeakable as if it were innocuous.

Once, I would have found it affirming to be in the company of others who had the courage to see the medical landscape as it is: a place where no birds sing and the sky is always gray, where treatment is administered with indifferent arrogance at best and cruel incompetence at worst. Once I would have found it a relief to immerse myself in pages that do not ask me to collude in the pretense that treatment equals care.

Once, these stories would have given voice to my anger; now, they exhaust me. Maybe I have been healthy too long. Maybe I have spent too much time with medical professionals who are both deeply caring and committed to changing medicine. In recent years I have been taken on more tours of clinics than I have sat frightened and suspicious in those clinics. Maybe I have gone over to the bright side.

I can imagine some readers, desperate to affirm the primacy of the bright side, reacting to these stories by shooting the messengers and dismissing these stories as doctor bashing (a preferred term of denial among professionals). "Doctor bashing" is another variation of old labels such as hysteria, used repeatedly throughout history to describe women who give voice to their frustration. The testimony offered in these stories and poems should not be dismissed. It's true. But no collection of texts contains the whole truth. The experience of illness has many facets; the practice of medicine includes moments of care. Reading these stories, people should be angry but neither discouraged to continue medical work nor fearful to become ill. The difficulty is to make the anger work for change, without allowing it to become a generalized fear of life.

## NOTES

1. Alan Radley, "The Aesthetics of Illness: Narrative, Horror, and the Sublime," *Sociology of Health and Illness* 21 (1999): 783.

2. Radley 783.

3. Martin Heidegger and David Farrell Krell, *Basic Writings: From "Being and Time" (1927) to "The Task of Thinking" (1964)* (San Francisco: Harper, 1993) 452.

4. Pierre Bourdieu, *Masculine Domination* (Stanford: Stanford UP, 2001) 35.

5. Bourdieu 62.

6. Bourdieu 75.

7. Bourdieu 49.

# Stereotactic Biopsy

### Amy Haddad

*Climb up here.*
The table is so high there are stairs.
*Lay down with your breast through the hole.*
The table is very hard.
I relinquish my right breast,
the tech pulls on it.
She raises the table even higher.

Face down, turned to the wall
arms straight by my side.
The bright light from a desk
traces my silhouette black against the white wall.
I can see the outline of my head, shoulders,
the dip of my back.

She tugs and adjusts.
*The site is close to your armpit.*
*We need as much breast tissue through the hole as possible.*
My breast does not cooperate.
After many X-rays, sighs of frustration,
the position is right.

I cannot move.
*Don't move.*
Her voice from somewhere below me.
A swish of air, the doctor enters.
No preliminaries to the tech or me.
Without warning,
a sharp burning in my breast.
I gasp.

*This will numb the site.*
*Now, this will be loud,*
*sort of a bang.*
*It won't hurt.*
*Don't flinch,* the tech warns.

Each time,
sixteen times,
she puts her hand on the small of my back
a warning touch
just before the gunshot sound.
The wide-bore needle pierces my breast,
taking a tunnel of tissue.

*Okay,* the doctor says,
*Let's see what we've got.*
A rustle of footsteps, the door opens and closes.
The room is absolutely still.
I stare at my outline on the wall.
Trapped.
Waiting.
Where did they go?

Thinking I am alone,
I start to cry quietly
then sob.
Between my first great gasping breath
and the next,
the doctor clears his throat.

# What If They Said?

AMY HADDAD

We have your breasts and lymph nodes. Now we want
your hair, all of it, brows, lashes, pubic hair,
the down that covers your arms and legs.
Hand over your strength and stamina,
no more walks. Give us your ability
to sleep and dream. Drop in the ink pens
and paper, you won't have the energy to write.
Surrender your books, where you seek solace.
Relinquish the pleasure of flowers' scent.
Lose your appetite for food, for sex.
Forget swallowing without nettles in your throat.
Abandon the clarity of your vision,
perhaps permanently.
Your wit, your ability to choose words,
play with ideas—
give us all of that as well.

After all,
we're trying to save your life.

# All Patients Are Political Women

JASMINA TEŠANOVIĆ

*Monday, 22 October 2001*
Today I woke up in the hospital. Last time it happened to me was when I delivered my baby. It was nice back then, I guess, not that it is bad now, just strange. I miss the baby. This is the other side of life, its downturn. I am not giving life, but losing it.

The woman lying in her bed on my right side lost her twin babies thirty years ago, the last time she was in the hospital. She is a professional nurse who also lost her mother fifteen years ago because they treated her for rheumatism instead of diagnosing her cancer. She nearly lost her only son, in the first of Milošević's wars, when he was missing for three months and found half crazy in a Croatian mental hospital. The Croats sent him back in a prisoner exchange. Then he was court-martialed by the Serb military because he killed a companion with friendly fire while falling wounded over barbed wire. Like one of the episodes from my essay on women in war, her life is so unusual and yet so common. The nurse is afraid. She is the most afraid of the lot who are due for operations today. She says, If I am lethally sick, I will sell all my belongings and just travel under a false name, alone, until my very end.

We are in the urgent department for operations on the head and shoulders. It is delicate surgery with uncertain medical results, fifty/fifty odds of survival. I look around me in wonder. Where are the thrown dice? What are the rules? I do not believe in destiny or gambling; I believe in science and coincidence. Now I am on the road, an actress and a spectator at the same time, both the horse and its jockey.

The woman in the bed in front of me is a recidivist case, cancer diagnosis, third operation. Her face is distorted and mutilated. She is elderly and well dressed, holding a mirror in her hand all the time and spreading cream over her scars.

The woman in the bed on my left is hysterical. Her husband was killed in the Bosnian war. She is a refugee from Bosnia with her nerves completely shattered, but somehow she remains under control. I have seen many such people in the past few years. I have written books for and about them. I know everything about her. Being a refugee is a specific, permanent state of stress. Like the homeless

Jews of old, modern refugees have their own laws and aesthetics. She is fighting with mosquitoes all the time—she needs an enemy. She talks all the time, to herself or to us. She has a beautiful soothing voice and is in fact a beautiful woman, but nobody can tell that at a glance. In the hospital, she dresses up as a refugee again: fancy nightgown, fancy slippers, brand-new, as if to disguise the fact that she has no property or papers. She is haunted by the half dead mosquitoes, muttering, Blood is all over the walls, all over me; all of them just want me, none of them want any of you. I have a feeling that she was raped.

The nurses, male and female, are handsome, dressed up, witty. We the sick, by construction, are the opposite. But we fight back. Most patients are dressed in their best underwear; they lick their wounds and try desperately not to be the Other. I am one of the few who knows that it is useless, so I am all in rags to consciously be the Other. By definition, the patients should come first in a hospital. Everything rotates around our illnesses: the gadgets, the doctors, the money, the politics, the science. Somehow the doctors are trying to take it all away from us, to make us objects, invisible, as in those nineteenth-century paintings in which twenty male doctors surround a hysterical woman, calling her a case and ignoring her, writing books about her and making careers without ever really hearing or seeing her. Now, in modern hospitals, all patients are political women.

I am waiting to be taken to the surgery room by a huge orderly dressed in green, a guy called "Ljuba the animal." His job is to carry the dead and the living from one place to another. He is extremely tender. I am listening to the small talk of men and women afraid to die. If I were at home, I would be the same. Here among the others, in the same boat, I want to be different, a heroine, an exhibitionist, ready to die for a change.

*10:30 A.M.*
I am alone in my small four-bed room, adapted for patients after the ceiling in the proper hospital ward caved in. Our beds touch each other. I have a feeling that we are all in the same bed.

Now the other women have been taken to surgery.

If you were alive, Mother, you wouldn't have let this happen to me. As a doctor, as a mother, you would have treated me properly and refused all this marring of the natural beauty of a body, its loss of integrity. My skin is perfect on my neck. My swollen gland is invisible; inside it is oval and calm. Why am I taking it out then?

*23 October 2001*
I dreamt of you, my dead, my beloved ones; you appeared as smiling angels in this miserable ward of lamenting, bleeding people. All of you were angels,

drinking *rakija*. My aunt was laughing, my cousin Biljana just being beautiful, and my mother was cleaning, preaching, demanding.

I am with you tonight, still half drugged, my whole head bandaged. More than in pain, I am in a floating trance, in a hallucinogenic open-minded state. Reality is confused with dreams, thought, and the past. My body is somewhere beyond me, out of my control, but I do not crave to get it back. I remember lying on the surgery bed, a huge metal table; six masked figures in green were hanging over my half-nude body. One tiny voice—was it male?—asked me, singing, are you Jasmina Tešanović? I was anointed in yellow, my long curly hair spread around me; I saw myself from somewhere above: a dead, romantic vampire. I said, I used to be Jasmina Tešanović. I meant it.

*24 October 2001*
The woman opposite me is falling apart, decaying. She has had three operations up to now—cancer is spreading all over her body and the last two operations were done one after another, so she has two wounds. She is losing hair and coughing incessantly, choking and spitting. I am torn between complete nausea and the urge to help her. But she is coping elegantly with her needs. I give her some medicines and advice, and she does the rest on her own.

Yesterday her two sisters gave two bottles of homemade *rakija* to the doctor who operated on her. He brought them back to her after a few hours with haughtiness and aggressiveness. He said, aiming his comment at all of us (even though he didn't operate on all of us): I refuse this.

The woman was hurt. Why didn't he give it back immediately to my sisters? she asked sadly. I am on pension and I live in a village. I have nothing else to give him. Is he angry because he wants more, something different, money? For her, this was not an issue of morality, bribery, or ethics. It is a Serbian custom to give a bottle of drink to the doctor or priest: very old-fashioned, and yes, perhaps immoral. But with the new forms of corruption floating around these days, it is relatively harmless. Some doctors ask for big money to perform their duty. In this case, I think she is just a nobody to him, becoming every hour even more of a nobody. She is going away, and he is an asshole who doesn't want to get compromised by a nobody, for nothing.

Somehow she is aware of it and ashamed of her illness and decay. To be sick in old inner Serbia was always a shame. Her shame is compounded by being childless and living with her sisters and their sons. She looks now at me, begging for tolerance.

My poor old girl, I have nothing against your death in our room-and-a-half our piece of corridor. It could have been me; I am just lucky and hopefully I will be out in a few days, with only this diary to remember the horror among us. But when we entered the ward, it was Russian roulette. We were equal, especially when we lay nude on the surgery tables, one next to another; the doctors jump from one table to another, speaking loudly of our bodies and laughing over drinks. You had your *rakija* under your bed. I bought a bottle of whiskey instead; I know the Serbian parvenus better.

My poor old girl, I know how you feel by now. I will open your window, let the fresh air come in and your breath go out. And I will take gladly your *rakija* with me and drink it with my friends in your honor.

The hospital ward is actually a beautiful building, an old Austro-Hungarian palace full of mosquitoes because of the damp and cracks in the walls. Our ward is just outside the proper cancer ward, as Dante's rings of inferno: the more lethal illnesses toward the center. All sick people are in one place, in the middle of downtown Belgrade.

The cleaning crew is cleaning all the time: all women, dressed in white. The surgeons are all men dressed in green. Thirteen of them visit us every day. M, the woman on my left, is in tears from her daily treatment. She is trembling, holding her hand over her face. She goes to bed silent, sobbing. The thirteen doctors come in right after for their daily visit. They are of different ages, statures, and cultures, but none of them say good morning, how are you? They only speak among themselves.

The doctor in charge today turns to M. Take away your hands from your face, he says sharply. We want to see your face. She pulls away her hands. Her blue eyes are popping out of her head dramatically; they are screaming as tears fall in showers down her wrinkled face. She says nothing. I am frozen. I sit on the edge of my bed when they come in and turn my side to them. I refuse to look at them or be exposed to their looks. But they dare not say anything to me.

Later, after the doctors leave, I ask, What is it, M? He called me a refugee, she said. It is not my fault, she screams; my husband was killed, my children scattered, and I had to leave everything. I am a refugee, homeless. Does it show in my face? He said, how come all refugees come under my knife? I answered, may you live through what I went through.

I gave her a pill to sleep. I know her story: she cannot stand the word *refugee*, in any context.

The dying woman needs something to stop coughing—no medicines here for bronchitis. She says I will trade my homemade *rakija* for a coughing pill. I take the deal; I want her to feel she owes me nothing. My friend will bring her pills.

Today they do not change my bandages or even look at my wound. They did it to my roommate and even offered her a drink, maybe because she is a nurse and knows how to behave with doctors. I ask the male nurse to change my bandages and count my stitches. He risks doing it. I give him some money and my signed book. He refuses the money but takes the book. So I give him the *rakija* bottle too. He says eight stitches. We both wonder why so many; the gland was so small inside my neck. Maybe because I paid no money. My father told me I must, but I was ashamed to be like him and humiliate the doctor, to take up the corrupt path of the past regime in our new democratic society.

Today I saw on TV that the medical staff is striking and demonstrating in the streets— simple staff, not the doctors. The insiders here explain why: the staff have no means to get bribed as the doctors do; they have only their small salaries that are not even under a collective contract. The new transitional regime is favoring the elite. Why am I again on the other side, in the gutters? I was on the winning team against Milošević, but somehow I am not in power again. Even now when "my people" are in power. Do my people really exist or just change when in power? The losers as well as the winners both seem to be mobile categories. My traumatized refugee in shiny, fancy pajamas but without a suitcase—a few years ago she was a rich woman in power, probably being cruel and intolerant to Muslims.

My family visits me on regular basis; they are classy, fancy, and happy guys. I see them as outsiders to me now. I am proud of them, but there is an abyss between us. I do not feel I am the black sheep or the outsider. I am now in a deeper reality than they will ever want to be. I am in a miserable ward fighting for my life. They are in fancy places with their whims and fears. The split is there. Will it ever heal, like my wound? It could happen to them too, but luckily it happened to me. I handle bad scenes even better than good ones: a professional survivor and a compulsive writer.

My father has a symbolic role in this new violence. He is an engineer, a man who resolves everything by action and intervention. He had his warlike way of dealing with my female body as his male territory. It is both a private and institutional violence, this radical, deep cut into my body to make sure it had no bad cells. I had to give a no cancer proof in blood, as a good female soldier. Well, now that we know it, I wear a scar, a battered woman.

My husband is angry with me for putting up with this social and paternal violence because I didn't say no. I couldn't. It was part of me, ever since I was born an only daughter to my violent father. I wasn't trained to say no to him or anybody else, just run and hide. But I am too old to run and hide; I have done it so many times, and I am tired now. My husband is a man; he cannot understand it. I love my husband better than my father and get along more with him, but I never could say no to any of them without risking death. So no more virginity; now I will wear the scar of the operated.

It seems I am in the winning lot. I actually forgot to ask the doctor the results, even though it was my main obsession before the operation. He was running after me to tell me I was okay. And I said, oh yes, my father will be very pleased, and I meant it. On the ground, in my ward in Belgrade, after a decade of sanctions, dictatorship, wars, and bombings, the score is harsher for losers.

A nine-year-old in the next room is supposed to be operated on today. Her mother is sleeping with her. The child has a harelip birth defect; she is the result being born in dark times. She is not in our game of malign or benign cells. She is hugging a teddy bear and a Barbie doll.

The rooms are not heated at all. Thank God winter is late because of the greenhouse effect. We do not have hot water, not even warm. The government said today they will find some humanitarian coal for the hospitals. But the European Union said only if the democratic coalition stops fighting among themselves. Now, whose is this democracy, Europe's or ours? And which democracy are we talking about here?

My friend brings me food from outside. And water. I am spoiled. My roommates eat the hospital food. I could. I love it, actually. It brings me back to kindergarten and boarding school, but I want to see my friends so I demand food.

My daughter kissed me as a bird, with her beak, a thousand times. What a pearl, what a bijou she is. She understood me standing there in rags and she said, you are just like grandpa, you like hospitals, and she flew away.

I asked her to come again and take photos of me in rags and bandages, smiling and posing. She did. Some patients refused, those who brought their best clothes and who feel guilty and ashamed of being sick. But their children faint on seeing them that way. I feel as they do, but as usual my exhibitionism helps me overcome my banality, and helps my daughter stay happy.

*11 A.M.*
The mother took her nine-year-old to the surgery room: mother went smiling and with a singing voice but came back with her own face completely deformed by pain and fear. Will her baby, first, come out alive, second, with a normal upper lip, and third, ready to grow up as a normal woman and forgive her?

I went through something similar back in 1993 when my daughter was extremely ill because of asthma. They extracted her tonsils without anesthetics. It was war, sanctions time, when people had no food, least of all drugs. She forgave me and got well.

*26 October 2001*
Going home: I won't be sleeping anymore in a corridor adapted to a room because the ceiling fell in the proper sleeping ward. Won't be sleeping anymore with four completely unknown women (one talks all night, another snores,

and the third one coughs and spits. And me, well, I do this—I write, an equally unpleasant trade, I guess, for the other three). We shared in three days just about everything we had. We become so intimate that we are ashamed of each other when our relatives come in the room. And the relatives sense it; they feel embarrassed and somehow, awkwardly, they hurry away.

It is not a male bonding as in army or gangs, nor a female one like we have in feminist workshops/schools of crying and healing, coming out; this is something specific I am trying to identify, but I am out of words. Life and death situations happen to me always in the Serbian language. Maybe that is what makes me Serbian, not my papers. I, who write and think in English and live and laugh in Italian, am actually silent in Serbian, as now, when I write but can't find the words. The awe, the abyss, the void—always in my mother tongue.

Feeling completely newborn, I am leaving my miserable ward. I leave my deep, true friendships without names or futures: only grimaces and medical results. I am leaving my books behind. Most people in the ward have read them. My books are definitely for miserable hospital/prison/concentration wards. Because they spring from wounds.

# Waiting for a Transplant:
# A Meditation

MARCY PERLMAN TARDIO

I sit at my desk by the window. Clouds fill the sky like clean, ruffled sheets. An icy chill lands on my left shoulder through a crack in the window. On my corner of Fifth Street and Seventh Avenue, men with beefy arms dig up the cement, like trenches; like graves. They are exhuming the bones of rusty water pipes, replacing them with clean ones. Like my doctor will do with my kidneys.

I don't mind it's cold. It's nothing an extra sweater can't insulate against. I eat oranges to keep myself pumped with vitamin C, my way to fight the microbes that nest on the computer keys and invisibly adhere to my fingertips. I dig for words, a shard of metaphor, some bottle caps of adjectives from my mind's ditch to describe this state of waiting.

This past year, I closed my homebirth practice due to my kidney failure, which ironically allowed me to return to college after twenty-two years. I've strained to recall fifth grade math to help my son Levi with his homework. I've toyed with different fingerings for my Bach French Suite. All of this was punctuated with dialysis. No saint, I've cried and readied myself for death.

But now I've achieved the coveted position of being *inscribed* in that great "Cadaver Kidney List" . . . *le-shanah tovah tikateivu*\* . . . may you be inscribed for a good year. . . . Now, the only thing left to do is wait—wait for a date when I'll be prepped, incised, planted with a recycled kidney, and stapled closed.

Outside, sledge-hammered cement dust flours up, caking people's shoes as they walk by. As the men dig the trenches, I reflect on my Jewish people, and their Arab cousins, both warriors in the Middle East who fight from their respective trenches. I think the acrid smell of spilled blood is the same, whether that person is Jew or Arab. Each war-ravaged person—splattered, dead, broken-hearted—could be that person whose kidney will be bequeathed to someone like me. I wonder whether the volume or color of my urine would be different if I received the kidney of a Jewish boy, a Muslim mother.

The high school across the street is letting out now. Teenagers yell and laugh as they duck through traffic and weave in and out of cars and mothers pushing

---

\* Greeting for Rosh Hashanna, Jewish New Year.

their children in strollers, women who wear their hair in dreadlocks or covered with *sheitels** or scarves. One of these kids or mothers crossing the street may get hit by a car, or even knifed by someone over a parking space. If that person dies, maybe he or she will leave a kidney for someone waiting for a kidney, like me.

But it's my elder son Java who's promised me his kidney. He's completing his first year as a teacher. It's also his first year as a husband, and he and Michelle are both in grad school. Amidst these challenges, he has added me to his list of complicated ventures. He'll teach till the end of June, and two weeks later he will entrust his body to the surgeon and his soul to Jesus and give me his kidney. My son's sacrifice will be my salvation. I will become free of belly tubes, clamps, and bags of dialysate; free from waiting for another mother's son or daughter to die so that a kidney can be "harvested" like a summer melon and repotted in my belly's soil.

Two men, arms broad and coppery as the water pipes they lift, guide the pipes into the completed trenches. The metal glistens in the afternoon sun like their sweaty skin, all flecked with a fine white dust. All labor is artistry. It's in a day laborer's arms, his muscles, a work of anatomic perfection as they glisten and strain while digging through concrete. It's how a surgeon cuts the precise millimeter of tissue with a scalpel, when the least jolt of his hand could mean the difference between Levi and I kicking around a soccer ball, or Java being propped with pillows and limb restraints in a wheelchair. It's the way my hands have helped women's vaginas stretch slowly to make room for their babies, and how my surgeon's hands will midwife my new life as the doctor places my son's kidney into me.

Still, all of this labor does not equal the strength and resiliency required by the body and the human spirit in order to heal. I look at a scab on my ankle, for example. It's about three millimeters round from a nick I got shaving my legs. It's remained the same for ten days: crusty, dry, unhealed. When I was a kid and fell off my bike while riding in our concrete backyard, knees sliced open, palms abraded, it would only take a little soap and water, a swab of Mercurochrome, a Band-Aid, and in three days it would be gone, leaving new pink flesh in its place. Now—with an autoimmune disease that causes my body to fight against itself, exacerbated by the long-lasting effects of chemotherapy and steroids—I do not heal.

Java is giving me his kidney with hopes it will save my life. The surgeon will put Java's kidney into my abdomen, somewhere near my bladder, and leave my own two desiccated kidneys in my flank to shrivel up. I will need to take high doses of steroids and immunosuppressive drugs. I will organize a welcome committee consisting of my heart, spleen, and pancreas. They will be responsible

* Ritual wig for Orthodox Jewish women as scarves are for Muslim women.

for making my new kidney feel at home. Perhaps my dormant uterus will wake up as she remembers this new kidney, a distant déjà vu sort of memory of the time she cradled it inside her nurturing walls thirty years before. Java's kidney, part of the duplicating cells that became him, released into one whole spirit and fleshy package that is my son.

Will my welcoming organs and the warm rays of my mind be able to convince this visiting kidney that it belongs with us, that we are now its home? Will it long for Java, whose young blood vigorously zooms like a falcon through his elastic veins? Will it miss the smell of testosterone?

Across the street, a bulldozer fills the trenches with dirt. The men put down large orange cones as a warning to pedestrians to watch their steps while they walk along the gristled pavement. They lift the old pipes and put them on the back of a flatbed truck. The new pipes, incandescent tunnels for clean, circulating water, are buried underground. We no longer see them, forget they are there; we take for granted that they will secure clean moving water into our homes.

Take for granted, as I did my birth kidneys, yet I cannot take my new kidney for granted. This fist-sized vital organ will be sewn into me, cradled somewhere in my pelvis just as Java was when he was cradled in my womb. As with the veiled heads of the pious, my kidney will be veiled in my hips, reminding me that that which is holy is also ordinary. Hidden from sight, it will call upon me to remember the sacred in the unseen.

# Pathology Report

VENETA MASSON

| | |
|---|---|
| The specimens | parts of me |
| are received | cut from their moorings |
| in two containers | floating placidly |
| specimen No. 1 | lifted out |
| labeled | by dispassionate hands |
| ovary | measured, weighed |
| the external surface | splayed on a countertop |
| distorted | so much |
| by a large | once secret |
| cystic structure | now exposed |
| filled with | old |
| dark | imperfections |
| reddish-brown | festering |
| material | like a failed heart |
| specimen No. 2 | large, scarred |
| labeled | utterly useless |
| uterus | no matter that |
| opening reveals | a creation of sorts |
| a mass | suggestive of life |
| with fleshy-pink | formed |
| whorled surface | inside |
| the cavity | which |
| is compressed | at last |
| by the mass | cut to the quick |
| representative sections | proved counterfeit |
| are submitted | stillborn |

# I'll Take Care of It

### JAN FELDMAN

I'll take care of it, the doctor said. And he took control.

He had me touch my right forefinger to my nose with my eyes closed, walk a straight line, and hold my hands extended. He delicately tapped my knees and ankles, producing uncontrollable jerks. He ordered blood tests and X-rays and EEGs and CAT scans. I was bled and photographed. Wires were fastened to my skull with sticky patches. Narrow sensors were placed inside my nose. My body was placed in a padded capsule with my head locked into place to obtain pictures of thin slices of my brain. I did not see any of the results.

"Good news," my doctor said when I reported back. "It is not a tumor."

"Oh," I said.

"What we have here looks like idiopathic adult onset seizure disorder. It is not uncommon," he said. "We have a number of approaches for controlling the seizures."

"Oh," I said.

The doctor prescribed pills. One the first day, two the second day, three the third day, then four, with food. He would monitor the serious side effects. The tired feeling, nausea, and dizziness would pass. "Get bloods drawn and call in three months," he said, showing me out of the office.

The reality of the diagnosis rattled my settled life like an earthquake. Everything shifted and some structures built on prior reality were tossed around and shattered. Others swayed and returned to place intact. Intact or shattered, impregnability was breached, control lost. Travel, jobs, friends, hobbies, sports, dreams—everything needed to be reexamined.

And with that insight, I settled back into comfortable, used ways of perceiving until the aftershocks rolled through. Mainly I denied and pretended I still perched on bedrock as I stumbled through drugged days. The doctor will take care of it was my mantra.

I wobbled and spun for three months, always tired or dizzy or slightly nauseated. I counted the days until I could report back to the doctor.

But first, the blood letting: surrendering my arm, breathing deeply as the vacuum sucked my blood into tubes, sliding my eyes away from the diagnosis written on each form and slip and chart, trying to look normal. I called the doctor. "Things look good," he said. "Your bloods are almost to the therapeutic level. Get more bloods and come in to see me in three months."

Three months to the next safe haven. I worried whether each spell of indigestion or dizziness was the flu or the medicine or a seizure. Timidly, I called the doctor for reassurance. After I had called a few times, the doctor sounded annoyed at my persistent questions and was brusque when I called to report another seizure. "We can take care of that," he said. I tried (needed) to believe the reassurance.

I returned to his office. I now had a chart plump with the results of blood tests, neatly filed X-rays, stick figures with pluses and minuses over different areas, and reports of how electricity traveled through my brain. "The bloods look good," he said. "We'll leave things as they are. Call me if you have another seizure." Bloods and return in three months.

My body continued its slip from self-harmony until its only certitude was my ability to touch my nose with my forefinger and to walk a straight line with my eyes shut. I gave up responding to unusual feelings, tried not to notice them, and certainly didn't bother the doctor.

Three more months. I spent the next office visit crying over my losses. "It's normal," he said, "everyone cries," and we talked beyond the ritualized testing of my reflexes. I was cautious in my tears not to say anything to bring disapproval. And I didn't have words for what the tears were really about.

When I started to cry during my next visit, three months later, he said, "More than once is unusual. Perhaps a psychiatrist . . ." and returned silently to our ritual: nose, reflexes, walk the line. I wanted to be normal in my abnormality, so I locked the tears inside. And eventually I didn't feel them anymore.

I no longer owned my sleep or appetites. Moods and pains could always signify something else. I felt my wit dull and my perceptions slow. Conversations seemed labored.

I started rooting around in old diaries and picture albums. I wanted to identify the real me from these snippets of the past and successfully rappel to the present, identity in hand. I was unsuccessful. I could not separate age and change from disease. I felt lost.

I remained, however, a compliant patient. Three-month visits widened to six-month phone calls. The side effects of the medicine were an accepted part of life, as was the occasional seizure. My chart was filed under "S" for success. My bloods were correct, my neurological markers were normal, and I appeared emotionally stable. The doctor had taken care of it as he said he would.

# White Coat Syndrome

Rebecca A. Pope

I don't go to the doctor very often—or at least not to the MD who, my insurance card tells me, is my "primary care physician." When I want a checkup, I visit Dr. Hu, OMD Lic. Ac. (Oriental Medicine Doctor, Licensed Acupunturist). She takes my pulses—I hardly feel her finely trained fingertips at three places on each of my wrists—looks at the color and shape of my tongue, and, with her needles and herbs, has fixed all the miscellaneous maladies I've brought to her, and even a few, like "low kidney chi," that I didn't know I had. Dr. Hu doesn't promise miracle cures. Like a good malt scotch, the bitter herbs are an acquired taste. They work slowly. I am patient, a good patient, for Dr. Hu.

When I, as I occasionally do, fear that I am suffering from something serious and horrible that might require treatments more high tech and invasive than Chinese herbs, I put off visiting the internist for awhile—which is often restorative in itself. If procrastination doesn't cure me, I reluctantly make an appointment. Four female internists, a physician's assistant, and a nurse-practitioner all see patients in this office. I noticed on my last visit that only the nurses, phlebotomists, and clerks wear white coats. I suspect this is an attempt to be politically progressive. I think of Dr. Hu's office; she wears a white coat, as do the slight and smiling man who boils the herbs and takes out the needles, and Cathy, who sits behind the desk with the appointment book, teaches Qigong with Dr. Hu, and whose real name can't possibly be Cathy. Dr. Hu's office is a democracy of white coats.

"We haven't seen you for a while," says the physician's assistant, a woman I have never met. She wears a bright purple shirt, gray trousers, and a stethoscope.

"I think the last time was three years ago. Stress fracture in my ankle. Too much running." I offer little else. I don't come in for regular checkups. I am not a good patient. She takes my blood pressure: 180 over 110. "Your blood pressure is really high."

"White Coat Syndrome. It's usually about 110 over 70."

I had hardly unpacked in Bethesda with my new life and new partner when the call from Chicago came. What my mother had for months been claiming was a bleeding hemorrhoid turned out to be the malignancy we had all been trying to deny. Surgery in a few days. I offered to fly home. "No, we can handle it," my father said.

"She was really lucky," the surgeon pronounced afterward. "The tumor was low, which inhibited metastasis. Everything looks fine, but she should have a course of radiation just to be safe. In case there are any stray cells." We exhaled; only a few wandering cells, and they could easily be mopped up with a little radiation. Of course the colostomy bag was unlucky, but there was a general air of reprieve and relief in which my mother, determined, as they say, to "put it all behind" her (a rather unfortunate phrase under the circumstances), participated. Without complaint she learned to manage the colostomy. She took the radiation treatments. We didn't think to question that recommendation; it came, after all, from the man in the white coat, and we were all amateurs at cancer then. She was compliant; she was a good sport; she kept her pain and fear and frustration to herself, which, I suppose, was lucky for the rest of us.

Of course the seven weeks of radiation burned her and made her sick, no doubt sicker than she allowed her children to see. But she soon regained her physical strength, and as the number of checkups and tests that pronounced her "clean" accumulated, we began to regain our faith in her body and in her continued presence. After five years without recurrence, she became a statistical "survivor" and we celebrated. How close she had come; how lucky we were. Time to forget.

Two years later pain returned. She had a hard time sitting. Probably scar tissue, the doctor said. The pain got worse. The MRI wasn't clear. Into the hospital for a biopsy. It took a few days to get the results: "good news, it's benign." The tightness in our shoulders, our heads, our stomachs, tightness we hadn't been conscious of, began to dissolve. We could celebrate again, even if she was still in pain. The next day another call: "We're really sorry; we don't know how this could have happened. There's been a mistake; it's malignant."

More appointments and consultations. More men in white coats. They were confident they could get it out. More surgery. My father, brother, and sister waited at the hospital ("No, you don't need to come," my father said again). I waited by the phone. This time the surgeon came out of the operating suite early, too early. He brought them to a small windowless room, the kind of room that is supposed to insure privacy and confidentiality but is really about shielding other waiting families from someone else's bad luck. He shut the door. My father knew. "Sorry. The tumor is resting up against her backbone. And up against the sciatic nerve. We couldn't get it. She's probably got a year, maybe a year and a half."

Later, one of the other doctors said that this new tumor was probably caused by the mop-up radiation after the first surgery, the radiation done "just to be safe." The doctors put a few radiation needles directly into the tumor before they closed, but that was all they could do because—and this was news to us—she had used up her lifetime allowance of exposure earlier. The maximum exposure guidelines are necessary, of course, because too much radiation can kill you.

My father forbade the doctors to tell my mother that she had twelve to eighteen months. Perhaps this was denial, perhaps a sense that no one, even someone in a white coat, can ever really know when someone else will die. Perhaps he knew of those studies that suggest that many people who are put on the clock die by the clock because they are so invested in being good patients. But then she didn't really need to be told. She knew that an inoperable tumor next to her backbone was serious trouble.

In times of catastrophe we fall back on what we know. The family academic, I know reading and research. I bought some books about alternative treatments and nutrition protocols for cancer and read them on the plane back to Chicago. I learned enough in a few hours to be appalled at what the hospital kitchen gave a cancer patient for Thanksgiving dinner and brought her organic yogurt with live cultures to replace the good bacteria that her superantibiotics destroyed. I read everything on cancer and nutrition I could get my hands on; some of it was quackery and junk. But I was surprised by how much good research was out there. You'd never know it talking to a conventional oncologist; in all the years of treating her, none of my mother's doctors had mentioned diet. I came up with a nutrition and supplement plan that corresponded to most of the more credible work I had read. It was not a program for the faint of heart or for the devotee of Domino's pizza: an organic whole food vegetarian diet supplemented with a little salmon. Lots of soy and garlic and greens. All very worthy, but lacking in the high fat and sugar that the standard American diet teaches us to associate with gastronomic pleasure, a lesson my mother had learned all too well.

In many ways it is easier to think of enduring all kinds of horrible treatments, treatments that will have an end, than to change permanently the bedrock habits of our lives. The hardest part for Mom was the no-sugar rule. Like people, tumors love sugar and grow fat and happy on it, and she was the sort of person who, on opening a restaurant menu, looked first at the desserts. I found a recipe in a Moosewood cookbook for an apple cake—all whole wheat flour and sweetened with maple syrup, not much fat. It didn't look like much, but it tasted remarkably good and seemed to palliate her craving for sweets. I knew she'd never bake it for herself—so I baked one for her once a month or so. It took most of a morning to make, and between organic ingredients and overnight delivery, the little cake cost nearly a week's pocket money, but it seemed a small price to keep her from the temptations of tiramisu.

A great believer in "mind over body," my mother was convinced that she would get well. She did visualization exercises every day and cultivated the positive "love yourself" attitude that all the feel-good cancer books recommend. I lamented the dualism of her paradigm, which seemed to encourage thinking about the ailing body as a hostile foreign country that must be subdued and conquered; but how can a cancer patient not on some level feel that the body has betrayed and must be made obedient again? And what woman who grows up in this culture manages to escape seeing her body, with its flesh and curves, as the enemy? Like her, I decided to concentrate on the positive and feel lucky that at least she was active and confident of her recovery, even if I, her overeducated daughter, didn't like her metaphor.

Like Dr. Hu's herbs, these methods of building the immune system take time. After about four months, though, her pain was nearly gone. At five months, her CEA test registered 0.1; 5.0 usually signals remission. Not bad for someone the white coats had written off. Relief, reprieve, we celebrated again.

The oncologist called her his "miracle patient." He must have meant this literally because he never evinced the least bit of interest in her regimen. Just as things were going, in his own words, miraculously well, the oncologist suggested that my mother try some chemotherapy. "I'd give it a 15 percent chance of wiping it out entirely," he said. I was appalled when my parents told me, and sick and panicked at the thought of it. I reminded them that chemo destroys the immune system, that to take it would put all the gains at risk. But I knew that I couldn't lobby too loudly. What if she felt coerced by me, skipped the drugs, and died anyway? Besides, I told myself, everyone has the right to make decisions about such grave matters without pressure.

The doctor prescribed a course of 5FU. I later learned that people in the cancer business sometimes refer to this drug as "Five Feet Under." I'm not sure if the phrase implies that the drug is so toxic that it can make you feel like you're dying, or that the drug is so ineffective that it won't save you from dying, or, most likely, that the drug will kill you more often than not.

The drug trashed her immune system, as I feared. She lost her appetite and was too sick to take the supplements. The tumor came roaring back—her CEA numbers climbed to 15—and so did the pain. When it was clear that the treatment hadn't worked and that my mother was sicker than ever, the oncologist shrugged his shoulders and said, "Actually, I've never seen it work in a case like this, but it was worth the chance."

When I tell this story people sometimes say that surely this physician should be sued for something. For what, I wonder, being unable to let a good thing alone? I paraphrase for them a passage from *Harrison's Principles of Internal Medicine*[1]: in those cases that do not lend themselves to easy solutions or for which no effective treatment is available, a feeling on the part of the patient that the physician is doing all that is possible is one of the most important therapeutic measures that can be provided.

The longer you linger over this passage the more stunning it becomes. It so casually licenses overtreatment. Here scientific medicine endorses the very "superstition" from which it claimed to save us. If all else fails, try the power of the white coat and the pointless treatment that you know won't work.

Perhaps cancer invites overtreatment and pointless treatment more than other illnesses. We have been engaged in a "war on cancer" since the Nixon administration. We die of cancer "after a long battle." War licenses extreme and aggressive and often hasty action. In times of war we are less critical of leaders and generals, more willing to go along with what they say must be done, feel greater pressure to fall in with the party line. We are more likely, in our fear, to mistake propaganda for sound and credible argument, the horrific for the reasonable. We let profiteers masquerade as patriots. We tell ourselves that we can't really concern ourselves about collateral damage.

And of course in a few months she died. An ugly and painful and excruciating death. The tumor pushed mercilessly against her sciatic nerve, and all the morphine—in pills, patches, and IV pouches—hardly took the edge off. She weighed less than a hundred pounds by then, but enough Ativan to down an elephant only rarely produced relaxation and the relief of sleep. Perhaps because she was a goner, the oncologist stopped returning my father's phone calls; Dad was left to guess at how much morphine he could give his wife of nearly fifty years without killing her. Finally the tumor grew so large that the blood in her legs could barely return to her chest to be pumped again. They swelled to three times their normal size and dripped so much fluid that she was constantly soaked—weeping they call it. When you pressed your fingers into those big boggy legs the indentations remained. Her toes began to blacken. She died by inches.

Cancer is insidious; you can think that it's dead, and like a vampire it returns to renew the parasitic feasting that leaves the patient bereft of flesh. I don't know for certain that Mom would be alive today if she had refused that chemotherapy. I do know that she died sooner because of it. And I don't know if the seven weeks of radiation caught those stray cells, but it certainly didn't keep her safe from anything. A few weeks after my mother's death, my father began to wonder why we hadn't been told at the time of her first surgery that the radiation treatments would use up her lifetime allowance. The trained accountant became suspicious. "Did she really need all that radiation, or was that more about keeping the machines, which must be paid for, busy and billing?" he asked one of the people at the hospital who had treated Mom. He got an awkward smile and shrug in response.

I told the physician's assistant a shorter version of this story (she was, after all, on the managed-care clock) as partial explanation of my raised blood pressure and

my air of I'd rather be anywhere else, even the dentist. She listened sympathetically, and her empathy was welcome. But I think in the end this narrative was to
her like the stories of so many disease-of-the-week movies and pulpy sentimental
novels: a sad story about the suffering of one person and the consequences of
cancer on those who loved her, consequences like a daughter's stress in the doctor's
office. It was a private story. It wasn't a story about the politics of medicine or the
economics of illness or the assumptions of the cancer establishment. Perhaps she
filled in the gaps of my narrative with the conventions to which those books and
movies have schooled us and imagined a mother who grows more noble as her
body declines, children who happily give up old resentments and lovingly bond
anew with parents and each other, good coming out of suffering, and healing
triumphing over death. She probably didn't imagine Mom's acid jesting in the
last week that the only doctor she was willing to see was Dr. Kevorkian.

These days I'm a medical refractory. The physician's assistant wanted to bring
me back into the fold of patients herded along from test to test and specialist to
specialist. This is, I recognize, what she understands good, and safe, medicine to
be. She thinks it's about submitting to regular medical surveillance, and I think
it's about exercising and eating organic and polluting the environment as little as
possible. She wasn't interested in the way constant testing for cancer and other
ills reduces the patient to a disease waiting to happen, or in the consequences of
that construction for the patient. ("I guess since I can no longer have children,
all I can do is have cancer" a friend described after a recent visit to the doctor).
She wasn't curious about the dangers of overtreatment that can result from all
the screening. She didn't want to discuss the values of a preventive medicine
that is less about prevention than detection. Cancer exists; we can test for it; it's
only sensible to submit because then you can feel safe—this seemed to be her
line of reasoning. It was black and white for her. White witches and wizards,
white hats, white coats, the good guys of fantasy and myth—their goodness is
always self-evident and unquestionable and without serious side effects.

It turned out that there wasn't much wrong with me the day I saw the physician's assistant, just a stage III panic and a hemorrhoid, probably the consequence
of bad form while lifting weights. She gave me a prescription, which I dutifully
filled. It cost twenty dollars after the insurance discount of forty dollars and
made me feel like I had a bad hangover. It didn't work. I went back to Dr. Hu,
who prescribed three-dollar ointment (available at your local Chinese grocery)
that smelled like Chinatown and felt good—and did the job.

Last week I read about a newly published study on white coat syndrome.
People whose blood pressures spike in the doctor's office are at higher risk of
heart attacks. I suspect—these articles are often frustratingly, even misleadingly
vague—the study concluded that white coat syndrome is a symptom of blood

pressure that tends to spike in response to stress. And such an irrational, even hysterical, stress at that—after all, it's not rational to have a fight-or-flight response in the doctor's office. But perhaps fight or flight is a reasonable response to the white coat: an alternative conclusion from the data might be that reducing the risk of white coat syndrome is as simple as avoiding the white coats.

## Notes

1. Dennis L. Kasper, Eugene Braunwald, Anthony Fauci, Stephen Hauser, Dan Longo, and J. Larry Jameson, *Harrison's Principles of Internal Medicine,* vol. 1, 14th ed. (New York: McGraw Hill, 1997) 3.

# Hospital Haiku

FRAN BARTKOWSKI

I held my own hand
while I slept
last night

to calm the pulse
of fear

# give my regrets

## DIANE DRIEDGER

I'm having a party
of third parties
you see they    keep coming
into my life
the physio  the acupuncturist  the herbalist
the GP too

it's called   see my body
it's not quite right
pin the tail on
the diagnosis

it's a formal affair
I'm usually dressed
in a paper gown
with a slit in the back

no need to call ahead
just show up
with several others in tow
ready to give a second opinion

# Doctor Patel Comes to Tea

### Muriel Murch

"Good morning, Jane." Dr. Patel strode past his secretary's desk without looking at her as he entered his office and closed the door behind him. The moments of transition, driving from the psychiatric hospital where he made rounds each morning, enabled him to shed the images, smells, and sounds that pricked at his senses and lingered in his clothes after leaving the wards. He loved the unknown, uncharted pathways that his patients seemed to be traveling back into their brains. Like an archaeologist surveying the workers on a dig, he would sometimes linger on his walk through his wards to search for the occasional shard of memory to be shaken free from the rotten decay of dementia.

He turned back to his desk and sat down with a sigh. He reached for his pile of correspondence for the day and began to read Dr. Frank's letter. Dr. Frank had written a brief outline and history of his care of Mrs. Andrews and asked would Dr. Patel be able to see her and sort out some kind of diagnosis and suggest some management. The letter closed with the normal thank you, and then Frank had added, *I think you will find her interesting.*

Patel put the letter down and thought about Frank. The two men had met when they were in their psychiatric rotation at the Clearwood Hospital. Their paths crossed often again as they set up practices in the same county. A friendship between the two men had begun to germinate in the hothouse enclosure of the locked male ward at Clearwood, but the exhaustion of the workload had thwarted their efforts and the budding companionship had no time to flourish. Besides, both men were somewhat shy and quiet. Frank was conscious that his comprehensive scholarship and brains had got him into medical school, while Patel was one of an ever-growing Asian medical presence that was still outside the core of young men and women who considered entrance to medical school theirs by right.

Patel swiveled his chair around to look back out of the window at the gray, cracked parking lot with the unshaded cars baking in the sunshine of this English summer morning. He saw his old Honda Accord and winced as he felt its paint blistering in the heat. It was a useful car for home visits, more functional than prestigious. He gazed over the flat roof of the old barracks that had fallen into civilian use. After fifty years nothing had been done to lift the austerity of a necessary postwar mentality. Even the buildings' names still conveyed their royal, nationalist origins: Alexandra, Victoria, Elizabeth. Funny, they are all women, all queens, he mused, though he had never bothered to explore why that was. He reached for his phone and dialed Mrs. Andrews's daughter, Susan King.

"Hello?" her voice a question.

"Hello, is that Mrs. King? This is Dr. Patel."

"Oh yes, oh, hello." He heard her surprise at his unfamiliar voice.

"I am phoning about your mother, Mrs. Andrews. Yes, I would like to come and see her today, this afternoon, after my clinic is finished. It would be about five o'clock. Would that suit you? I am sorry it would be so late." He spoke quickly as he always did when he had already decided what would work for him.

"Actually, it would work out quite well." Not very well—don't sound eager and say very well, Susan thought to herself.

"It might be between five and six tonight. You are sure that is not too late?"

"No. That will be fine. Look out for the beech hedge, that is the entrance." But it won't be fine, Susan thought.

Sadly she realized that Dr. Patel was right to visit her mother in the evening and see her at her worst. A night's rest allowed oxygen to flow to her mother's brain and bring brief moments of clarity and articulation in the morning. But as the day wore on and she struggled to stay mobile, to stay in control, the synapses of thought and speech closed like flowers at the end of the day and could connect no more, leaving her brain to strike out on its own down the pathways of old memories and new paranoias.

Susan knew that the woman Dr. Patel met that evening would not be the same one who would come to greet her when she arrived to visit in a half hour's time.

Susan and her mother began their visit, as they always did, with a catch-up cup of coffee. Susan cupped her mug in both hands and said casually, "A Dr. Patel is going to come and see you this afternoon."

Mrs. Andrews moved a little forward in her chair; no longer relaxed, she was watchful, wary, and a little bit excited. "Who is this doctor?"

"Do you remember Dr. Frank wanted another doctor to come and see you? This is the one. He phoned to say he would like to come today, after he has finished his clinic, so I don't expect it will be before five, probably closer to six, but he still might like a cup of tea." Susan stressed the time of his visit and knew that she would have to repeat it again during the day if her mother was not to feel surprised by his arrival that evening.

Her mother sat back in her chair and took it all in. She sensed another challenge, another predator coming to stalk her in her nest. Why couldn't they leave her alone, she thought, both women thought. Why must she be hounded and hunted, flushed out into the open to be sniped at as she stood vulnerable, old, and losing her mind.

Susan said nothing more about the new doctor's visit, for the moment.

Instead she asked, "What shall we do about lunch? Would you like to go out?" Susan was relieved that she could provide some distraction to the challenges that lay ahead.

The fish pie at The Princess was always hot, cheesy, and comforting. They both sipped their half pints of cider like a last drink before the execution. These chaperoned lunchtime outings to the pub were the only time that Mrs. Andrews now allowed herself to drink. Fearful of losing control, she guarded every porthole to the open seas of her mind.

While her mother napped at home after lunch, Susan walked into the village to do the errands of shopping, the post office, and the cleaners. She stopped at Brown's, the bakers, and bought a coffee cream cake for her mother's tea and they sat down together a little after four. By the time five o'clock arrived without Dr. Patel, Mrs. Andrews was fretting. At five thirty the phone rang sharply, breaking into their expectant silence. It was Dr. Patel, lost as he never thought he would be, somewhere along the road outside the beech hedge.

"Stay where you are. I am going to walk out into the road to meet you." Susan left the front door open and walked down the driveway to the beech hedge. Immediately she saw the scruffy car with a neat man on the phone inside.

"Hello, Dr. Patel." Her voice smiled into the phone and caused him to look up, caught, as it were, in the headlights of her welcome.

"Hello there." He snapped his phone shut, reached for his bag, and almost sprang out of the car. Fumbling with his keys and phone and locking the car, he tried to get everything in his left hand to shake Susan King's extended right one.

"You did find us then. Well done. It is not always easy. Let me show you the way." She turned to walk in front of him down the narrow pathway that led to the front door where Mrs. Andrews was standing, head cocked to one side, watching and fixed.

Dr. Patel was surprised at his own quickening heartbeat and eagerness when he saw her and simultaneously breathed in the intoxicating evening air.

"Good evening, Mrs. Andrews. I'm Dr. Patel, a consultant psychiatrist for people over sixty-five. I believe you might qualify for my attention." He looked up at the tall older woman and for a long moment they stared deep into each other's eyes before Mrs. Andrews straightened her back and raised her head once more.

"Don't you count on it," she replied before turning to face the open doorway and leading the way into the house to begin this closing battle. Susan and Dr. Patel both extended their arms out, beckoning the other to follow Mrs. Andrews before Susan led the way and Dr. Patel followed her. Mrs. Andrews turned to face them when she reached her chair, as if at bay.

"Darling," Susan said, "why don't you sit down? Dr. Patel, would you like this chair? May I get you some tea?"

"Yes please, that would be nice. Thank you." Susan turned back to her mother.

"Any more for you, darling?"

"No thank you. I've had my tea." Her mother was poised between tea and supper, a restless time that always now brought fearful wonderment of imagination and terror. Dr. Patel was waiting for her to sit down in her chair before quietly lowering himself into the matching one by the stairs. He sat still for a moment. Slowly he breathed in the room and the home. He smelt the faint but deep odor of urine that he guessed, correctly, was coming from upstairs and Mrs. Andrews's bedroom.

She absorbed and drank up the modern, urbane smoothness that covered his handsome, dark good looks like a stream of fluid silk. She took in his neat navy suit, his blue and white striped shirt with its stiff white collar and red tie. He allowed her this time of watching, as an honest hunter is still while his prey searches for danger.

Susan came back into the room with two mugs of tea and placed one in Dr. Patel's hand while gently setting out a small coaster on the little table beside his chair.

"Thank you." Dr. Patel glanced at Susan and politely waited until she sat down, perched on the edge of the sofa, across the room. She leaned forward holding her mug of tea. All three paused for a moment. Dr. Patel leaned forward also, managing to make his posture deferential and not threatening. Mrs. Andrews relaxed back in her chair, but her head was cocked and raised. She was smiling now, thrilled at the engagement with the younger man and yet cautious, cautious, as a mouse is mesmerized by a coiled and silent snake.

"Mrs. Andrews, to help me get a better understanding of who you are, I am going to ask you a few questions about your life. Please stop me—" Here, Dr. Patel held his hands up, palms facing her, and, waving them from side to side, he repeated, "Please stop me if they are too personal or you do not wish to answer."

He gave another, less benign, pause before adding, "for any reason." Susan sat back on the sofa, trying to relax as a parent would watching her young child's first performance in a school play. She too sensed the danger that was waiting for her mother.

Dr. Patel started slowly with the questions when and where were you born? Mrs. Andrews answered slowly and correctly. The next few questions were general and allowed her to answer from her current reality. Susan listened, heart-stoppingly aware of how many lapses of memory her mother was covering with a weak effort of being obtuse and vague. What Susan didn't know yet was how aware Dr. Patel was of this also. She watched him follow her mother down the path of her life, and it was not until her mother lost her way and took Dr. Patel to a landscape that was not in her mother's reality that Susan interrupted.

"Do you know the area well?" She spoke quickly in her urgency to head him off from any wrong assumptions he might make about her mother.

"Yes, I live in Hazelbush."

"Do you know the Fernwell Road that now leads to the motorway?"

"Yes," he began, but she carried on.

"The big house, Fernwell Hall, with the old run-down garden and the eggs for sale. That is where my mother lived since she was very young." Susan added the last hesitantly before continuing. "After my father died she moved to a new house, and then came here closer to the village when she was sixty-four. She has lived here, alone, ever since." Dr. Patel blinked, excited by this connection. He couldn't help himself as he leaned forward eagerly.

"I know Fernwell Hall well. Why, we are almost neighbors. I live in the Chestnuts, just two doors away, on the other side of the farm."

Susan too leaned forward, anxious to give him any information, any connection that would cause him to cleave to her mother. She poured out her words quickly in a protective wave with which to shield her mother, to give her a rest from the questions and probings of Dr. Patel's searching.

Dr. Patel listened with interest as Susan told him the history of his home before; catching his eagerness to belong, he pulled himself back to his purpose.

"This is fascinating. I would love to hear more. Maybe we can talk about it again." He stood up. Susan looked at his upright presence and knew a transition was in progress. For a moment his slight, dark, masculine frame was the central point of the room. He moved behind Mrs. Andrews and drew out one of the large mahogany dining room chairs and placed it just behind her, glancing, as he did so, at the heavy needlepoint seat covers. He sat down and propped an elbow on the back of her armchair. She tilted her head back, as if ready to listen to him but the half smile of her face told Susan that she was remembering the cradling of a man's arm.

"Now, Mrs. Andrews, I would like—if you will permit me—to ask you some more questions. And I am going to give you three objects to remember. While I ask you questions, I will come back to the objects and ask you to tell them to me again. Would that be all right with you?"

She nodded. How could she refuse? She was too excited to speak and tremulous at the thought of this engagement. He began by giving her three simple objects to remember, two were visible from her chair—a clock and a tree—but the third, a dog, was not. He repeated the words clock, tree, and dog, and she repeated them after him with a hesitant confidence: clock, tree, dog. Susan watched as Dr. Patel leant back in the chair like a cat pulling back on its haunches. He asked more seemingly simple questions and encouraged her mother with her nearly, and sometimes even completely, correct answers.

"What day is it? Who is the prime minister? What is your phone number? Can you repeat the three objects I gave you?" Four times he did this and each time the objects became more distant and harder for Mrs. Andrews to recall from the ebbing streams of her memory. She was busy trying to play the question game and dismissed Susan's fearful look as she had always dismissed Susan's concerns for her. Dr. Patel gently continued with his questions, repeating some he had asked before but in a different way. "What year were you born? What is the date today?" Why, we could all be hesitant and muddled answering such questions, Susan thought to herself. But she knew she was searching to buy time for her mother, time that was not for sale.

At last he was satisfied. Gently, as at the end of a waltz, he let go of Mrs. Andrews's mind with a small bow.

"Thank you very much. You have done very well and been very helpful."

He stood up and put the chair back at the dining room table, noticing again the set of needlepoint chair covers. An industrious and diligent lady, he thought to himself. He did not touch Mrs. Andrews as he turned back to her but said, in a manner she recognized from her own long-ago guardianship of her deceased husband, "I want to have a word with your daughter now and then I will come back and say good-bye to you."

"We can talk in the garden," Susan broke in. She turned to her mother. "I will bring you some supper, darling, and then we will be back inside." Susan went into the kitchen and quickly put together a small salad and sandwich. It took no time, this repetitive routine she had done almost every day for over two years.

She returned, hoping that the time she had given her mother alone with Dr. Patel had been enough to satisfy her mother and not too long for him. She put the supper tray in front of her mother and ushered Dr. Patel out of the door.

"We will just be outside, darling." They went out and around the back of the house into the little garden and sat on the old bench her mother had dragged from home to home. Dr. Patel spoke first.

"You are dealing with dementia of course." His "of course" struck Susan as swiftly as a French executioner's sword; the cleanness of his strike and professional assessment severed the reality she had been trying to maintain and left it rolling away on the grass in front of them. The trial had been swift, seemingly fair, but the conclusion had been forgone, and she knew it. Before she could utter a word in this new afterlife, he continued.

"We no longer talk about treatment but about management, you understand that?" A statement, a question, a pause? Susan sat up from her curled position as straight as she could to meet him without actually standing up.

"A vascular dementia," she replied, also a statement and a question.

"Um hum, multifaceted," he acknowledged—and corrected, "Of course, you want to know how long for: two, three, maybe five years. It depends on the care. I have seen one patient go on for fifteen years. And your mother's heart is strong."

Susan's own heart sank at the words. Fifteen years of slow erosion. How could her mother bear it, and there would never be enough money for that, three to five years maybe. But she shook herself away from those distant practicalities and returned to Dr. Patel and what he had to say about the here and now.

"She cannot stay here of course—even with what you have put in place, she is no longer safe alone. I wonder if she would come to my day hospital? I think not. No, she is too proud a woman. This will come and go you know. Some days will be better than others but always it will continue to get worse. You need to be thinking now of where would be right for her." He paused here, like a doctor giving a diagnosis of terminal cancer. He did not tell her all he knew of the road ahead for her mother: the evaluation based on cold clinical assessment, the nursing homes who put these women to one side, the small wards for the elderly mentally infirm that smell like slowly swirling, blocked toilets. Instead he waited to hear what he knew she had begun to think about. After the diagnosis he could do no more than guide, counsel, prescribe, and remember, as best he could, the woman he had just met before she disappeared. Sitting on the old bench for a moment, he imagined what she must have been like as a young woman living in that old rundown house when both the Hall and Mrs. Andrews were young and glorious. He began to go over in his own mind the marks of her personality that he remembered, her flirtatiousness, her effort, the photographs of her family, her pride. He brought himself forward to listen to Susan.

"I have begun to talk with my mother about Beach Grove. It is just up the road, close enough for her friends to visit. She remembers it as the old hotel it used to be. I have also begun to bring people from Beach Grove's outreach program in three evenings a week and they are getting to know each other. She didn't like it at first but now seems to be accepting them. We go to lunch there once a week together, which she hates. I don't know what else to do. This house is too small for someone else to stay with her all the time. She would drive them crazy and . . ." she paused to draw breath, searching for the next words, "anything might happen."

Dr. Patel nodded his head. Good, he thought, she has already made the decision. Mrs. Andrews would be an appropriate candidate for Beach Grove. She just needed to be encouraged and carry on that path. He sensed Susan's relief at his assent. Susan could not think what else to say. She wanted to ask for reassurance that her mother would be all right but knew that all he could give her now would be platitudes. There was no longer any safety.

At that moment Mrs. Andrews appeared from alongside the house. She had only eaten half of her supper, so anxious was she not to let them be alone together for too long. Dr. Patel and Susan both looked up. Susan sat, numbed, not wanting this time where she still might gather some comfort from his words to end. It was Dr. Patel who was able to smile up at her mother.

"Hello, Mrs. Andrews. We were just coming back in."

"Oh yes." Mrs. Andrews tried to make a joke of her words but all three of them felt the fear in her. Dr. Patel rose to his feet. Susan followed and they both moved toward Mrs. Andrews as she made her way unsteadily on the grass towards them. The sun had dipped down behind the trees that bordered the small communal garden, and the first hint of evening cool reminded him he was ready to go home to his supper. Together the three of them walked the short distance back to the door and stood for a moment. Dr. Patel offered his hand first to Mrs. Andrews.

"Goodbye, Mrs. Andrews. It has been a pleasure to meet you."

"Goodbye." As Dr. Patel held her hand, he felt it tremble like a wounded, captured sparrow and he acknowledged, with a slight squeeze of his fingers, that he understood the fear she felt in his presence. He turned to speak to Susan, whose face had lost much of its composure.

"Goodbye. I will be back in touch with Dr. Frank."

"May I call you too?" Susan spoke quickly, not quite pleading but wanting to make sure there was a doorway still open to him.

"Yes, of course. That is no problem. If we need to I can see your mother again. Goodbye."

Susan put her arm around her mother as Dr. Patel turned on his heel and walked away from the house and down the driveway to his car. The two women stood watching as he unlocked the old Honda and climbed in. He turned the car out of the driveway and eased forward into the street. The women stood arm in arm together, waving until he was out of sight.

# Narratives of Womanhood: Social Constructions of Body, Sexuality, and Reproduction

৪১

THIS SECTION ADDRESSES the essential question: how much does being a woman have to do with the unique image and function of the female body? The works included in this section highlight questions regarding the construction of women's physicality. Are women's identities, self-image, and social worth intrinsically tied to their uniquely female organs? The first essay in this section, introduces this idea of the female body part separated from the whole. Anne Wenzel's "The Placenta, The Pancake" discusses the historic and cross-cultural construction of this temporary organ. The placenta, argues Wenzel, has crossed the line in Western cultures from contested territory to medical property—tissue to be sampled, analyzed, and discarded as waste, no longer even remembered as belonging to the female body. She writes, "Out of the mother's 'neglect' of the placenta has risen the intense gaze of the physician. In America, as women have placed less emphasis on the placenta . . . physicians have placed more weight on its knowledge." It is perhaps the paradigm for other body parts excised from the female body—no longer lost parts of self, they become privileged over their owners as repositories of secrets about the body, medical texts to be read in their own right.

A portion of this section addresses lost body parts and body/self fragmentation. In the context of a friend's post-mastectomy reconstruction, Maureen Tolman Flannery describes the role of her "symmetrical breasts" in her self-image and role as a mother. Bushra Rehman's poem locates "All my unborn children / my mother's smile, my father's laugh / my sister's tongue and my crooked teeth / but also the potential for genius" in her lost reproductive organs. Lynne Sharon Schwartz puts this experience in a social context in her short story. Her protagonist mourns the loss of her reproductive organs through surgery and rails against the medical system that both pushes her into an unnecessary oophorectomy and ill prepares her for the emotional results.

Elissa Meites's story about abortion, "Choose," and Joan Baranow's "Watching the Laparoscopy" and "Follicles," further illustrate the medicalization of women's reproductive lives. For an infertile woman, is infertility an "illness" that is "curable" through medical technology? Is the then pregnant woman "well"? For a woman with an unwanted pregnancy, is that same pregnancy an "illness" that abortion "cures"? We include contributions about both in this collection because, regardless of the answers to these questions, it is clear that women's relationships to their reproductive selves are mediated by a medical establishment that defines "illness" and "wellness" for us.

The social construction of the damaged female body is another theme of this section. Marissa Bois and Edith Wypler Swire each write about bodies whose very nature as female are threatened as a result of illness and its medical treatment. Turning the accusatory gaze of the voyeur upon her/himself, Bois writes, "The scar. . . . Uncomfortable? Look, go ahead, *see: this* is me. . . . I watch your eyes linger on the naked space in between my jeans and tee shirt. Hmm . . . you think. Is that really . . . ? When we speak eye to eye, I see you glide your gaze down to my exposed stomach. . . . I flirt with actually lifting up my shirt, pulling down my pants, and screaming at you, 'Here, wanna see the whole damn thing? Stare all you want, honey!'" Similarly, Swire discusses the experience of a colostomy as a defeminizing experience. "I couldn't eat," she writes, "knowing the food would end up in the bag. I was filled with disgust and self-loathing. . . . The fear of cancer was nothing compared to the fear of living with the bag that threatened my very identity as a woman." Regina Arnold, who passed away shortly before publication of this anthology, discusses the impact of chemotherapy-induced hair loss. Hair is not just a symbol of femininity but a signifier of culture and politics. Arnold describes her mother's resistance at her 1960's Angela Davis–like Afro, and her own desire at one time to shave her head as a feminist gesture. Enforced baldness from cancer, however, challenges a woman's status in her gender.

These works deal with body parts removed, bodies damaged as a result of illness. Three contributions to this section deal with female bodies changed, devoured, and marked as a result of not illness, but social victimization and violence. Here, suffering is imposed upon bodies not because of illness, but to cause illness. In Cortney Davis's "Anorexia," we the readers view a young woman's eating disorder through the eyes of her mother—and are left to wonder about cycles of gendered expectations. Dawn McGuire's "My Brown Daughter Wants to Know" deals with clitoridectomy—which has become a highly contested gender-based cultural practice. The adoption in the poem—the saving of a brown daughter from the practices of her "brown mommy"—parallels the power discrepancy inherent in Westerners condemning the body-altering practices of other communities. Simultaneously, the poem parallels the struggles of two mothers—brown and white—to keep their daughter safe from literal and social mutilation. Suffering based on gender violence is imposed from forces within the family in Andrea Nicki's "Adventures of Amelia." A father's sexual abuse creates sickness, such that, "Amelia went to the doctor's / every day, hopeful for a cure. / The doctors said there was /nothing wrong, / but she could not agree." The reader is left wondering about the responsibilities of "the doctors" and the relationship between biologically and socially caused suffering.

# The Placenta, the Pancake: Metaphor in Medicine

## ANNE WENZEL

In every birth, there are two births. First, the infant arrives, shuddering and squawking, and it is to the infant that most in the delivery room attend. The second birth occurs when the bloody residue called the placenta, or afterbirth, detaches from the uterus and must be gently pulled from the vagina and collected. The placenta then makes its descent from labor and delivery to the morgue.

Each night, OB nurses placed the placentas, contained in thick white plastic buckets, at the door that divided the morgue from the lab. My father, a pathologist for whom I worked as an assistant during the summer, referred to them as "groceries" because the buckets were discreetly placed into brown paper bags and delivered to our doorstep. It was my job to haul the bags in, remove the placentas, and prepare them for midmorning gross examination.

One by one, I would pull off the lid of each bucket and take a long, deep look at the contents. I held my breath to avoid smelling the metallic and sweet stench of blood. Though called "afterbirth," the placenta's purpose is much more vital than the term would suggest. The placenta is a temporary organ that the woman's body builds from scratch from the contact of the chorionic sac (which holds the fetus) and the uterus. The placenta performs all of the fetal organ functions—with the exception of the central nervous system—while the fetus is in the uterus. It also forms a barrier between the mother's circulatory system and the fetus's. Most placentas are perfectly round, about the size of a dinner plate, thick as a rib eye and with a similar meaty grain. With gloves on, I reached into the bucket and picked up the soft, dark-red placenta, pulling pieces of the sac and umbilical chord away to expose the meaty membrane. Then, I placed it gently back into the bucket and took the bucket to a spigot attached to a vat of formalin, a mixture of formaldehyde and salts that would "fix" the placenta, making it firm, easy for the pathologists to cut pieces that—through a delicate process involving wax, chemicals, and incredibly sharp razor blades—would be turned into slides. As the formalin splashed into the bucket and crept up my nostrils, the smell of blood disappeared.

Placentas were ubiquitous in the morgue. It was not unusual to have seven bags blocking the door every morning. And for this ubiquity, as well as their general messiness, they were despised by most of the doctors, the techs, and especially lowly scrubs like me, who had the task of cleaning the buckets. We'd listen for warnings during the day: a soft jazz version of Brahms's lullaby, broadcasted through the PA system every time a baby was born, perhaps providing proof for apprehensive family members in waiting rooms all over the hospital that life was continuing its routine, circular course. In the morgue, there would be heavy sighs all around.

Providing some relief was the fact that not all placentas had to be given equal scrutiny. With each bucket came a slip of paper that designated the placenta either as NPLAC, not to be examined by the pathologist, or EPLAC, to be examined. NPLACS had come after uncomplicated births of healthy babies with high Apgar scores. These placentas were round and red and healthy. All I had to do was fix them in formalin and stack them on a shelf, where they waited out three weeks before going to the garbage can. EPLAC placentas were about half that size and tapered at the edges. Often they were crumbling to pieces and discolored: blue gray or purple or meconium stained, from the infant's first bowel movement discharged in utero.

Not all women's placentas came to the morgue, either. Four or five times in the course of his practice, my father told me, a woman asked to have the placenta sent to a facility to be frozen. Should the child one day require stem cells, undifferentiated cells abundant in the umbilical cord that might be useful in some kind of therapy, they would be available in the frozen placenta. Some also asked to keep them for their own personal use. But in our hospital, as in most American hospitals, women signed a blanket consent form that gave the hospital control over the placenta. Over 70 percent of the time, my father estimated, the placentas were waiting for him at the morgue's door.

Curious about how women regard their placentas, I recently asked a friend who is six months pregnant and having a midwife birth what she was planning to do with it. Shocked by the question, she said, "To be honest, I hadn't even thought of it!" This response, I gather, is consistent with most modern American experiences of birth. Unless something goes wrong, the placenta doesn't often factor in: afterbirth, afterthought. In many cases, the very idea of it seems to disgust women.

It does not help that doctors tend to choose food metaphors when describing the specimens they examine. My father would often point to the lining of a gallbladder with his scalpel and say "strawberry gallbladder," which meant a heavy amount of cholesterol had deposited inside the organ and given the surface the grainy appearance of the inside of a strawberry. Cutting the brain or heart into heavy slices during an autopsy was "bread-loafing." And so on, interminably—nutmeg liver, anchovy-sauce liver, sugar-coated spleen. "Pancake" was his nickname for placenta, a name in which I always detected a bit of affection, in the way a teacher will love most her most troublesome student. "How many pancakes have we got today?" my father would ask entering the morgue, unbuttoning his shirt cuffs and rolling up his sleeves.

As with my father's pancakes, the placenta seems to excite the metaphoric imagination across cultures. Anne Fadiman reports in her book *The Spirit Catches You and You Fall Down: A Hmong Child, Her American Doctors, and the Collision of Two Cultures* that the Hmong, a Laotian tribe, call the placenta the "jacket." "It is considered one's first and finest garment," Fadiman writes, that in the course of one's death must be returned to and donned again.[1]

> Only after the soul is properly dressed in the clothing in which it was born can it continue its dangerous journey, past murderous *dahs* and giant poisonous caterpillars, around man-eating rocks and impassable oceans, to the place beyond the sky where it is reunited with its ancestors and from which it will someday be sent to be reborn as the soul of a new baby.[2]

In Laos, the Hmong buried their "jackets" in their homes, girls under their parents' bed, boys "in a place of greater honor, near the base of the house's wooden pillar" that held up the roof and held a male guardian spirit who watched over the house and its inhabitants.

As metaphors, "pancake" and "jacket" are striking in their differences. Each suggests a different function of the placenta, one that nourishes and one that contains. The biggest difference, though, seems to be one of permanence. We eat pancakes. They pass through our bodies and are eventually discarded as waste. In contrast, we claim a jacket as our own; a jacket holds us, stays with us. It is something to which we return.

In the hospital, a placenta is, in a sense, devoured. When my father carried the placenta, dripping from the bucket, and placed it on the paper towels, he regarded it with extreme care. I watched him cut the amniotic sac from around the base of the placenta, then wrap it like a wet towel around his scalpel, making it into the shape of an eggroll so that when he cut it, he knew he was getting a good cross-section. I watched him slice randomly the placenta's parenchyma (its meat), checking for infarctions, or clots, and calcifications. When he sliced a portion of the umbilical cord, he counted the number of vessels, looking for three: two that provided blood to the fetus and one that removed waste, though sometimes only two vessels have developed. He recorded everything on a Dictaphone, his foot pressing on and off the pedal between the efficient work of his scalpel and his gross examination. When the examination was complete and specimens had been gathered for the slides, the leftover shreds of the placenta were placed back in the bucket, the bucket stacked on a shelf, and three weeks later I threw the placenta into a large, yellow biohazard trashcan that sat in the middle of the room. Perhaps, then, the terms the placenta is framed in either reflect or determine how it is used.

Like the common American parlance of pregnancy and birth that removes the mother from the experience—a child "is delivered" or a mother "is expecting"—the term "placenta" (or the Hmong's "jacket" for that matter) does not reference the mother who has created the organ from the stuff of her own body. Language of birth is framed around the fetus. Historically, too, it seems most cultures have framed the afterbirth in terms of the fetus. In her book *Anthropology of Human Birth,* Margarita Kay writes that among Guatemalans, "the placenta is thought to have a special relationship to the child, sometimes referred to as the second child."[3] Guatemalan midwives thus ensure that the afterbirth is properly disposed of by burning it and burying its ashes. Similarly, in the Nigerian Onitsha Ibo tribe, the afterbirth is buried along with a banana stem. The child's name is then given to the banana tree that grows from that stem. Kay adds, "Onitsha people say that to kill a banana tree is to kill small children."[4] In the births of Seri Indians, once the placenta is expelled, midwives wash, salt, and rub it with ashes "to make the baby strong," then bury the placenta at the base of a cactus outside the village.[5] In her book, *Listen to Me Good: The Life Story of an Alabama Midwife,* Linda Holmes writes that afterbirth in Alabama in the 1950s was called the "life of the mother" and—after its expulsion from the mother's body—was salted, buried near the house, and the place of its burial marked with a rock or piece of tin.[6] But rarely is the mother's relationship to the placenta acknowledged, and one might say that taking the mother out of the language of birth and afterbirth might put the placenta that much further out of her concern.

To most mothers, placentas are a subject of great concern. Mothers of all mammal species, excluding humans, eat their placentas, a practice that might hint at the term's gastronomic origin. There is some dispute whether this practice, called placentophagy, was once common in human cultures, though the number of recipes and personal testimonies now abounding on the Internet suggest a recent burgeoning trend (placenta lasagna an apparent favorite). Jacques Gelis, in *History of Childbirth: Fertility, Pregnancy, and Birth in Early Modern Europe,* writes that in premodern Europe, the placenta was used medicinally and therapeutically on problems from infertility to freckles until the eighteenth century. Even Hippocrates writes about placenta as being part of the pharmacopoeia, he adds. As doctors replaced midwives and the process of birth became medicalized, however, common practice and use of the placenta simultaneously became "primitive." When "the medical profession showed signs of rejecting" the placenta as therapy, he writes, it became something "repugnant," something "to be gotten rid of," the waste of the birth.[7]

Dealing in specimens, the morgue is akin to a reliquary. Stacks of removed or discarded human parts line the walls: a child's tonsils, a woman's left breast tissue, a man's severed toe peppered with gun powder, swollen prostates, gallbladders, wedges of kidney or liver, all floating in preservative while the occasional corpse sits in the freezer or on the table in the center of the room, a room that can feel at times like one sick aquarium. Most of these specimens (except the toe) have been removed for good reason: cancer, disease, abnormality, or simply the threat of it. Most of the placentas, however, are NPLACs, "not to be examined." They are normal. So how do they find their way to the morgue's door?

Out of the mother's "neglect" of the placenta has risen the intense gaze of the physician. In America, as women have placed less emphasis on the placenta, ceremonially, therapeutically, or otherwise, physicians have placed more weight on its knowledge. Indeed, if my father were to choose a metaphor for the placenta besides "pancake," it would be something along the lines of "book" or "encyclopedia." From the size, shape, and makeup of the placenta, a doctor can read the entire gestational story, a story to which the woman might find little access. The placenta could become a means by which the physician's gaze is able to "read" the body and life of a woman patient.

Like children, placentas themselves are unique. So if asked why—when the bags are at the door—the pathologist needs to receive them all, even the normal ones, my father would reply, "Because there is such a wide range of what is normal that to know what is abnormal requires constant and consistent observation of as many placentas as possible." This becomes even truer with increases in litigation on behalf of children with malformations or complications such as cerebral palsy, where the placenta becomes the key specimen in determining where these abnormalities came from, whether from the doctor's practice (or malpractice) or from within the mother's body.[8] That these abnormalities could show up later, not during or immediately after the birth, is cause, pathologists would argue, for all placentas to be kept in the morgue for reference.

I look in the dictionary. I find that the term infant means "incapable of speech." Fetus means "fruit," placenta "flat cake." A pancake! The placenta can be devoured or cherished, scrutinized, wondered at or discarded, familiar and still chillingly foreign to observe. It is a momentary part of the woman's body, which becomes richly contested territory in the delivery room. In the course of "giving birth" she is also assumed to be giving away this "temporary organ" for the knowledge and care of others, and—my father would add—for her own knowledge of the care she has received. Perhaps such an assumption should not be so easily made; a placenta is truly something worth its own consideration, whether therapeutically as in stem cell research or placenta pizza or even symbolically as in burial or placental art, and not to be simply breezed by with a blanket consent.

Eventually, I began to look forward to my daily offices as a scrub: counting the placentas in the morning, holding the soft tissue, knowing just how much formalin to splash into the bucket to fix the placenta without being wasteful, and delivering it safely to my father's hands later that morning. At the end of a long week, I would take the cleaned buckets on my hip—stacked five feet high like a Mad Hatter's hats—onto the elevator to the second floor, where the warm and busy mess of birth was taking place. The buckets went to the floor of a closet filled with diapers and formula. On my way out, I always lingered a while to watch the infants behind the quiet glass walls, making their first rough movements into the new world.

## Notes

1. Anne Fadiman, *The Spirit Catches You and You Fall Down: A Hmong Child, Her American Doctors, and the Collision of Two Cultures* (New York: Farrar, Straus, and Giroux, 1997) 5.

2. Fadiman 5.

3. Margarita Artschwager Kay, *Anthropology of Human Birth* (Philadelphia: F. A. Davis, 1982) 243.

4. Kay 184.

5. Kay 227.

6. Margaret Charles Smith and Linda Janet Holmes, *Listen to Me Good: The Life Story of an Alabama Midwife* (Columbus: Ohio State UP, 1996) 40.

7. Jacques Gelis, *History of Childbirth: Fertility, Pregnancy, and Birth in Early Modern Europe* (Boston: Northeastern UP, 1991) 169.

8. Kurt Benirschke and Pete Kaufmann, *Pathology of the Human Placenta* (New York: Springer-Verlag, 1990).

# Anorexia

## CORTNEY DAVIS

Still, I'm the only one who might tell her—
*Look at your thighs! Skinny as toothpicks!*
She laughs me off, her thick-soled combat boots too big for her legs.
The whole of her maybe, *what, a size two?*
And the hair, long ringlets she dyed the color of eggplant.
*Hungry?* I ask, clattering dinner dishes, fanning the smells her way.
I'm offering dark bean soup, nachos with yellow cheese melting over the plate.
She stands like a sliver festering in an open wound.
When she turns to lift the kettle, to pour tea, add Nutrasweet, she almost
    disappears.
*Where did you go?* I shout.
The hot liquid gives her cramps.
She runs to the bathroom, comes back chewing Tums, Maalox, complaining.
*It's hunger,* I tell her, *not disease,* but she knows as well as I do.
I sit down, mouth watering, take large spoonfuls of soup, dip my bread.
She reads a magazine: mannequins thin as endive, their skin the color of cream.
When she turns to look at me again, I see scooped out gourds where her eyes
    should be.
A smooth, domed skull like the fragile skin of an egg.
She yawns, and I invent exotic desserts hidden inside her mouth.
One has thin pastry in layers, honey flowing.
The other is aflame—vanilla ice cream, cherries, chocolate sauce, a rich biscotti.
When she swallows, she makes glugging noises in her throat.
Dinner's almost over.
She goes to the refrigerator, opens the door.
*Just looking?*
She decides to brew more tea, turns the burner up until the kettle screams.
Frugal, she takes the used tea bag, dips it over and over into the new, boiling
    water.

# My Brown Daughter Wants to Know

### Dawn McGuire


Definitely, you've noticed.
I knew something was up when you turned four
and you changed your name to "Acacia."*

You wanted to ride the brown pony.
You asked for a brown Barbie.
You asked
   *Where is my brown mommy?*

Hana—your birth name
to which we added Hope.
   *Hana Hope!* you say proudly
when you're not being Acacia—

When it is safe, when the newest war ends,
when there is food again, then you and I
will go to Addis. You will meet her.

*I am so glad,* she wrote,
*that Hana is your daughter now,*
*and you and I are sisters.*

By now you would have had the *sunna.* At four
or five, a girl from your tribe must have her clitoris removed.
Otherwise, no man will marry her.

This is considered less extreme. Not the whole
vulva cut away, the gash stitched tight
or held together by thorns.

---

*Acacia is a common tree in sub-Saharan Africa and almost iconographic of the East African
savannah.

You would sit on a stool and someone would hold your legs apart.
Crying would bring shame. You would not cry.
A razor, glass, or the midwife's teeth are used.

It seems a small thing in the world, I know—
my daughter
delivered, with all your hungers, whole.

Yet I look into your eyes and I think
I am peering over the rim
of the world's wound.

I am small before it, shallow.
A brown mother peers back,
equal in bafflement.

When I am old and maybe even paler
and this belly that did not carry you
is wound round some hard infirmity,

I want my daughter to comfort me.

Even if so many vows I will have broken,
have broken,
I want you here, to heal me

as you did last evening
singing your Acacia song to your dolls
the brown ones and the white ones
all in the one bright circle.

# Adventures of Amelia

ANDREA NICKI

*Injuries*
Amelia's father locked her
in the garage after church.

She knocked and knocked
on the window until it broke,
and cut her wrist.

Her mother told her
to soak her blouse
so that it wouldn't stain
permanently.

Amelia made painting
after painting all in red.

*Fathering 1*
Amelia's father said
he noticed she was developing

and perhaps he should
buy her a girdle?

Amelia ate ten peas
for dinner
and prepared for the worst.

*Fathering 2*
Amelia lay asleep
as her father undressed
and came into her bed.

He was so heavy
she couldn't breathe.
She thought he was trying
to kill her with his spear.

Amelia unzipped her skin
and got out,
watching the mad beast
prey on the smaller animal.

She tried to scream
but she had no mouth or throat.

The mad beast left
and Amelia got back
into her body,

but she could not understand
why she so ached.

She must have had a bad dream,
she thought.

*Fathering 3*
At dinner Amelia stared
at the blackness
of her father's pupils,

which seemed to blot
everything out,

widening and contracting
from some weird inner light.

Suddenly a spasm
gripped her whole body,
and she lost consciousness.

*Sickness*
Amelia began to have

terrible headaches
and stomachaches
and earaches and backaches.

Amelia went to the doctor's
every day, hopeful for a cure.

The doctors said there was
nothing wrong,

but she could not agree.

# The Bag

EDITH WYPLER SWIRE

I wasn't in charge of my body anymore. Following emergency surgery for a perforated colon, I didn't know what to expect. The indignity of a colostomy was hidden from me for a day or so. Then came the moment when a nurse undid the dressing and there it was—a hole in my body where none should be. The nurse called it a fistula. When she began cheerfully explaining how to change the colostomy bag, I couldn't listen. My mind had gone far away in horror. Attached to me was this foreign appendage, the bag with its revolting contents. I shivered at the weight of it lying on my belly.

They had cut an opening in my abdomen and then stuck on a bag. Why? The answer was surreal, obscene, and embarrassing. I was a woman who prided herself on her aesthetics, her dignity. I had been a concert viola player and my life had been filled with the elevation and delicacy of music. Base bodily functions were something I had always considered to be very secret and private. The doctors had given me a way to bypass an intestinal obstruction/perforation, and the nurse said I should be very grateful and happy that my life had been saved. I wasn't glad or grateful at all.

I was ashamed of the bag and tortured by a nagging pain that teased and taunted me to remember. "There's something wrong . . . there's something terribly wrong." To make matters worse, I could see the bag in broad daylight resting on my stomach. In the weeks to come, I underwent many tests to discover what the mass was, and still no answers. I suffered the indignities of each procedure, having to drink liquids past the point of being full, holding my breath until I panicked for air, or being knocked out by drugs that allowed them to do what no conscious body would permit. A few months passed and I grew thinner. I couldn't eat, knowing the food would end up in the bag. I was filled with disgust and self-loathing.

The doctors were looking for cancer. I didn't think for one second about having cancer until they told me what they were looking for. I held myself in numb misery, realizing I had already arrived at the most dreadful outcome for me; to live with a bag of waste hanging from me, forever. The fear of cancer was nothing compared to the fear of living with the bag that threatened my very identity as a woman.

I wasn't able to articulate my feelings until, one day, a wonderful doctor asked me how I was doing. I allowed that I was weary of hurting and horribly ashamed of the bag. Ashamed is too benign a term to describe how I felt. I told him I was revolted having my own waste on the outside. He looked right at me and didn't interrupt. He didn't poke and prod me while pretending to listen. He acted as if he really cared and I began to believe he really did. The doctor told me he had surgery recently and thought maybe all surgeons would be better for going through some of what their patients went through. He touched me gently and ignored the bag that I fixated on. He gave me hope that one day I could be whole and normal again. I believed he could help me because he knew from experience the helplessness of not owning your body anymore.

After three surgeries and much time spent with this kind man, I was pronounced cured. That mass was not malignant after all, and my doctor rejoiced with me that I would no longer need the bag. As time went by, I stopped needing to touch my abdomen to check if the bag was okay. Then I stopped needing to touch myself to make sure the bag was really gone. Eventually I threw out the saved colostomy dressings and tape. I belonged to myself again. Finally, I wore a bathing suit.

# Distant Scars

## Marissa Bois

It is long and jagged, extending in a sloping line from three inches above my navel to below my pelvic bone. Thin and threadlike in some areas, in others it bleeds outside the line, puckering the flesh here, smoothing it there. This blemish of skin meanders around my belly button, as if wishing to maintain its perfect shape. There are places along this erratic braid where one line becomes two, and then three. An overlap of many scars, a scalpel's slow slice traced and retraced again where numerous operations meet before parting once more. There are more scars. Different shapes and colors, contorting the flesh of other body parts. But this is the one that occupies the most space.

There was a night when I stood completely naked in front of the bathroom mirror. This was the last night that the skin on my stomach could claim smooth flawlessness. I lifted my shirt partway up, exposing my stomach under the blaring overhead light. Tentatively I exposed my skin inch by inch, until I stood there with nothing to hide under. I stood and stared until I knew I would remember my body *before*. My naked body burned my eyes as I stared, determined to brand my reflection into memory. Before the mirror I stayed until my eyes tired and closed.

The scar is the mark and reminder of my disease, the way invisible pain has carved its slow tattoo so others may see. Uncomfortable? Look, go ahead, *see*: *this* is me; *this* is a part of me that, no matter how hard you try, you will never know, never understand.

Before you turn away, I watch your eyes linger on the naked space in between my jeans and tee shirt. Hmm . . . you think. Is that really . . . ? When we speak eye to eye, I see you glide your gaze down to my exposed stomach. How many glances do you need to answer your questions? *Yes, it is.* Another downward cast of the eyes. *Do you wonder what it's from?* You could try asking. But you never do. Instead, when you think I'm not watching, that I am ignorant of your curiosity, you stare. I flirt with actually lifting up my shirt, pulling down my pants, and screaming at you, "Here, wanna see the whole damn thing? Stare all you want, honey!"

Lying in bed I take one finger and follow the scar as it curves around my navel. I know this path well by now. After eight years, I am familiar with every fleshy dent and crevice. Here. This is one place where three lines run alongside each other, briefly separating before they converge once more. It's bumpy. A place that cannot fool my finger into thinking it is normal skin, unblemished and scar free. There are tiny mounds that cling to the underside of my skin, forming little lumps that stick out awkwardly. These appeared one day when I was tracing the same line over and over again in nervousness. I looked down as if I were touching a part of someone else's body, foreign and unfamiliar. At first I was repelled by their obscenity, their foreign and unwelcome appearance on my body. But over time, this mountain landscape of scar tissue became another path in my scar, another detour my finger could trace and retrace.

"Well, that's the end of your bikini-wearing days." She said it as though my ten-year-old life were about to end. The nurse was busying herself around the room, occupying her hands and eyes so she could pretend not to see my exposed abdomen. Days after the operation, the tiny rectangular strips still clung in a neat, vertical line over my stomach. They formed a railroad rusted with red-stained strips of gauze. The line of the scar stretched from below my pubic bone up over my navel, splitting my stomach into two asymmetrical halves. I periodically fingered the corners of these strips with the same intensity one plays with barely healed-over bug scabs. Some of the edges unstuck from my skin, but I never took them off voluntarily, never touched the place where the gauze met the line of my scar. I liked looking down and seeing that mysterious dirty trail. I didn't need to see what was underneath.

Yet it was inevitable, unavoidable. I discovered that beneath their neat covering, the red line of the scar was crude and abrupt. It protruded rudely, demanding recognition. I could see the dark red that collected in some places, clinging to the gauze and making the strips hold on even tighter.

When they began to fall off I mourned their loss. One gauze strip washed away while I was in the shower; three were slyly ripped off when I struggled to put on my first pair of jeans after the operation. Days passed and I shed the strips like tired old skin. One morning I awoke to discover the last five strips lying in a litter of dirtied petals beneath me. The scar glared up at me, in all its rawness, reminding me of its newfound permanence. It wasn't going anywhere. I wrapped the remains of the gauze strips in an old handkerchief and stuffed it into my going home bag.

# Hair Matters

Regina A. Arnold

"You will probably lose your hair." This is one of the first things my male oncologist says to me about the chemotherapy treatments he will be administering. He quickly points out, with a smile, that some women don't lose their hair. What he doesn't tell me is that I will not only lose the hair on my head, but my pubic hair, underarm hair, and any other hair on my body.

When it comes to talking about the effects of chemotherapy treatments, hair ranks right up there at the top, particularly for women. It's normal to see bald heads on men, but not on women—unless you're Sinéad O'Connor. I will never forget the first day I dared to dress up and walk into my office without one of my African print scarves wrapped around my bald head. I thought I would be daring, strut my stuff. Hadn't I always talked about going bald? And then a friend and colleague stopped by to chat with me and the other two academic deans in the office. "Are you comfortable like that?" she asked, alluding to my bald head. "Yes," I replied with a smile, and some other small talk I don't recall, but . . . the office staff has never seen my head bald again. My baldness was making others feel the way only my friend had the nerve to verbalize—uncomfortable. And since I wanted to interact with people without a stigma being attached to me, I bought more scarves from the African bazaar in Harlem and later, two very good wigs from the Town Wig Shop in Hackensack, New Jersey.

There are lots of wig shops around, and lots of wigs to choose from. I looked at curly Afro wigs, long, straight-haired wigs, and short pixie wigs, all in a variety of price ranges. Dismissing the shabbily made curly Afro wigs, I settled on a Tina Turner look. Hey, why not? I also bought their best-selling (and more expensive) "Raquel Welch" signature wig, which was short, with highlights, and tapered. I alternate between them, depending on how I feel—funky and wild or soft and subdued.

It is not lost on me—this switch from my own tight curly hair (which I had worn in an Afro, in braids, and in African locks) to straight hair like I had worn (straightening it with a hot comb and later, processing it with the latest commercial relaxers) prior to the 1960s and the Civil Rights and Black Power movements. My mother, with her relaxed hair, never approved of the Afros I wore. She saw them as a liability, as the way not to get ahead, as going against the system. The whiter you looked and acted, the more likely you were to be successful (in spite of skin color) in white America. Her reaction to my first Afro, in the 1960s, is something she doesn't like to be reminded of. She literally disowned me: "You're no child of mine! Don't come home! I don't want to see you!" It took me years (and a lot of therapy) to realize my mother's actions were not a rejection of me, that it was not about the hair at all but about black radical politics. What my hair meant to her was that I was identifying with Angela Davis and the Black Power movement. Straightened hair was a symbol of how far we had progressed. Why would I want to go back to our African roots—roots from which she had struggled to disengage? But she was a child of the '40s and I was a child of the '60s. That was the difference.

I used to talk about shaving my head, about baldness, as a feminist statement (or perhaps it was just to annoy my mother). That was before the decision was no longer mine to make. Now, my clean-shaven head is a cancer marker, a symbol of loss and illness instead of attitude and freedom. I remember the day I sat at my dining room table and, with the help of my friend Clifton and my son Philip, cut off my African locks after seven years of growth. It was not an occasion for celebration; but cutting them off was preferable to having them go thin at the roots and fall off when I least expected it.

I've been in and out of treatment for the past three years—trying to keep these runaway cancer cells in check—and in and out of my signature wigs, African print scarves, and an occasional pink baseball cap from Martha's Vineyard. Just when my hair starts making itself into a small Afro and I remove the scarves and wigs—starting to feel light and free again—it's time for treatment and back to baldness.

A few weeks after he helped cut my hair, my son sent me a card: I pulled it out of the envelope to see a wide-eyed African girl-child with a head full of wild black hair, not combed or braided. Inside, Philip had written, "That gal sure got some hair on her head!" I loved it.

# Symmetrical Breasts

MAUREEN TOLMAN FLANNERY

It had been a long haul,
but my friend was thrilled,
her zest unchecked by repeated attempts
to realign her breasts.
After malignant mass, mastectomy,
a tram flap, a tattooed areola,
and surgery to recreate an inframammary fold,
this, the second larger implant, had given her
a reconstructed breast
nearly symmetrical with the old one.

And I knew, as I heard her extol
the praises of her plastic surgeon,
that I would have gone home and coveted
my daughter's small, firm buttocks,
her waist indented like a new paragraph,
would have stood in the shower
and made new exercise resolutions,
looking down at the full belly
of a Rubens nude,
nostalgic for the graceful well of toned flesh
that once stretched between protruding pelvic bones,
and lamented my gender's monopoly on cellulite,
hardly having given a thought to the two tight breasts,
sagging only slightly after nursing four,
worldly wise and worse for wear,
but still soft, warm, and nearly the same size.

# A Dream of Living Coal

## Maureen Tolman Flannery

*for my grandmother, Maggie Hopkin Tolman*

It was black, they told her,
shriveled, necrotic,
dead inside her for weeks
and poisoning her system like nightshade.
She'd have died within days, the doctor said,
had she stayed on the mountain with the sheep.
She owed her life to the team and rig
that rumbled her delirium down
the rutted trails to town.
For years she would dream
of grabbing from the fire
a glowing cinder
in the shape of a baby.

# Ovary

BUSHRA REHMAN

I left my ovary on the subway last night.
Stepped out. Felt light.
Heard the door close behind me
and then realized I had left my ovary behind.

If there was an honest person left
in New York, maybe they would return it.
But you can get 2,000 dollars for an egg,
at least that's what the *Village Voice* says.
And with enough eggs in there
to last me a lifetime, whoever found it
is going to be rich.

I reported my ovary lost the next day.
The woman who answered the phone said,
"We've got lots of hearts, livers, kidneys,
and brains, but no ovary."

"No ovary?" I said. "Please
would you look again?"

She sighed, but then being a woman
I guess she did understand.
"What did it look like?"

"Like a walnut, kind of shriveled and red."

"What did it contain?"

"All my unborn children,
my mother's smile, my father's laugh,

my sister's tongue and my crooked teeth,
but also the potential for genius . . ."

There was a pause on the other end,
then she said, "I'll be right back."

But when she returned, she said
there was nothing like my ovary
there, but that I should call back.

I called the next morning.

"You again? Well, today
I have one limb and one liver
in pretty bad condition."

"Anything else?"

"A handful of fetuses like a bucketful of shrimp."

"Anything else?"

"A human head."

"Is it Leary's?"

"Yes, he's dead."

"But I've got no ovary,
no ovary," she said.

If there was an honest person left
in New York, maybe they would return it.
But you can get 2,000 dollars for an egg,
at least that's what the *Village Voice* says.

But still I call every morning
and it's always the same woman.
She tells me about all the pieces of people she finds missing
and I tell her about all the pieces of me I have lost
and have not found yet.

# *So You're Going to Have a New Body*

LYNNE SHARON SCHWARTZ

I

Take good care of yourself beforehand to be sure of a healthy, bouncing new body. Ask your doctor all about it. He can help.

Your doctor says: "Six weeks and you'll be feeling like a new person. No one will ever know."

Your doctor says: "Don't worry about the scar. We'll make it real low where no one can see. We call it a bikini cut."

He says: "Any symptoms you have afterwards, we'll fix with hormones. We follow nature's way. There is some danger of these hormones causing cancer in the lining of the uterus. But since you won't have a uterus you won't have anything to worry about."

He says: "There is this myth some women believe, connecting their reproductive organs with their femininity. But you're much too intelligent and sophisticated for that."

Intelligently, you regard a painting hanging on the wall above his diplomas; it is modern in aspect, showing an assortment of common tools—a hammer, screwdrivers, wrenches, and several others you cannot name, not being conversant with the mechanical arts. A sort of all-purpose handyman's kit. You think a sophisticated thought: *Chacun à son goût.*

You are not even sure you need a new body, but your doctor says there is something inside your old one like a grapefruit, and though it is not really dangerous, it should go. It could block his view of the rest of you. You cannot see it or feel it. Trust your doctor. You have never been a runner, but six weeks before your surgery you start to run in the lonely park early each morning. Not quite awake, half dreaming, you imagine you are running from a mugger with a knife. Fast, fast. You are going to give them the healthiest body they have ever cut. You run a quarter of a mile the first day, half a mile the second. By the end of two weeks you are running a mile in nine minutes. Pretty soon you can run three miles in twenty-three minutes. From the neck down you are looking splendid. Perhaps when you present your body they will say, Oh no, this body is too splendid to cut.

II

You will have one very important decision to make before the big day. Be sure to consult with your doctor. He can help.

He says: "The decision is entirely up to you. However, I like to take the ovaries out whenever I can, as long as I'm in there. That way there is no danger of ovarian cancer, which strikes one in a hundred women in your age group. There is really nothing you need ovaries for. You have had three children and don't intend to have any more. Ovarian cancer is incurable and a terrible death. I've seen women your age . . . However, the decision is entirely up to you."

You think: No, for with the same logic he could cut off my head to avert a brain tumor.

Just before he ushers you out of his office he shows you a color snapshot of some woman's benign fibroid tumors, larger than yours, he says, but otherwise comparable, lying in a big metal bowl wider than it is deep, the sort of bowl you often use to prepare chopped meat for meat loaf. You nod appreciatively and go into the bathroom to throw up.

III

Your hospital stay. One evening, in the company of your husband, you check in at the hospital and are shown to your room, which is not bad, only the walls are a bit bare and it is a bit expensive—several hundred dollars a night. Perhaps the service will be worth it. Its large window overlooks a high school, the very high school, coincidentally, that your teenaged daughter attends. She has promised to visit often. Your husband stays until a staff member asks that he leave, and he leaves you with a copy of *People* magazine featuring an article called "Good Sex with Dr. Ruth." This is a joke and is meant well. Accept it in that spirit. He is trying to say what he would otherwise find difficult to express, that your new body will be lovable and capable of love.

Your reading of *People* magazine is interrupted by your doctor, who invites you for a chat in the visitors' lounge, empty now. He says: "You don't have to make your decision about the ovaries till the last minute. However, ovarian cancer strikes one in a hundred women in your age group." Hard to detect until too late, a terrible death, etc., etc.

As he goes on, a pregnant woman in a white hospital gown enters the visitors' lounge, shuffles to the window, and stares out at the night sky. She has a beautiful olive-skinned face with high cheekbones, green eyes, and full lips. Her hair is thick and dark. Her arms and legs are very bony; her feet, in paper slippers, are as bony and arched as a dancer's. Take another look at her face: the cheekbones seem abnormally prominent, the eyes abnormally prominent, the hollows beneath them abnormally deep. She seems somewhat old to be pregnant, around forty-five. When she leaves, shuffling on her beautiful dancer's feet, your doctor says: "That woman has ovarian cancer."

The next morning, lying flat on your back in a Demerol haze, when he says, "Well?" you say, "Take them, they're yours."

You have anticipated this moment of waking and have promised to let yourself scream if the pain is bad enough. Happily, you discover screaming will not be necessary; quiet moaning will do. If this is the worst, you think, I can take it. In a roomful of screamers and moaners like yourself, baritones and sopranos together, you feel pleased even though you have only a minor choral part. Relieved. The worst is this, probably, and it will be over soon.

A day or two and you will be simply amazed at how much better you feel! Amazed, too, at how many strangers, men and women both, are curious to see your new bikini cut, so curious that you even feel some interest yourself. You peer down then up into the face of the young man peering along with you, and say, "I know it sounds weird, but those actually look like staples in there."

"They are," he says.

You imagine a stapler of the kind you use at home for papers. Your doctor is holding it while you lie sleeping. Another man crimps the two layers of skin together, folds one over the other just above where your pubic hair used to be, and your doctor squeezes the stapler, moving along horizontally, again and again. Men and women are different in this, if you can generalize from personal experience: at home, you place the stapler flat on the desk, slide the papers between its jaws, and press down gently. Your husband holds the stapler in one hand, slides the corner of the papers in with the other, and squeezes the jaws of the stapler together. What strong hands they have! You think of throwing up, but this is more of an intellectual than a physical reaction since your entire upper abdomen is numb; moreover, you have had almost nothing to eat for three days. Your new body, when it returns to active life, will be quite thin.

No one can pretend that a postsurgical hospital stay is pleasant, but a cheerful outlook should take you far. The trouble is, you cry a good deal of the time. In one sense these tears seem uncontrollable, gushing at irregular intervals during the day and night. In another sense they are quite controllable: if your doctor or strange men on the staff drop in to look at your bikini cut or chat about your body functions, you are able to stop crying at will and act cheerful. But when women doctors or nurses drop in, you keep right on with your crying, even though this causes them to say, "What are you crying about?" You also do not cry in front of visitors, male or female, especially your teenaged daughter, since you noticed that when she visited you immediately after the surgery her face turned white and she left the room quickly, walking backwards and staring. She has visited often, as she promised. She makes sure to let you know she has terrible menstrual cramps this week, in fact asks you to write a note so she can be excused from gym. Your sons do not visit—they are too young, twelve and nine—but you talk to them on the phone, cheerfully. They tell you about the junk food they have been eating in your absence and about sports events at school. They sound wistful and eager to have you returned to them.

## IV

At last the day you've been waiting for arrives: taking your new body home! You may be surprised to learn this, but in many ways your new body is just like your old one. For instance, it walks. Slowly. And if you clasp your hands and support your stomach from below, you feel less as though it will rip away from the strain inside. At home, in the mirror, except for the bikini cut and the fact that your stomach is round and puffy, this body even looks remarkably like your old one, but thinner. Your ankles are thinner than you have ever seen them. That is because with your reproductive system gone, you no longer tend to retain fluids. An unexpected plus, slim ankles! How good to be home and climb into your own bed. How good to see your children and how good they are, scurrying around to bring you tea and chocolates and magazines. Why is it that the sight of the children, which should bring you pleasure, also brings you grief? It might be that their physical presence reminds you of the place they came from, which no longer exists, at least in you. This leads you to wonder idly what becomes of the many reproductive organs, both healthy and unhealthy, removed daily: buried, burned, or trashed? Do right-to-lifers mourn them?

You sleep in your own bed with your husband, who wants to hold you close, but this does not feel very comfortable. You move his arms and hands to permissible places, the way you did with boys as a teenager, except of course the places are different now. Breasts are permissible, thighs are permissible, but not the expanse between. A clever fellow, over the next few nights he learns, even in his sleep, what is permissible.

Although you are more tired than you ever thought possible, you force yourself to walk from room to room three times a day, perhaps to show this new body who is in control. During one such forced walk . . . Don't laugh, now! A wave of heat swirls up and encircles you, making you sway dizzily, and the odd thing is, no one has mentioned this—it pulsates. Pulses of heat. Once long ago and with great concentration, you counted the pulses of an orgasm, something you are not sure you will ever experience again, and now you count this. Thirty pulses. You cannot compare since you have forgotten the orgasm number; anyhow, the two events have nothing in common except that they pulse and that they are totally overpowering. But this can't be happening, you are far too young for this little joke. Over the next few days it is happening, though, and whenever it happens you feel foolish, you feel something very like shame. Call your doctor. He can help.

A woman's voice says he is extremely busy and could you call back later, honey. Or would you like an appointment, honey? Are you sure she can't help you, honey? You say yes, she can help enormously by not calling you honey. Don't give me any of your lip, you menopausal bitch, she mutters. No, no, she most certainly does not mutter that; it must have been the tone of her gasp. Very well, please hold on while she fetches your folder. While holding, you are treated to a little telephone concert: Frank Sinatra singing "My Way." Repeatedly, you hear Frank Sinatra explain that no matter what has happened or will happen, he is gratified to feel that he did it his way. Your doctor's voice is abrupt and booming in contrast. When you state your problem, he replies, "Oh, sweats." You are not sure you have heard correctly. Could he have said, "Oh, sweets," as in affectionate commiseration? Hardly. Always strictly business. You were misled by remembering, subliminally, "honey." "Sweats" it was and, in the plural, a very hideous word you do not wish to have associated with you or your new body. Sweat, a universal phenomenon, you have no quarrel with. Sweats, no.

Your doctor says he—or "they"—will take care of everything. For again he uses the plural, the royal "we." When you visit for a six-week checkup, "they" will give you the miraculous hormones, nature's way. In the meantime you begin to spend more time out of bed. You may find, during this convalescent period, that you enjoy reading, listening to music, even light activity such as jigsaw puzzles. Your twelve-year-old son brings you a jigsaw puzzle of a Mary Cassatt painting—a woman dressed in pale blue, holding a baby who is like a peach. It looks like a peach and would smell and taste like a peach too. At a glance you know you can never do this puzzle. It is not that you want another baby, for you do not, nor is it the knowledge that you could not have one even if you wanted it, since that is academic. Simply the whole cluster of associations—mothers and babies, conception, gestation, birth—is something you do not wish to be reminded of. The facts of life. You seem to be an artificial exception to the facts of life, a mutation existing outside the facts of life that apply to every other living creature. However, you can't reject the gift your son chose so carefully, obviously proud that he has intuited your tastes—Impressionist paintings, the work of women artists, peachy colors. You thank him warmly and undo the cellophane wrapping on the box as if you intended to work on the puzzle soon. You ask your husband to bring you a puzzle of an abstract painting. He brings a Jackson Pollock puzzle that you set to work at, sitting on pillows on the living room floor. Your son comes home from school and lets his knapsack slide off his back. "Why aren't you doing my puzzle?" "Well, it looked a little hard. I thought I'd save it for later." He looks at the picture on the Jackson Pollock box. "Hard!" he exclaims.

V

Your first visit to the doctor. You get dressed in real clothes and appraise yourself in the mirror—what admirable ankles. With a shudder you realize you are echoing a thought now terrible in its implications: no one would ever know.

Out on the city streets you hail a taxi, since you cannot risk your new body's being jostled or having to stand up all the way on a bus. The receptionist in your doctor's waiting room is noticeably cool—no honeying today—as she asks you to take a seat and wait. When your name is finally called, a woman in a white coat leads you into a cubicle just off the waiting room and loudly asks your symptoms. Quite often in the past you have, while waiting, overheard the symptoms of many women, and now no doubt many women hear yours. As usual, you are directed to an examining room and instructed to undress and don a white paper robe. On the way you count the examining rooms. Three. One woman—you—is preexamination, one no doubt midexamination, one is post.

When your doctor at last enters, he utters a cheery greeting and then the usual: "Slide your lower body to the edge of the table. Feet up in the stirrups please." You close your eyes, practicing indifference. It cannot be worse than the worst you have already known. You study certain cracks in the ceiling that you know well and he does not even know exist. You continue to meditate on procedural matters, namely, that your doctor's initial impression in each of his three examining rooms is of a woman naked except for a white paper robe, sitting or leaning on an examining table in an attitude of waiting. He, needless to say, is fully dressed. You contemplate him going from one examining room to the next; the devil will not have to make work for his hands. After the examination you will be invited, clothed, to speak with him in his office, and while you dress for this encounter, he will visit another examining room. It strikes you that this maximum-efficiency setup might serve equally well for a brothel and perhaps already does. This is a brothel surrealized.

Your doctor says you may resume most normal activities, may even do some very mild exercise if you wish, but no baths and no "intercourse." "Intercourse," you are well aware, stands for sex, although if you stop to consider, sex is the more inclusive term. Does he say "intercourse" because he is unable to say "sex," or thinks the word "sex" would be too provocative in that antiseptic little room, unleashing torrents of libido, or is it his indirect way of saying that you can do sexual things as long as you don't fuck? This is not something you can ask your doctor.

The last item of business is the prescription for the hormones. He explains how to take them—three weeks on and one week off, in imitation of nature's way. He gives you several small sample packets for starters. At home, standing at the bathroom sink, you extricate a pill from its tight childproof cardboard-and-plastic niche, feverishly, like a junkie pouncing on her fix. Nature's way. Now, no more "sweats," no more tears. Your new body is complete. What is this little piece of paper in the sample packet? Not so little when you open it up, just impeccably folded. In diabolically tiny print it explains the pills' bad side effects or "contraindications," a word reminiscent of "intercourse." Most of them you already know from reading books, but there is something new. The pills may have a damaging effect on your eyes. Fancy that. Nature's way? You settle down on the edge of the bathtub and go back to the beginning to read more attentively. First, a list of situations for which the pills are prescribed. Funny, you do not find "hysterectomy." Reading on, you do find "female castration." That must be . . . yes indeed, that's you. You try to read on, but the print is so terribly small, perhaps the pills are affecting your eyes already, for there is a shimmering film over the fine letters. Rather than simply rolling over into the tub, go back to bed, fully dressed, face in the pillows. No, first close the door in case the children come in. Many times over the past weeks you have lain awake pinched by questions, pulling and squeezing back as if the questions were clay, weighing the threat of the bony-footed woman pregnant with her own death—an actress summoned and stuffed for the occasion? part of a terrorist scheme?—against your own undrugged sense of the fitness of things. Now you have grasped that the questions are moot. This is not like cutting your hair, and you have never even had a tooth pulled. The only other physically irreversible things you have done are lose your virginity and bear children. Yes, shut the door tight. It would not do to have them hear you, hysteric, *castrata*.

But of course the sun continues to rise, your center is hardly the center of the universe. Over the next few weeks you get acquainted with your new body. A peculiar thing—though it does not look very different, it does things differently. It responds to temperature differently and it sleeps differently, finding different positions comfortable and different hours propitious. It eats differently, shits differently, and pisses differently. You suspect it will fuck differently, but that you will not know for a while. Its pubic hair has not grown back in quite the same design or density, so that you look shorn or childlike or, feeling optimistic, like a chorus girl or a Renaissance painting. It doesn't menstruate, naturally. You can't truthfully say you miss menstruation, but how will you learn to keep track of time, the seasons of the month? A wall calendar? But how will you know inside? Can it be that time will feel all the same, no coming to fruition and dropping the fruit, no filling and subsiding, moist and dry, moving towards and moving away from?

## VI

At nine weeks, although your new body can walk and move almost naturally, it persists in lying around the house whenever possible. And so you lie around the living room with your loved ones as your daughter, wearing an old sweater of yours, scans the local newspaper in search of part-time work. Music blares, Madonna singing "Like a Virgin," describing how she felt touched as though for the very first time. Were you not disconcerted by the whole cluster of associations, you might tell your daughter that the premise of the song is mistaken, the very first time is usually not so terrific. Perhaps some other evening. Your daughter reads aloud amusing job opportunities. A dental school wants research subjects who have never had a cavity. Aerobics instructor at a reform school. "Hey, Mom, here's something you could do. A nutrition experiment, five dollars an hour. Women past childbearing age or surgically sterile."

A complex message, but no response is really required since her laughter fills the space. Your older son, bent over the Mary Cassatt puzzle, chuckles. Your husband smirks faintly over his newspaper. He means no harm, you suppose. (Then why the fuck is he smirking?) Maybe those to whom the facts of life still apply can't help it, just as children can't help smirking at the facts of life themselves. Only your younger son, building a space station out of Lego parts, is not amused. Unknowing, he senses some primitive vibration in the air and looks up at you apprehensively, then gives you a loving punch in the knee. You decide that he is your favorite, that one day you may run away with him, abandoning the others.

## VII

The tenth week, and a most important day in the life of your new body. Your doctor says you are permitted to have "intercourse." If your husband is like most men, he can hardly wait. Proceed with caution, like walking on eggs, except that you, eggless, are the eggs on which he proceeds with caution. Touched for the very first time! Well, just do it and see if it works; passion will come later, replacing fear. That is the lesson of behavioral science as opposed to classical psychology. But what's this? Technical difficulties, like a virgin. This can't be happening, not to you with that hot little geyser, that little creamery you had up there. Come now, when there's a will . . . Spit, not to mention a thousand drugstore remedies. Even tears will do. Before long things are wet enough, thank you very much. Remember for next time there's still that old spermicidal jelly, but you can throw away the diaphragm. That is not the sort of thing you can hand down to your daughter like a sweater.

## VIII

Over the next month or two you may find your new body has strange responses to your husband's embraces. Don't be alarmed: it feels desire and it feels pleasure, only it feels them in a wholly unfamiliar way. In bed your new body is most different from your old, so different that you have the eerie sensation that another woman, a stranger, is making love to your husband while your mind, your same old mind, looks on in amazement. All your body's nerve endings have been replaced by this strange woman's; she moves and caresses the way you used to, and the sounds of pleasure she makes are the same, only her apparatus of sensation is altogether alien. There are some things you cannot discuss with your husband because you are too closely twined; just as if, kissing, your tongues in each other's mouths, you were to attempt to speak. But you cannot rest easy in this strangeness; it must be explored, and so you light on an experiment.

You call an old friend, someone you almost married, except that you managed in time to distinguish your feeling for each other from love. It was sex, one of those rare affinities that would not withstand daily life. Now and then, at long intervals, a year or more, you have met for several hours with surprisingly little guilt. This is no time for fine moral distinctions. He has often pledged that you may ask him for any kind of help, so you call him and explain the kind of help you need. He grins, you can see this over the telephone, and says he would be more than happy to help you overcome the mystery of the sexual stranger in your new body. Like Nancy Drew's faithful Ned.

You have to acknowledge the man has a genuine gift as regards women. From the gods? Or could it be because he is a doctor and knows his physiology? No, your knowledge of doctors would not bear out that correlation, and besides, this one is only an eye doctor. In any case, in his arms, in a motel room, you do rediscover yourself, buried deep, deep in the crevices of hidden tissues and disconnected circuits. It takes some time and coaxing to bring you forth, you have simply been so traumatized by the knife that you have been in hiding underground for months, paralyzed by any kind of penetration. But you are still there, in your new body, and gradually, you feel sure, you will emerge again and replace the impostor in the conjugal bed. You feel enormous gratitude and tell him so, and he says, grinning, "No trouble at all. My pleasure." Perhaps you will even ask him about the effects of the pills on your eyes, but not just now.

"Do I feel any different inside?" you ask. He says no, and describes in exquisite terms how you feel inside, which is very nice to listen to. This is not in your husband's line or perhaps any husband's—you wouldn't know. After the exquisite description, he says, "But it is different, you know." You don't know. How?

He explains that in the absence of the cervix, which is the opening of the uterus, the back wall of the vagina is sewn up so that in effect what you have there now is a dead end. As he explains, it seems obvious and inevitable, but strange to say, you have never figured this out before or even thought about it. (It is something your doctor neglected to mention.) Nor have you poked around on your own, having preferred to remain ignorant. So it is rather a shock, this realization that you have a dead end. You always imagined yourself, along with all women, as having an easy passage from inside to out, a constant trafficking between the heart of the world and the heart of yourself. This was what distinguished you from men. They were the walled ones, barricaded, the ones with such difficulty receiving and transmitting the current running between the heart of the world and the heart of themselves. It is so great a shock that you believe you cannot bear to live with it.

Watching you, he says, "It makes no difference. You feel wonderful, the same as always. You really do. Here, feel with your hand, so you'll know." With his help you feel around your new body. Different, not so different. Yet you know. Of course, with his help it becomes an amusing and piquant thing to be doing in a motel room, and then it becomes more love, wonderful love, but you cry all the way through it. A new sensation: like some *Kamasutra* position, you wouldn't have thought it possible.

"At least you don't have to worry about ovarian cancer," he says afterwards. "It's very hard to detect in time and a terrible way—"

"Please," you say. "Please stop." You cannot bear hearing those words from this man.

"I'm sorry. I know it's hard. I can't imagine how I would feel if I had my balls cut off."

With a leap you are out of bed and into your clothes while he looks on aghast. How fortunate that you did not marry him, for had you married him, after those words you would have had to leave him. As you leave him, naked and baffled, now not bothering to inquire about the effects of the pills on your eyes yet thanking him because he has done precisely what you needed done. It will be a very long time before you see him again, though, before the blade of his words grows dull from repetition.

IX

Months pass and you accept that this new body, its torso ever so slightly different in shape from the old one, is yours to keep. Not all women, remember, love their new bodies instinctively; some have to learn to love them. Through the thousands of little acts of personal care, an intimacy develops. By the sixth month you will feel not quite as teary, not quite as tired—the anesthetic sloshing around in your cells must be evaporating. You resolve to ignore the minor nuisance symptoms—mild backaches, a recurrent vaginal infection, lowered resistance to colds and viruses . . . Now that the sample packets of hormone pills are used up, you are spending about fifteen dollars a month at the drugstore, something your doctor neglected to mention in advance. Would he have told you this, you wonder, if you were a very poor woman? How does he know you are not a very poor woman? Foolish question. Because you have purchased his services. The pills cause you to gain weight, jeopardizing the thin new body and the ankles, so you run faster every morning (yes, it runs! it runs!), racing nature's way. One very positive improvement is that now you can sleep on your stomach. Your husband can touch you anywhere without pain. When he makes love to you you feel the strange woman and her alien nervous system retreating and yourself emerging in her place. You will eventually overcome her.

And before you know it, it's time for your six-month checkup. You do not respond to your doctor's hearty greeting, but you comply when he says, "Slide your lower body to the edge of the table. Feet up in the stirrups please." He does not know it, but this is the last time he will be seeing—no, seeing is wrong since he doesn't look, he looks at the wall behind your head—the last time he or any man will be examining your body. There is nothing he can tell you about how you feel, for the simple reason that he does not know. How can he? Suddenly this is utterly obvious, and as you glance again at the painting of assorted tools, the fact of his being in an advisory capacity on any matter concerning your body is both an atrocity, which you blame yourself for having permitted, and an absurdity, such an ancient social absurdity that you laugh aloud, a crude, assertive, resuscitated laugh, making him look warily from the wall to your face, which very possibly he has never looked at before. How can he know what you feel? He has never attempted to find out by the empirical method; his tone is not inquisitive but declarative. He knows only what men like himself have written in books, and just now he looks puzzled.

Why not tell your doctor? That might help. In his office after the examination you tell him—quite mildly, compared to what you feel—that he might have informed you more realistically of what this operation would entail. Quite mild and limited, but even so it takes a great summoning of strength. He is the one with the social position, the money, and the knife. You, despite your laugh, are the *castrata*. Your heart goes pit-a-pat as you speak, and you have a lump in your throat. To your surprise, he looks directly at your face with interest.

He says: "Thank you for telling me that. But not everyone reacts the same way. We try to anticipate the bright side, but some people take it harder than others. Some people are special cases."

X

A few months later, you read a strange, small item in the newspaper: a lone marauder, on what is presented as a berserk midnight spree, has ransacked the office of a local gynecologist. She tore diplomas from the walls and broke equipment. She emptied sample packets of medication and packages of rubber fingers and gloves, which she strewed everywhere, creating a battlefield of massacred hands. She wrote abusive epithets on the walls; she dumped file folders on the floor and daubed them with menstrual blood. As you read these details you feel the uncanny sensation of déjà vu, and your heart beats with a bizarre fear. Calm down; you have an alibi, you were deep in your law-abiding sleep. Anyhow, you would have done it quite differently—not under cover of darkness, first of all, but in broad daylight when the doctor was there. You would have forced him into a white paper robe and onto the examining table, saying, "Slide your lower body to the edge of the table. Feet up in the stirrups please." Not being built for such a position, he would have found it extremely uncomfortable. While he lay terrorized, facing the painting of common tools, you would simply have looked. Armed only with force of will, you would have looked for what would seem to him an endless time at his genitals until he himself, mesmerized by your gaze, began to look at them as some freakish growth, a barrier to himself, between the world and himself. After a while you would have let him climb down untouched, but he would never again have looked at or touched himself without remembering his terror and his inkling that his body was his cage and all his intercourse with the world was a wild and pitiable attempt to cut his way free.

XI

A year after your operation, you will be feeling much much better. You have your strength back, or about eighty percent of it anyway. You are hardly tired at all; the anesthetic must be nearly evaporated. You can walk erect without conscious effort, and you have grown genuinely fond of your new body, accepting its hollowness with, if not equanimity, at least tolerance. One or two symptoms, or rather habits, persist: for instance, when you get out of bed you still hold your hands clasped around your lower abdomen for support, as if it might rip away from the strain inside, even though there is no longer any strain. At times you lie awake blaming yourself for participating in an ancient social absurdity, but eventually you will cease to blame as you have ceased to participate.

Most odd, and most obscure, you retain the tenuous sense of waiting. With effort you can localize it to a sense of waiting for something to end. A holdover, a vague habit of memory or memory of habit. Right after he cut, you waited for that worst pain to end. Then for the tears, the tiredness, and all the rest. Maybe it is a memory of habit or a habit of memory, or maybe the blade in the flesh brought you to one of life's many edges and now you are waiting, like a woman who after much travel has come to the edge of a cliff and, for no reason and under no compulsion, lingers there too long. You are waiting for something to end, you feel closer than ever before to the end, but of what, you do not push further to ask.

# Watching the Laparoscopy

## Joan Baranow

You wouldn't guess how clean it looks—
white and rosy, the ovaries
globular, like scrambled egg whites,
the uterus dark and firm as a plum.
I could see now what they meant
in the medical texts, in those inadequate
drawings—only more lush, soft,
each organ self-contained.  Strange,
I had imagined the gut was contiguous.
When the instruments entered in, the clamps
and probes, the pencil-like laser, I
did not feel sick, even when blood
pulsed from the split tubes, even
when he snipped them into petals
and crimped them back with a hot stick.
I wanted only to understand.  My illness
had gone through the body thoroughly,
touching everything, and I had not known
how my own flesh had suffered, how it
had sought to protect itself, without help.
And now scar tissue, thick, milky,
glimmers in the surgical light
like something poured from a basin,
a rich glue.  When he slid the clamps
through my belly's incisions,
they went straight down, they closed
like clam shells on the stuck organs.
We could see the adhesions then, shining
curtains under the hot blue flare,
before the laser split them
and the bowel fell back, the tubes

came loose, as if the surgeon
had snapped a puzzle apart.
I wanted to see it again, to know
where each piece of me went
after the surgery, how I would be whole,
but he fast-forwarded to the last
procedure—the Bruhat technique—
and then the screen regained its blank blue.
*I don't want to paint a rosy picture,*
he said, *your chances are slim,*
and he used numbers and percentages
to prove I was as well as could be made.
*Your eggs would've had to solve a maze*
*to get in.*  And now…
            We got up to go,
*I hope to hear some good news.*
But already I saw the next surgery,
my children born in a sterile dish.
And now you ask what else I might do
to bear a life.

# Follicles

## Joan Baranow

Like blackberries
on the gray screen.
We counted three,
the unripe one
slipping
inside the flesh of ovary.

I felt the needle, pressure,
its thin incision,
the doctor's voice
when she said,
"Let your legs fall to the side now."
I was nowhere but here,
entered.
When the embryologist
found the first egg,
he shouted through the glass.
After that, a whir
in the clouded dish,
a being, brief.
Then the cells stopped.

And I saw myself retract,
the name *Mother,*
that little boat,
pushed off.

# *Choose*

## Elissa Meites

Let's play a pretend game.

Imagine you're on winter break. You've just finished a set of exams for your graduate degree. It's been the hardest couple of weeks of your life, and you're proud of yourself for doing everything right; little do you know. Let's say your family is all out of town. Your parents are someplace ancient without you, like Damascus or Timbuktu, a place full of musicians and foreign photojournalists. And your boyfriend's off somewhere partying too; Miami, maybe, or Cancun. So you're all alone. You sleep luxuriously late and spend a lot of time playing realistic new video games on the computer.

One afternoon, instead of playing video games, you look dreamily at diamond rings on the Internet and decide you might like an oval cut instead of the traditional round, or maybe you like the marquise better.

Your period's late but that's easy to explain: too much stress, or too much relaxation, and anyway, your breasts are tender, so that means it'll come in the next day or two. You're not stupid, so of course you think maybe you're pregnant, but that's ridiculous because you're not stupid, so of course you always used a condom.

Nicholas comes home, or Ahmed or Jose or whatever his name is, the boyfriend, and brings you wrapped presents and kisses and stories. Let's pretend he is the most wonderful person in the world and you have never been so happy to see him. Now that he is back everything is going to be fine since he will take care of anything that needs taking care of, like you.

You drop hints.

There's not much to do over break but notice that it still doesn't come. It's maybe a week or two late, you can't exactly remember. But now you're sure it's late, probably.

You say it in a whisper in the middle of the night, maybe I'm. When you touch your belly Nicholas reacts with honor and humor. You joke about what it would be like to be parents together: you could run away and start a little family, scrape to make ends meet, you and Nicholas wouldn't have to finish grad school after all. It's funny because you both know it is just a joke. Before you fall asleep, you are arguing about important details like stroller colors. It is all very abstract.

The obvious thing to do is buy a test, just in case. The two of you decide how the test is going to work. Even though you both like the optimism of the test that shows a "+" sign for "pregnant," you choose the one where the two stripes show up in separate windows because there is less chance of confusing the control strip with the test strip. You are not taking any more chances. You are supposed to pee on the plastic stick for five seconds then wait three minutes for the results. It would also be okay to dip the stick in a clean container of your urine, but you can't find a new tupperware in the kitchen and don't want to pee in the used yogurt container. Nicholas wants to come in the bathroom with you, but there is no way you are going to let him do that. You want to look at the test by yourself, but there is no way he is going to agree to that. Finally, you pee on the stick (not on your hand) while he waits outside your bathroom door, and then you bring it outside in your fist, wait three minutes, and turn it over together.

Nicholas asks you to marry him. You say of course, and you put your arms around his shoulders and wonder how to position the hand holding the test stick, since technically it is covered with urine. You don't have any rings, but anyway you don't need them because they are oppressive capitalist symbols that wouldn't jibe with your new bohemian life as poor, unmarried dropout parents. You act confusedly delighted and gay, pretending that these are the circumstances under which you always thought you would decide to get married. You put on your favorite record and dance together, like you are supposed to.

That evening you wake to the sound of him gnashing his teeth. You cry silently. You feel awful. It is the night of your engagement and you feel awful.

You have to start telling people, because you're responsible like that and you're making a mature decision. Your families react like this:

"Heavy." (Your brother.)

"Oh." (Your father.)

"You two really need to set your priorities." (His mother.)

"I hope you make the right choice." (Your mother.)

"I'm happy." (His father, in response to Nicholas's plaintive question, "Isn't anyone happy about this?")

You are disappointed in every one of them.

It is the end of break and you have to go back to school. You had been looking forward to seeing your friends, but they have all gotten so much younger in just a few weeks. Their vacation stories are all about playing video games or other immature pursuits not involving pregnancy.

No matter what, the first thing to do is call for an appointment. It is the first time you have called the student health clinic and the receptionist wants to know how to direct your call. You feel awfully exposed.

"Thinkimpregnant," you whisper.

"Ohhhhhhhhhhhhh," she says, "You need to speak with a nurse."

You're on hold.

Now the nurse answers, asks what the problem is.

"I think I'm pregnant," you say.

There is a long pause. A really long pause.

"My planner's not working, let me transfer you," she says.

You're on hold again.

Someone else finally picks up.

"I think I'm pregnant!" you announce cheerily, hoping she will finally be the one to offer you some encouragement.

"Oh dear," she says.

You can come in after hours tomorrow.

At the clinic you see one of your classmates in the waiting room. You don't ask her why she is there and she doesn't ask you. Here at the clinic they are stocked with disposable tupperware cups for urine tests. You go to the clinic bathroom, use the packet of towlettes to wipe front-to-back like it says on the written instructions they handed you, and then you expertly catch your pee in the cup midstream as if you'd had practice. A little while later the doctor comes in and gives you a business card for the ob/gyn specialty clinic.

You've only wondered for two weeks, but you're already four weeks pregnant. Actually you're officially six weeks pregnant because it turns out they count pregnancies as starting two weeks before the day you actually have the sex that gets you pregnant.

You are trying to make an appointment at the ob/gyn clinic where someone can talk to you about your options. You have classes from nine to five with a ten-minute break every hour, when you dash to the phone. The clinic puts you on hold and tells you to wait ten minutes. You keep hanging up and calling back during your next break, when the same thing happens. When you finally get through to the gynecology clinic, the automated message tells you, "If you are pregnant, call the obstetrics clinic." Finally you skip class and go to the obstetrics clinic in person. It is here that you have to say out loud, "YES, MY FIRST PREGNANCY." You have an appointment in three weeks.

Let's pretend Nicholas takes you to the jewelers and buys you a modest diamond ring. You don't want to spend too much on something so impractical when you might need to sell it in a few months to pay for daycare. You both agree that your decision to get married has nothing to do with the baby. He puts the diamond ring on your finger. You feel like Cinderella at the end of the movie just before the screen goes black and the credits start to roll.

These days there are babies and pregnant ladies everywhere you look. Everywhere: the grocery store, the laundromat, the gas station. You and Nicholas make a great game out of it. When you see a baby you point to it and say, "baby."

The day of your appointment at the obstetrics clinic comes and the nurse escorts you into a little room to talk about your options. You say you haven't been sick at all and she says, "That's because you are young and healthy and pregnancy won't be hard on your body." You shut the door.

"Do you have any questions?" She finishes her presentation and sits back in her chair. Later you think this action was deceptively relaxed, a snake coiling before she strikes. "I think you've laid out one option very clearly," you say bravely. "Can we discuss the others? We still aren't positive it's the right time for us to have a baby." The obstetrics nurse cocks her head. She doesn't understand your question. Then she lunges. "Oh, it's not the right time for you to have a baby? Then let me ask you one thing: WHAT WERE YOU DOING HAVING UN-PROTECTED SEX?"

You can't believe she sounds so hostile. You can't believe she's never seen this before since almost half of American women get an abortion at some point in their lives. You stare at her and mumble, "We weren't." You can't wait to leave. The obstetrics nurse snorts and says, "Didn't work, huh?" She starts shuffling papers. She answers the telephone. You feel like you are in a school principal's office, in trouble for doing something awful. You try to remember what it was like to have your dignity.

The next day you are sick.

Nicholas likes to say he's pregnant too. Your replies are not very generous.

You drop neuroscience class because you just can't deal with higher brain functions right now when you are busy reproducing. Thank God you have the wedding plans to distract your nosier classmates.

You understand now that you were wasting your time with the psychotic nurse at the obstetrics clinic, and you stay home from school to call the gynecology clinic. You explain you're ten weeks and three days pregnant and you need to talk to somebody about your options. "Call the obstetrics clinic," the receptionist says. You want to smack something. Instead you explain that you already visited the obstetrics clinic and want to discuss a broader range of options. She transfers you to a gynecology nurse, who asks you, "So, do you want to be pregnant?" You don't know how to answer.

You wonder what this would be like if you didn't speak English or couldn't add to twelve weeks. You wonder what this would be like if you didn't have health insurance. You wonder what this would be like if you hadn't learned in reproductive health class that twelve weeks was an important deadline. You wonder what would happen if you weren't so determined to get an appointment to talk about your options, or if you lived in a less liberal, less urban part of the country. You don't really wonder; you know.

You are back on the line with the gynecology clinic receptionist, who types something into her planner. "We can see you in three weeks," she says. You think, but that's too late. You think, Jesus, I'm killing my baby. You're crying because you're killing your baby even though you can't kill your baby because they won't give you an appointment.

You and Nicholas are making wedding plans, scouting locations and sketching out a guest list. You want it to be a beautiful day. You think about how you will wear your hair, and what an adorable couple you will make in the photographs. You spend hours looking at photographs of dresses without knowing if you should go for the slim fit or the empire waist.

They find space for one more gynecology clinic appointment after all, on Monday. Before you can discuss options he has to do an ultrasound. You cannot look at the screen. It is too early to tell the sex of the baby, but it is growing appropriately and has a good strong heartbeat. If there are any devastating malformations caused by the glass of wine you didn't know you should have avoided two months ago, the doctor doesn't see them on the ultrasound.

Your options, as you know perfectly well, are these: to go through with the pregnancy and either keep the baby or give it up for adoption, or to end the pregnancy with drugs or with a surgical procedure. And actually, it's too late for the drug option because you are past the seven-week point, a deadline you wish the very first doctor had mentioned. This doctor says he can't tell you which choice is right for you. You realize you were kind of hoping he would.

You're going to need an appointment before the end of the week, just in case you decide that's what you want. You can always cancel it at the last minute. But Lois the scheduler has already gone home for the day. She'll call you tomorrow. Or you can call her, either way. The doctor gives you a stack of papers to take home: a sheaf of information on induced abortion, a sample consent form, a pamphlet on the Pill, four small prescription papers to take to the pharmacy, a carbon paper lab request to take to the lab, and a Post-it with Lois's phone number on it.

You don't want to go to the pharmacy, but Nicholas takes you in the car, just in case, and buys you all four prescriptions. One is an antibiotic to take twice a day for five days starting one day before the procedure so you won't get bacterial infections in your vagina. Another says it is for preventing stomach ulcers, which makes no sense, but you're supposed to take one pill six hours before the procedure, with food, except the other paper says you're not supposed to have any food on the day of the procedure. The third is a muscle relaxant so the doctor will be able to get his abortion tools into your cervix with less difficulty; you are supposed to take one tablet every six hours for 48 hours, but you can't remember when those 48 hours are supposed to start. The last orange bottle is a pain medication to take "as needed." There are twenty pills. You wonder if twenty would be enough to kill you.

Nicholas has stopped talking to the baby and you never started. When you look at your belly and try to find the words they don't come.

Tuesday goes by. Lois doesn't call you, but your hippie aunt does. She says the way to talk to a fetus is to tell the hovering baby "being" that you need to break your agreement with it. She e-mails you an article about psychic abortion. You print it out but stuff it on the bottom of your growing to-do pile. You haven't done any homework in a couple of weeks.

You're proud of your body for being able to do the magical feminine baby-making thing, but you're kind of surprised it would betray you by doing something so important so unexpectedly. Sometimes you feel angry with the baby for its nerve in moving into your body uninvited, but you love it anyway because it's made from you and Nicholas and you both spent all last night in the bookstore looking up possible names for it.

Wednesday a baby hypnotizes you in the hallway. It can't stop staring ac-cusingly.

Wednesday afternoon you call Nicholas about the wedding and you end up talking about whether you should raise the baby after all. You can't imagine having Nicholas's baby and then giving it away. Nicholas says that if he can't have the baby he doesn't want anyone else to have the baby either. You wish you could stay secretly pregnant for like five years so you could finish school and get married and take your vitamins every day and get a job first and still do right by your baby.

You call Lois to get it over with. She asks why the doctor wanted you to make an appointment. This is the first time you say the word abortion out loud to a health care worker. You're tired. You try to modulate your voice to sound sad instead of crisp and efficient. Let's say she reacts with great surprise: "He DID?" and after another moment, "He just told me to close out Friday's clinic." She says, "He already has two scheduled for that day." She hangs up. Guess you're having a baby.

Half an hour later she calls you back. You have an appointment for Friday after all. You've got it and you're not sure you want it. That's how you feel about the baby too. At least you have two more days to decide.

Thursday is a blur. There are still people at school learning about your engagement and you are still getting surprised congratulations.

Friday comes. You take your prescriptions, just in case. In the shower you cry and pray to every deity you can think of for strength and comfort. Nicholas is on his way over to take you to your appointment.

You walk up the stairs to the clinic, diamonds weighing down your hand. You're still not sure what the right choice is.

Let's pretend there is such a thing as a right choice.

At least you know you have a choice.

# Narratives
## of Family Life
## and
## Caregiving
ফ৯

THIS SECTION OPENS with Penny Wolfson's "Space and Absence in Muscular Dystrophy." Wolfson, the mother of a son with Duchenne muscular dystrophy, approaches the issue of caregiving by exploring the impact that a chronically ill child has upon his family, home, and siblings—quite literally the space he physically and emotionally occupies. In her essay, Wolfson is critically aware of the power of narrative writing for a caregiver, of the "voice" that emerges from the relationship of caregiving.

Like Wolfson, both Joan Milano and Maggie Hoffman's narratives deal with the experience of parenting a severely ill child. Milano's diary excerpts describe the ordinary activities of family life as stark contrast to the final days of her adult son's life. Hoffman's tale spans her daughter Molly's brief life as well as her own advocacy for her daughter—from day-to-day advocacy for care to larger, philosophic questions of the meaning of a worthwhile life. Her narrative documents the struggle of a parent advocate to justify—to family, friends, insurance companies, and the medical establishment—the continued provision of care for her severely disabled child.

A number of works in this section discuss the caregiving that adult daughters give to their elderly parents, and the theme of role reversal is a poignant and powerful thread between them. In Gail Rosen's "My Mother Is Cleaning," a mother's household cleaning, once a symbol of the "perfection / of her home / her shrine," disintegrates into a symptom of her growing dementia. Donna Henderson's "Vigils, III" chronicles a dying mother's gradual separation from her family during hospice care. "Oh . . . of course," utters the mother "dismissively" when she is reminded about her interest in her family members. The narratives in this section not only illustrate the ill parent's loss of role, but the guilt, family conflict, and isolation faced by family caregivers of all ages. The young protagonist in Suzanne E. W. Gray's "Blister" cares for her ill grandmother's bedsore, all the while torn between resentment at the role she is forced to play and guilt that she may have caused the injury through neglect.

The narratives in this section echo the suffering experienced by the caregiving witness. As readers, we also stand as witness, expanding the oftentimes invisible concentric circles of connection around those who experience illness.

# Space and Absence in Muscular Dystrophy

PENNY WOLFSON

*Duchenne muscular dystrophy (DMD) is an inherited neuromuscular disorder that annually affects approximately one in 3,500 male newborns worldwide. The disease is caused by a dysfunctional gene that normally encodes for an essential muscle protein called dystrophin. In children with Duchenne—nearly all are boys, since the gene is carried on the X chromosome—an exon deletion or duplication occurs, and as a result none of the protein is manufactured. The mutated gene causes widespread progressive muscle wasting and ultimately, usually by the end of the second decade, death from respiratory or cardiac failure. Although the steroid prednisone is now routinely prescribed to slow muscle degeneration, there is no cure for DMD.*

I have been a writer most of my life—poet, journalist, essayist—and in some ways it is only an accident that my writing has been largely about muscular dystrophy. But I have become a kind of lay expert out of need: almost twenty years ago, my son Ansel, then three, was diagnosed with the Duchenne form of dystrophy. I knew from that day I would document his disease in writing. As I noted in a recent essay, "Voice Lessons":

> I wrote about Ansel immediately, the day after his diagnosis, at the counter of a coffee shop a block away from his special education nursery school. I wrote about him furiously, in a way I never had written about anything. I wrote about him to create art from his small existence, which I was told would be short. I wrote about him because I thought I would drown in the identity of disabled-child's mother, in the endless cycles of doctor's appointments and the ugliness of clinic corridors and the devastating prospect of my child in a wheelchair. I wrote about him because I knew my own life would be limited by this disease, by this increasingly dependent child, and writing was something I could do, at home, where he needed me. I wrote about him to savor his life, to save his life; I wrote about him to save mine.[1]

The idea for this essay grew not out of some internal mental dialogue but from a concrete experience: A woman from a neighboring village has a son with

Duchenne; he is now a teenager. I had met them both years ago, when he was first diagnosed, and had now and then wondered about them. She was calling me now—this was in late February 2004—because her son was having some serious social problems and was, like many other teenagers with Duchenne, very angry. She wondered, could Ansel and I come by and visit? She thought Ansel would be a good role model for her son, perhaps help him get through these difficult years. Ansel agreed, and so we went.

And what really struck me immediately, even before I noted the depression of the mother and the anger of the boy, which were both substantial and real, even before I met the two younger brothers, who seemed swept aside by the centerpiece of this disabled brother, all the mother's focus and worry and frustration being on her boy with Duchenne—what really struck me was the space this boy took up, physically, in this household. It was an attractive, relatively new house, and many renovations had been made to accommodate the boy. Everything related to him and his disability was big: his spacious room, all his own, on the first floor; his wheelchair; the tub with its mechanized chair that swung him in and out; the doorways of the rooms in the house; the space between furniture—itself a sort of absence—the big-screen TV he had in his bedroom so he could play video games. The whole time I was there, an hour or so, all I could think about was the physical centrality of this boy in this family, the way he, through no fault of his own, swallowed up space, time, attention.

Anyway, after we left I pondered this for a long while, and I thought, yeah, *space;* that's what the experience is like: the wheelchair; sometimes the second, backup chair; the scooped-out minivan; the big aisles between the furniture; the charger; the bath chair; the physical therapy balls and weights—don't forget the splints!—and the heavy suitcase ramp we keep in the back of the van. Some families have stair climbers or an elevator. Maybe a Hoyer lift. A respirator at some point. And just—space. The bulkiness of everything. The width of the sneakers that have to accommodate the braces. That damned huge turning radius of the wheelchair.

The space taken up by the chair—and the damage wrought by its relentless power, the way it barrels into everything—was the subject of a passage in my 2003 book *Moonrise: One Family, Genetic Identity, and Muscular Dystrophy,*[2] from a chapter originally entitled "Chaos":

> It is the house itself that finally does me in. "I feel like I live in a slum," I tell my children one day, and they protest, quizzical and hurt.
>
> This is the state of my kitchen: Two cabinet doors have been torn off their hinges. I have placed the doors, white Formica slabs, at the bottom of the stairs, where a

beautiful Navajo rug hangs and where there is a landing that is a repository for junk. Now two rectangular holes display the jumbled contents of our kitchen.

"Open cabinets," Joe says. "That's what you wanted, wasn't it?"

The refrigerator bears several deep horizontal scratches in its pebbly white metal; the bottom of the long, fake-wood handle is awkwardly, dangerously bent because it has been pulled out from its lower screws. A few months ago I spent hours on the phone with GE ordering parts for this handle, which consists of seven interlocking pieces; Joe spent several maddening hours fitting the pieces together.

The short wall that separates the kitchen from the living room—a two-foot-long piece of fiberboard between two open doorways—is gouged and scarred from repeated blows, and now glaringly reveals the metal structural ribs beneath. The electrical plug for the telephone has been yanked out over and over again, and some of its prongs are bent; the outlet plate itself is chipped at every edge.

This is to say nothing about the rest of the downstairs. If the closet door in the hallway is left open—it's the kind with a folding door that runs along a track—Ansel will almost certainly slam into it. The hardwood door of the supposedly handicapped-accessible bathroom has borne so many blows that it is cracked through; a piece of the baseboard heating next to the toilet is dented or pulled off its base almost daily. The antique pine lowboy in the hallway has been sideswiped and now sports a scratch across one door. Both this cabinet and the grand cherry desk we bought for the hallway have each lost a corner—a small chunk of solid wood—to the wheelchair. One day last week Ansel drove past the "entertainment center" in our living room, caught a wheel on the brushed metal knob to the bottom drawer, and embedded it sideways. It wasn't his fault, but I lost my temper with Ansel: "Can't you be more careful?"

Joe tries to fix the damage. On Saturday morning he buys a jumbo-size jar of putty, takes out a knife, and goes to work. He sands, he patches, he tidies, he scrapes, he smoothes. He straightens out the refrigerator handle as well as he can. He takes the rusted piece of baseboard and carries it down to the utility room and pounds out the dents. He realigns the broken closet door. Shaking his head when he examines the hinges on the kitchen cabinets—"I don't think this will work"—he nevertheless fills in the holes and jimmies the hardware. The door hangs a bit askew, leaving an empty space like a knocked-out front tooth, but for the time being it stays in place. We keep our fingers crossed.[3]

Of course this physical taking up of space is in some ways the least important, though most tangible, element of the experience of living with DMD. But it is in many ways symbolic: Mary-Lou Weisman, in her memoir *Intensive Care: A*

*Family Love Story,*[4] talks about her insomnia during a night in which her son Peter, in the late stages of muscular dystrophy, has awakened her to turn him over in bed. She's unable to go back to sleep, exhausted from caring for her child, who at this point cannot bathe, dress, or feed himself, who interrupts her sleep several times a night, and who is approaching the moment of not being able to operate the joystick on his motorized chair. Sitting alone in the living room at 3 A.M., she observes the uninhabited wheelchair in the living room, "plugged into the wall, recharging, sucking up electricity." It's a metaphor for what she feels the disease is doing to her and her household, really, sucking up the limited energy and resources she has to give.

"Chronic illness has a way of taking over family life," Joan Patterson and Ann Garwick note in their excellent article, "The Impact of Chronic Illness on Families: A Family Systems Perspective."

> [These] families face . . . the same kinds of challenges other families face, plus an added set of demands. . . . In our study of medically fragile children living at home, families identified a number of . . . sources of strain and demand: a) financial strains relating to a parent leaving the work force, costs for home modifications and non-reimbursable medical expenses, and worry about losing insurance coverage; b) losses of family privacy, spontaneity in life, time for other family members, and work opportunities; c) problems with service providers and third-party payers and d) personal distress from caregiving strains, worry about the future, and the pressures of constant decision-making.[5]

And when the chronic disease is progressive, they note, as the symptomatic person becomes increasingly less functional, the family is faced with increasing caretaking demands and uncertainty about the degree of dependency, as well as numerous losses and anticipation of early death. All these add up to what the authors call a pileup of demands, which, in eating up family space and time and pleasure, create a state of constant, inescapable stress.

The disease is ever present in the family's midst, Patterson and Garwick go on to say. "It affects them emotionally, cognitively and behaviorally, often changing day-to-day routines, plans for the future, feelings and meanings about the self, others, and even life itself."[6]

Siblings bear many burdens too; sometimes it feels as though every decision, every action, every resource is directed at their disabled brother or sister, and they often feel neglected, perhaps not receiving whatever resources, love, or time that they ought to or deserve to.

I remember my daughter, Diana, who is very close to her older brother, at the age of fifteen walking out of a therapist's office for the first time and saying with a huge sigh of relief, "I didn't have to talk about Ansel at all!" as if she had never had that open space before, just to talk about herself. I remember her resentment even as a very small child when her dad carried Ansel but she had to walk; I remember her annoyance at the way we customized the wheelchair van by removing the favored, center seat; I see her anger when she sometimes has to perform household tasks that Ansel, her older brother, cannot.

It is not just in the present that children feel their disabled or chronically ill siblings taking up their own critical space; it is in the future as well. Many of these brothers and sisters see themselves or are seen by their parents as keepers and caretakers when and if their parents die. Paul Monette, who wrote a beautiful and bitter memoir, mostly about his emerging homosexuality, called *Becoming a Man: Half a Life Story,* had a younger brother named Bobby who had spina bifida. Monette remembers the moment when his parents asked him, Paul, what he planned to do after college:

> "I'm going to write."
>
> A pause, in which you could hear the fizz of the lights on the Christmas tree.
>
> "But that's not a job," my mother finally sputtered. "It's—it's a hobby. Paul, don't you understand? If something happens to us, you'll have to take care of Bobby."[7]

Despite the love he felt for Bobby—he saw his brother as spirited and independent, a kid with his own opinions, unbowed by life in a wheelchair—Monette experienced this pronouncement by his mother "like a prison gate clanking shut." He writes, "I suppose it must have made me angry, the prospect of giving up my own life to take care of his."

Though their caretaking may not extend into an endless future—unlike those of other chronically ill children, boys with Duchenne nearly always die young—the impact of the genetic aspects of the disease, especially for female siblings, can be an even more profound and perhaps incalculable burden. My daughter has for years said she will not bear any children of her own, and I wonder if it is the possibility of being a carrier that makes her afraid. But even without the genetic piece, it is a terrible burden to know you will surely lose your brother at an abnormally young age.

I know that Diana and my younger son, Toby, have a more balanced view of their brother and much more love than many siblings have for their brothers and sisters—and rightfully so, since living with him has many positive aspects—but anger is a big part of DMD, and my other children do resent Ansel's terrible anger. As I note in a 2003 article called "Watching Out for Ansel":

> Both Diana and Toby would say that it isn't the physical disability that's hardest to take: it's the anger that goes along with it. Perhaps because he takes prednisone, known to be a mood destabilizer, or perhaps because of the frustration he feels at not being able to use his body, Ansel sometimes expresses anger on a level that can seem absolutely ballistic. It frightens Toby—he can still remember Ansel throwing the M volume of the encyclopedia at him—and infuriates Diana. This summer we were at a national park visitor's center outside of Albuquerque, and Ansel, hearing from a ranger that the trails at the site weren't wheelchair-accessible, threw a fit, knocking over a display of decorative magnets. Diana, hugely embarrassed, fled, vowing she'd never speak to him again. It blew over, [and] by the end of the hour they were back to their usual bantering relationship, but such conflicts linger.[8]

But let's face it. The irony of all this space grabbing, both physically and mentally, present and future, the irony of the way this disease sucks up everything in its path and pushes aside the needs of all us others in the family, the irony of this, and the paradox of muscular dystrophy, is that the lives of those with DMD in the family are, after all, often filled with loss, the expectation of greater loss, that is to say, the space of future absence.

What will happen when Ansel dies? In *Moonrise,* there is a section where Ansel is absent from the house for a weekend, and this is how it plays out:

> Ansel has been away from the house for almost the entire weekend, attending a model UN at a nearby high school Friday night, all day Saturday, and Sunday morning. We are not used to his being away, and Diana and I feel his absence. The question doesn't seem to be, "Is this what it will be like when he's away at college?" but "Is this what it will be like when he is dead?"
>
> "Ansel is what makes the house happy," says Diana later that week, and I think back to the moment of his birth, when I heard a sound that reminded me of the popping of a champagne cork. Diana and I try to think about what makes Ansel fun. "He's just a very up person," she says, which is odd, because he is also a big complainer, a class-A kvetch. "Puns," I say. "Remember when he wrote that story about the teenage monster who wasn't frightening enough because he didn't have enough 'scaritonin'?"
>
> "Non sequiturs," Diana offers, and it's true. I used to call Ansel the king of non sequiturs. We all might be having a conversation about, say, the fact that the Lobster Roll is the only restaurant worth going to in the Hamptons. The

rest of us might consider the topic exhausted and move rapidly on to another subject. We might be talking about the book I am reading for my graduate psychology class, or about how boring Toby finds second grade. And then maybe half an hour later, sometimes a day later, Ansel will pipe up with, "There *is* that Mexican place in Easthampton," as though there has not been even a tiny break in the conversation. His neuroses are funny, too, I say: For instance, he worries about global warming every time the temperature in winter is above average. Everyone else is enjoying the sun, but Ansel is worried! And he always worries about being worried: "Should I be worried?" He is so much like me, and like my father was, that I can't help laughing at the reflection.[9]

In some ways because of the constant undercurrent of loss, Duchenne muscular dystrophy can't help but be a sad topic. But I want to end not on the negative aspects of space and absence finally, but on Ansel, our joyful presence, a boy who has surpassed every expectation the doctors and his parents had of him, perhaps through luck, perhaps, I hope but doubt, through something we did—maybe the prednisone, maybe the splints—and through his own drive and splendid stubbornness. He—and I hope our family—has turned our losses and his future absence, which of course we all fear terribly, which we can't ever imagine, into a positive and very full life. At twenty-two, he is flourishing. We keep our fingers crossed.

NOTES

1. Penny Wolfson, "Voice Lessons," *Sarah Lawrence Magazine* (Spring 2003): 14.

2. Penny Wolfson, *Moonrise: One Family, Genetic Identity, and Muscular Dystrophy* (New York: St. Martin's, 2003) 243.

3. Wolfson, *Moonrise* 207–8.

4. Mary-Lou Weisman, *Intensive Care: A Family Love Story* (New York: Random House, 1982) 306.

5. Joan Patterson and Ann Garwick, "The Impact of Chronic Illness on Families: A Family Systems Perspective," *Annals of Behavioral Medicine* 16 (1994): 135.

6. Patterson and Garwick 131.

7. Paul Monette, *Becoming a Man: Half a Life Story* (New York: Perennial Classics, 2004) 159.

8. Penny Wolfson, "Watching Out for Ansel," *Good Housekeeping* (Feb. 2003): 196.

9. Wolfson, *Moonrise* 220.

# Remembering Dan:
# Excerpts from My Journal

## Joan Milano

Dan was twenty when he was diagnosed with Ewing's sarcoma. He'd come home from college for Thanksgiving vacation and complained of back pain. Two days later a biopsy showed evidence of a malignancy. Within a week he'd begun a course of treatment, which included surgery, radiation, and aggressive chemotherapy.

The first recurrence was diagnosed three-and-a-half years later, just after Dan submitted applications to medical school. More chemo, more surgery, more radiation, and an autologous bone marrow transplant absorbed six months but gave him another year of remission. Ten days after a second recurrence was diagnosed, Dan married Laura, his college girlfriend and soul mate.

Dan died on the day after Thanksgiving, exactly six years to the day of his original diagnosis. At the time of Dan's first recurrence, I began to jot down thoughts in a small red notebook I carried in my purse. The following are excerpts.

*Three Weeks before Dan's Death: 11/5/97*
I arrive at 4 p.m. Dan is very uncomfortable. He has edema and swelling of his liver and has gained eight pounds since last week. His body looks more distorted every time I see him. The tumor is visible now and protrudes from his lower chest and abdomen. He's taking his meds when I arrive, removing each bottle from the plastic medication box where the entire collection is stored and carefully examining every label. He's been on the phone with Dell ordering the new computer we'd promised as a wedding present.

Laura and I visit. She's excited about her job. They want her to begin next week. It's a bad time for Laura to begin a new job, but it's a good opportunity. She asks to see the clothes I brought for Dan—a choice of sweat pants and underwear in sizes ranging from XL to XXXL; clothes I hated buying, having had to repeat over and over to myself that Dan would be more comfortable in these "loose fitting clothes." Laura reviews all of them, hesitating over the Hanes boxers. "Hmm, sort of dull. How about something a little more sexy," she suggests. Dan says he'll try on one pair each day—that's all he has the strength for.

Dan is waiting for a call from Ramon, the salesman he's been dealing with to finalize the computer order. Impatient, he calls back and gives the order to Richard, as Ramon is unavailable. He decides to opt for two-day Federal Express delivery, a rare indulgence for him. I pick up the hospice folder that's on the table. We begin to talk about the services available while waiting for the fax copy of the order to arrive. Dan wants to make sure he won't be separated from his doctors by hospice. Dr. B. has been coming to the house to visit him, and these visits are important. He wants to remain as independent as possible, and help from family and friends will make him less dependent on hospice. He's trying to get on top of things, so that Laura can work.

"This is a wonderful opportunity for her," he says. The salary is good, and she needs to be able to focus on working without worrying about him. He'll miss not having her at home. She's patient with him. She knows him well and is able to push him in helpful ways. But maybe, if he has enough help in place, he can manage without her. He's hoping he will stabilize, but if not and he dies, he wants to be sure she will have an apartment and an income. He doesn't want her to have to worry about anything—at least not for the next two years. Being without him and grieving will be hard enough. Having this job will help her a lot.

"She needs to feel we're all behind her," he repeats, "and believe she's doing the right thing." As Dan is talking—and I am weeping—the phone keeps ringing and faxed papers from Ramon arrive and fall from the fax machine. Outrageously, this conversation is now intermingled with answering the phone and checking the faxes. Then the machine runs out of paper, and Dan gets up to replace the paper roll. While he is adjusting the paper, it slips and rolls onto the floor. Dan bends over to pick it up. He's obviously in a lot of pain and it is an extraordinary effort for him to manage this. But it's clear he must do it himself. I wait and watch, desperately wanting to bend for him but knowing not to interfere.

The computer order is finalized. I prepare dinner to be eaten later in the evening. Laura returns from her break. Four hours have passed, my shift is over, and I leave.

Once again, I am awestruck by Dan's resilience, focus, and fierce commitment to living. Yesterday the news about his medical condition was devastating. Today he spends his day engrossed in buying a computer and cheering Laura on in her new endeavor. Dan's beautiful, thick, wavy hair has been replaced by stubble. His tall, lean, handsome body is twisted, swollen, and weakened. Trying on one pair of sweatpants or bending to pick up a paper exhausts him. We speak of his future, not as a researcher or the doctor he planned to become, but of his death and how Laura, his bride of barely six months, will grieve for him. Despite the unrelenting progress of his disease he remains Dan; so unquestionably Dan.

Nothing makes sense to me. I want to scream, to laugh, to cry. I am lost. There are no maps or signposts I can follow. But there is Dan, his body decaying, his soul soaring, leading the way. How will I manage without him?

*Recalling a Day One Week before Dan's Death: Written November 19, 1999*
I'd slept next to Dan the night before. I tried not to think about what it meant that my six-foot, married, twenty-six-year-old son asked me to sleep next to him but focused instead on hoping my presence would comfort him. He was having trouble breathing. A hospice nurse had begun staying at night. Though kind, she seemed nervous and was of little help. I spent the night listening to Dan breathing, helpless, fearful of the sounds I heard, terrified by thoughts of what lay ahead. Finally, his breathing became easier, and we both drifted off to sleep.

Dan spent the day preoccupied with regulating his pain medications. He was taking solid doses of Oxycontin and Dilaudid. He fought the sedating effects of the drugs but needed the relief they provided. The medication would overpower him and he would nod off and sleep. Minutes later he'd jolt himself back to consciousness and want to know how long he'd slept. I desperately wanted him to rest, but he was too frightened to allow himself to sleep. The best I could do was to help him cat nap, and we agreed I would let no more than ten minutes pass without arousing him. The medication slurred his speech, and his thoughts were slowed. Nonetheless he kept track of everything he needed to do—when to take which of what seemed like hundreds of medications, how to time eating with taking his meds, and what he could manage to eat. He even called Laura at work just to see how she was doing. He was determined to get the dosage of his pain meds right and was on the phone with anyone who was likely to have something to offer him. I dialed the numbers, he handled the calls. As always, he was in charge.

I can't imagine how I kept going. I looked for ways to occupy myself. I felt better when I was moving. I hoped that hearing me puttering around the apartment might comfort Dan as I remembered being comforted by the sounds of my mother's household routines when I was sick and in bed.

By late afternoon everyone began arriving: Amy from school, Eric from work, Laura from her job, and Andy from his. Laura was struggling. Dan was slipping, and nothing she did or didn't do could stop the process. She needed to get away but also felt guilty. Despite the tension that had grown so thick between us, we stood in the hallway and talked; two despairing women trying to steady a universe spinning out of control.

I remember Dan greeting everyone who came into the apartment. Talking was helping him stay awake and alert, he said. But as he spoke he'd drop off to sleep then rouse himself—over and over. At dinnertime Dan was hungry and we consulted the familiar take-out menus, Dan ordering his usual sushi deluxe and miso soup. He played UNO with us while waiting for dinner to be delivered—and to our surprise, won two games. After dinner Amy remembered the term paper she was writing for school. Dan recalled having written a paper on the same topic, and Eric was able to retrieve it from Dan's old computer. So we sat around, the six of us and the hospice nurse, eating, talking, and reading and discussing Dan's college paper.

We left Dan's apartment around 10 P.M. As we drove home we spoke of the attunement we all felt that night—silence when Dan was silent, speaking when Dan could speak—a kind of dance: a beautiful, glorious, precious dance that never stopped, never left our collective attention, even as the theater in which we danced seemed to burn in flames around us. What some call denial is nothing of the sort but rather the strongest affirmation of life I can imagine: normality and ordinariness against a background of absurdity. On this day two years ago, Dan refused to withdraw from life: his vitality and his commitment to remain connected to the people he loved survived the day. Death would have to wait.

# And Then She Died

MAGGIE HOFFMAN

Limitless potential, that's what a newborn baby is. A poet, astronaut, gymnast, president—a baby can become anything. The concept of "pure possibility" is intoxicating for new parents. So it was difficult for me to comprehend, hours after Molly was born thirteen weeks prematurely, the huge limitations on her future. Molly was blind. Molly had cerebral palsy. Molly had a seizure disorder. Yet she wanted to live as furiously as any baby. I have always thought that Molly's eagerness to live was so intense that she pricked a hole in her sac, causing first a trickle and then a gush of amniotic fluid draining out of me.

Molly's brain hemorrhaged, and I couldn't grasp the severity of her brain injury or the concept that she was so damaged, that much of her body's normal functioning was destroyed. Molly didn't understand either, apparently, because she fought so hard to learn to breathe without a ventilator; spunky kid.

Her tenacity forced me to focus on *her,* not on her problems. I needed to connect with her in a special way, not just as another pair of latex-gloved hands; she had to know I was her mother. So I sang to her. Every day I scrubbed my hands, carefully donned a sterile gown, stood next to her IV-line-crowded body, and sang to her. For hours and hours every day: "You are my sunshine, my only sunshine. You make me happy, when skies are gray. You'll never know dear, how much I love you. Please don't take my sunshine away."

I could swear that she would relax when she heard my voice. I was entranced by the strength in her tiny two-pound body. My God, her determination to live made me proud; she was mine and she knew my voice and she wanted to live. I was in love. When the doctors and nurses in the intensive care nursery called me unrealistic, a parent living in denial, Molly contradicted them by fighting to live each day.

Molly was ill at some point every single day. I figured she could live that way for many years. The first serious threat to her life came at nine months. She couldn't drink and swallow, so I would carefully snake a thin feeding tube down her tiny nose, into her stomach. She vomited after every feeding and could not gain weight. I was exhausted from feeding her every two-and-one-half hours, around the clock. Just as I got the last of her formula into her, she'd start to scream, retch, bring it all back up, and then scream some more. She was in constant pain. It was interminable, this cycle of feeding, throwing up, and screaming. I started screaming too: when was this going to end? After months, Molly was starting to bring up blood. Her doctor scheduled extensive surgery to put the feeding tube directly into her stomach and to close off her esophagus so that she could no longer regurgitate her meals.

My mother suggested, the week before surgery, that maybe Molly had lived the natural course of her life. Maybe medical science was not going to improve Molly's life by prolonging it with artificial technology. Maybe we shouldn't "save" her.

I howled, banishing her arguments. How could I deny Molly a lifesaving procedure and end her life?

Unfortunately, the only change was the entry point of the feeding syringe; now I was "snapping" it onto her stomach tube, but she was still in terrible pain. Months later, after realizing that Molly's stomach still could not absorb nutrients, her doctors surgically inserted an intravenous line near her heart. Molly was saved.

Life evened out once again. Now that Molly was out of pain, her disabilities seemed trivial to me: after all, she would never live independently, and she was blissfully unaware of her deficits. Molly enjoyed her brother and sister, giggling whenever she heard their voices. Each morning, when Molly turned two, she boarded a bus with a nurse and her IV pump, and went to school. There she crooned to music and began to learn rudimentary sign language; she could "ask" for music and signal to be turned over. Molly's skin was soft, her laugh full bodied, and she was my perpetual baby, thrilled to be cuddled and kissed.

When Molly was three, I met my husband Darryl. I lived two separate lives: mother extraordinaire and eager lover. Planning a date was akin to military maneuvers: secure a nurse for Molly, a babysitter for the other kids, and time it between IV bag changes. Six months into my relationship with Darryl, Molly became critically ill and I "disappeared." I couldn't expend any energy on him.

Molly had been very ill, running a fever that her doctors couldn't explain. Blood tests were run repeatedly, but nothing was diagnosed. I was in the bathroom when Molly's nurse burst through the door, holding the phone out to me. "Get her to the emergency room immediately. NOW!" one of her pediatricians ordered. Debbie was not warm and fuzzy, never called me just to "check in," so her words jolted me into action. "She has an infection and could go into shock any minute. Leave your house this instant." An ambulance would have taken too long; I didn't bother with the wheelchair, just strapped her into a car seat and drove to the hospital, too frightened for prayer. Within moments, I was consenting to put her on a ventilator—life support. She was sedated and paralyzed with medication so that she wouldn't fight the ventilator. She lay as if asleep—my mom and I called her Sleeping Beauty.

The nurses let me sleep in her intensive care room—something only allowed if a patient is expected to die. Doctors explained that she had "shocked lungs" and that she had less than a 10 percent chance of survival. As days turned into weeks, her GI (nutrition) doctor pulled me into a conference room. He wanted to explain that Molly's biological father had requested that she be taken off the ventilator. I went wild, insisting that I was the custodial parent. "He left the kids eighteen months ago. He can't make that choice." The next bit of information inflamed me further. The doctor stated that a number of nurses and residents (physicians-in-training) had asked to be taken off her case. They felt precious resources were being wasted on a child with "such a poor quality of life." Molly's doctor was trying to be kind. He wanted to give me a choice as well as explain the cool reception I was receiving from some of the hospital staff.

The conflict was moot; after sixteen days, Molly started to recover and could breathe on her own.

I felt vindicated when, weeks later, I wheeled her into the ICU for a visit, Molly dressed up with ribbons in her hair, laughing and cooing and demanding to be heard.

Darryl demanded to be heard too. He wanted to be legitimate, to be acknowledged as part of my life. I introduced him to all three children. He felt great affection for Jacob and Rosie, but while he admired my devotion to Molly, he found her hard to love. She didn't look at people, as she was blind. She didn't speak; one had to learn her crude signs. She didn't walk or feed herself. Molly was an acquired love, if one put in the time. I couldn't separate myself from her long enough to view her through an outsider's eyes. Molly's teachers and nurses shared the same love, emanating from awe at her very existence and at the fact that she enjoyed her life.

Molly began to experience bouts of pneumonia, easily treated, but the reality of her scarred lungs was apparent—she kept having respiratory problems. She was taking steroids daily to help with her breathing. One unexpected side effect was that the medication lessened the inflammation around her brain—Molly started to talk. Just a few words, "More." "Music." "No." "Mom."

Jim, the senior pediatrician, asked me to come into his office, alone. He told me that Molly had "six to nine months to live." I was stunned. Molly didn't have a specific disease, I reminded Jim. He explained that Molly's body was being supported by medical technology, which had its own consequences. Some of her medications weakened her ability to fight infections, and she was being fed artificially. What this meant, Jim implied, was that she was living past her "natural" life cycle. Jim had an agenda. He wanted me to contemplate the future:

what if Molly developed another serious infection—would I want her placed on a ventilator? "She would not be able to be taken off it again," said Jim.

Her voice. What would her quality of life be without her voice? Molly now communicated largely through her vocalizations: her sounds conveyed desires and feelings. Life without a voice would be too cruel. I agreed to a Do Not Resuscitate (DNR) order; Molly would not be placed on a breathing machine.

When I told Darryl about my decision, he said, "How can you give 90 percent of your time to the child with no future and deny Jacob and Rosie your attention? They need you more." Did they need me more or was he really saying that *he* needed more attention? I wasn't sure.

Darryl and I married, but he was living in Pittsburgh while I stayed on Long Island. Every two or three weekends, I'd fly in to visit him. Molly was having seizures frequently, but in every other way her quality of life was at its best. Her kindergarten teacher tutored her at home. "Molly," she'd say, "turn on the teddy bear's music" and she'd crack up as the bear beat his drum. So when snow was forecast, I left for Pittsburgh anyway, knowing that I had babysitters and nurses all lined up.

And then Molly got sick. And twenty-two inches of snow shut down the airport. And I left Darryl to take an anxiety-filled, all-day train ride, confined and out of control, inching my way back to my baby. I walked from the train station, forcing myself through the hip-high snow banks. Molly had a fever but she responded as I rocked her. I took her to the doctor. Again her blood tests were negative, but her fever started to rise. Another of her constant pediatricians let my mother drive to his home to retrieve liquid Motrin, because the drugstores were all closed by the blizzard. That night I sat, all night, with Molly in the bathtub filled with tepid water, willing her fever down.

The next morning, as I walked from the bathroom back into her room, I saw her, purple and seizing. I knew. I called her doctor and told him, "This is it." I described her condition and asked if I could bring her to the emergency room. He reminded me of my decision and I affirmed it. Carrying Molly, who was limp and barely breathing, I ran into the hospital. I saw a resident coming at us with an ambu bag and mask to assist her breathing in preparation for a breathing tube and a ventilator. "She's DNR," I spit out, haltingly.

"I needed to hear you say that; otherwise, I'd have to place her on the breathing machine," the resident calmly answered.

Her doctor came to the hospital and tried all the possible medications; Molly was under an oxygen tent, but her blood gas readings were as bleak as she looked.

"Now would be the time I would put her on a ventilator," he said. "You may still change your mind."

"Her brain has been without oxygen for so long now; she can't possibly live her life in any meaningful way."

"I can't comment on that," he stated unhelpfully.

I heard myself speaking as if I was discussing some routine academic "case," and yet, my heart was racing and I could not believe that I could speak in such a practiced way about my girl.

"Do I have to take her home to die? Do you need this bed for another child?" I desperately wanted to stay in the hospital, didn't want her to die in front of her brother and sister, didn't want to remember this horror every time I walked into her room.

Once in the ICU, I had to keep repeating the DNR request. The state has very stringent laws, intended to help, but the system is barbaric. The strength necessary to keep repeating "DNR," literally ordering a death sentence, is soul destroying. At first, she seemed to be a bit better. Then her body started to shut down. Her kidneys stopped working. It was happening. My breathing was shallow. Crying raggedly, I lay with her, stroking her beautiful hair, kissing her soft-as-a-baby's skin, my baby's skin. And then she died.

# Vigils, III

DONNA HENDERSON

1.
They call what she's dying of now *multi-system decline.*

We are twelve in the living room, plus two hospice staff.

The room is vibrant with sunlight, anxiety, the delicious
absence of beeping chrome.

Heather's made muffins. Whole grain, with chocolate
chips thrown in: a brilliant, needful touch.

Outside, mowers' reassuring, order-promising drone.

We are wearing our "solidarity badges":
squares of adhesive tape with safety pins stuck through.
The hospice worker, writing, asks about these.

"For the tape and pins that kept her tube attached,"
one of us explains, "Yesterday, when she had it pulled,
we put these on."

"That's *good!*" the hospice worker approves,
writing something down, "We encourage ritual."

2.
"What are your interests?" the worker asked our mother,
filling out her form. And mom has taken this literally,
thinking the worker means not what *were* they,
which were countless (just five months ago!),
but what are they *now*, which are zero.
Well, dying's one.

As mom struggles through something thick & slow
to answer, Bonnie starts pointing dramatically
toward herself, nodding at mom with a goofy
smile of encouragement.

Some of us—getting it—join in.

"What," mom slurs, gradually noticing, "are all of you doing?"
"Us!" Bonnie chirps, "One interest is us, *your family!*"

"Oh . . . of course," mother utters dismissively,
"That goes without saying."

Closing her eyes again, turning away.

3.
*Family uses humor to cope,*
concludes the worker on our *Plan of Care,*
left for our reference after hospice goes.

# My Mother Is Cleaning

GAIL ROSEN

My mother is cleaning.
Ruthlessly eliminating any stain or spill
   or messiness
that interferes with the perfection
   of her home
   her shrine.
Dust would not dare settle.

My mother is cleaning.
A half apron, made by her mother,
   edged with lace.
Pushing the vacuum, canister following
   like the dog I longed for
   but could never have.
Too messy. Too unpredictable.

My mother is cleaning.
Wiping sink, counter, cabinet,
   sink again. Forgetting.
Counter again. Forgetting.
Cabinet, sink,
counter, sink.
Wringing the cloth, hands still strong.

My mother is cleaning.
Bent in half, pointed finger seeking out the crumb
   rudely lying on the tile.
Two steps forward, another crumb,
   two steps forward, another,
   like Hansel and Gretel's trail.
But they do not lead her home.

My mother is cleaning.

# In the Dream

LYN LIFSHIN

My mother says, look,
I'll show you why I
can't go to the party
tonight, takes off
her blouse, back
toward me. I see no-
thing, a dime-sized
bump I never would
have noticed with a
cut across it. My
mother, who never
complained, cooked
venison when the
hurricane blew a
roof off a friend's
house and thirteen
people slept in our
beds the day some
thing was cut out
of her, blood still
dripping. My mother
who could open jars
no one else could,
who never stayed in
bed one day, says
the small circle
hurts. I press her
close, terrified
I'm losing what
I don't know

# *Blister*

SUZANNE E. W. GRAY

The small stone house stands alone beneath the tremendous desert light. The heat has bleached the roof silver, buckled the shingles. When she was young and hale, Midge would join her husband on the roof every spring to replace the shingles torn off by the wind or deformed by the sun. Now they go unmended. Behind the house looms a dirt mountain littered with boulders; across the valley larger mountains scratch the sky. The highway runs next to them. At night, from inside the house, the faraway string of headlights can be seen, and the faint wash of light in the sky, emanating from Barstow.

Elsa wrangled her grandmother's difficult body into the bathtub. The nurse was coming and Elsa was anxious, but even in her haste she stared at the tile to avoid looking at the old woman's body. Elsa didn't want to see her grandmother's skin, mottled and dull, like dirty linoleum. She didn't want to see her bare, hanging arms, her curled feet, her obscene little paunch, the stringy place where her thigh attached to her pelvis.

Elsa wetted her grandmother's scraggly hair and scrunched it full of lather with one hand, steadying her skinny frame with the other. Sometimes she was glad that Grandma couldn't talk, that the disease that had paralyzed her limbs had progressed to her throat. At least Elsa didn't have to make conversation with someone she barely knew. Two months ago, when she had taken over the daytime care of Grandma so that her mother could work—just until school started, her mom had promised—Elsa had talked her way through the day, asking about the spoon collection, the antique sewing machine, the threat of rattlesnakes. But Grandma only sat, looking out at the spiky limbs of the Joshua tree and the valley beyond it, and Elsa soon tired of her own monologue. Now she labored in silence.

Elsa's mother planned to buy a computer that would allow Grandma to type by blinking her eyes, once she had saved enough money. Until then, Elsa and her grandmother communicated through indistinct noises and guesswork. Sometimes Elsa wondered if Grandma was insane. According to the doctors, her mind would remain whole until the disease stopped her from breathing and she died. Elsa thought that insanity was a reasonable response to spending every day immobile, sweating, staring at an endless landscape of sun and dirt.

Elsa soaped the washcloth and scrubbed Grandma's back but hesitated when she came to her rear, bending down to peer at the sullen curve of the blister that had appeared there last week.

"Sucks," Elsa muttered. The blister was big now, two inches across. She dabbed at it. It bulged. Elsa winced, jerked her hand away and gripped the washrag with both hands. The blister was her fault. She was the one who watched Grandma all day, the one who strategized her pillow placement and kept her from sinking in her seat. Elsa's mother had said nothing, but Elsa feared the nurse's expert condemnation. She was a specialist.

Grandma started to tilt forward and Elsa grabbed her before she could collapse. Elsa's cheeks tingled with panic. "Sorry about that," she said, her voice echoing off the tile. She rubbed her face and finished washing Grandma without touching her rear.

Elsa scowled as she thought of the pamphlet her mom had given her, which claimed it was an honor to care for a dying family member. She didn't see how. She hadn't even met her grandmother until she was seven. Elsa remembered Grandma striding through the yard, visoring her eyes with one hand, pointing at the vegetable garden, the windmill, the well. That Grandma was a different person than the one she was washing now. This Grandma was hardly a person at all.

Elsa dried Grandma sloppily and stepped into the wet bathtub to lift her out of her bath seat. She deposited her grandmother, still naked, in her chair, and wheeled her into her bedroom to get dressed.

The nurse was late. Elsa darted about the living room, towing a garbage bag, trying to clean up. The room was littered with soda cans and junk mail and magazines and pill bottles and ponytail holders and sandals and bedclothes. She grabbed the soiled paper plates from last night's dinner and threw them in the bag. Before she had started taking care of her grandmother, she had enjoyed picturing herself as a tender saint dabbing the forehead of a grateful old woman, but a week or two of wading through trash that she never had time to clean had quickly bleached that image.

Grandma lay face down on the couch, ready for inspection. Her calves and feet stuck up at an angle because her knees could not straighten all the way, and the hem of her polyester pants slipped toward her knees, exposing her bony ankles. Elsa had to exercise her daily to make sure that the rest of her joints didn't freeze. Grandma watched Elsa hurry about the room, her mouth open, the side of her face pressed against a needlepoint pillow.

Elsa paused before a cluster of empty glasses on the windowsill, ducking her head to wipe her face with her shirt. Outside, on the rise near the old garden, a cottonwood tree marked the spot where her grandfather was buried. Its dry leaves rattled in the wind. Elsa had watched the neighbors dig the grave, when she was small, standing in the shade of the porch with her mother and grandmother. "Should have put him in Forest Lawn—this just isn't right," her mother grumbled. Grandma leaned on a table laden with food. "Sure it's right, Jan. It's right. Fruit leather, Elsa?" She held out a plate of purplish strips. Elsa had backed away, afraid of the wildness in Grandma's face.

Elsa picked up the dirty glasses and held them against her belly. "Why the heck do you live out here, Grandma? Mom said this is where they dispose of nuclear waste."

From the couch, Grandma made a noise.

"What?"

Grandma made a noise again, louder.

Elsa sighed. The doorbell rang and she quickly returned the dirty glasses to the windowsill. The wind jerked the door wide when Elsa opened it.

"Hi, I'm Yolanda Mierez, the wound-care nurse—I'm here to see Midge?" Curly brown hair blew around the woman's face; a piece caught on her lipstick and she brushed it away.

"Hi," Elsa said. She hoped the nurse didn't notice how messy the house was.

Yolanda bustled past Elsa into the living room, spotted Grandma on the couch, and cocked her head to the side to align their faces. "How we feeling today, Midge?"

Grandma groaned.

"She can't really, like, talk," Elsa said, feeling embarrassed.

"I see. Does she usually lie in this position?"

Elsa grabbed a magazine from the coffee table. "Uh, I thought you would like her that way so you could, you know, examine her." She sat down and opened the magazine in front of her face.

Yolanda spoke to Grandma. "Well, I'm sure you'll be happy to know that I will be doing more than looking at your buttocks today. Would you like to sit up for a while?"

Grandma looked pleased. Elsa hauled Grandma into a seated position, bolstering her listing posture with the couch cushions. "We should be getting one of those special eyeball computers for her soon. Just a few weeks. My mom's really excited about it."

"I'm sure that will be very helpful." Yolanda pulled a stethoscope and blood pressure cuff out of her bag. The house was hot and quiet. "Big breath . . . again . . . again . . ." She pulled the stethoscope around her neck and glanced at Elsa. "Are you still in school?"

"I'll be a senior this fall."

"Congratulations. Barstow High? You like it?"

"I've only been for a couple months. We just moved in April, to take care of Grandma."

Yolanda turned to Grandma. "That's lovely. I'm sure your granddaughter works very hard to keep you comfortable." She snapped a sterile cap onto her electric thermometer and stuck it into Grandma's ear.

Elsa concentrated on the magazine. She wondered what Yolanda would think of her caregiving once she saw the blister. There would be a lecture, of course. She might even call Jan at work and demand that she supervise Elsa more carefully. Then Jan would have to quit working in order to take care of Grandma, and Elsa would be stuck in the house with both of them, all the time. She cringed.

Yolanda wrote something in her folder. "Your mom said that Midge has a blister on her bottom? Midge, do you mind if Elsa lays you down, on your side?"

Elsa bit her lip. She lowered Grandma, rolled her to face the back of the couch, and worked the clothing down to her knees. Elsa stepped back. The blister spread across the lower part of Grandma's left buttock, so that it capped the knob of her seat when she was sitting down. Its surface was pale and taut. The surrounding skin was bright pink and lined with cracks; the pink part consumed most of the left cheek. The rest of Grandma's skin hung loose, minutely wrinkled. Elsa pressed her teeth together and looked away.

Yolanda wriggled her fingers into a pair of gloves, wiped the blister clean, and measured it with a flimsy plastic ruler. "Four centimeters," she said, her face expressionless. She produced a camera. "Now, Midge. I'm going to take a picture of your wound, if you don't mind."

Elsa inhaled sharply. "That bad, huh?"

"Oh, this is just for her records. We need to document our progress." Yolanda wrote something on the ruler, posed it next to the blister, and took a few photos. Then she announced, "Midge, you have a stage two pressure ulcer."

Grandma blinked. "Okay," Elsa said warily. "Okay." She crossed her arms, jamming her thumbs into the creases of her elbows.

Yolanda faced Elsa, raising her penciled eyebrows in encouragement. "You know how when you're sitting still for a long time, you have to change positions or your bottom goes numb? Stay there long enough and your skin will die. Too much pressure, not enough blood. That's why it's important that Midge get help changing positions on a regular basis."

Elsa paced into the kitchen and blindly started piling dirty dishes into the sink. She didn't want Yolanda to see her face.

"But to look at it brightly, the skin is not broken. I'll give you some skin protectant—that'll toughen the surface and make it resistant to water. Pressure and liquid, the two worst things for a wound." Yolanda hoisted her bag to the chair and dug through it. Elsa pressed her thumbs against her eyelids and quickly wiped them on her shirt. My fault, she thought. My fault.

Yolanda called Elsa back to the couch. She handed Elsa two bottles and a gauze pad and explained how to clean the bulging sore, swab it with skin protectant, and tape the bandage to Grandma's skin.

"What happens if it doesn't work?" Elsa asked as she slid her arm underneath Grandma's legs and pulled her pants back on.

"Then the blister will turn into an open sore—stage three, where underlying tissue becomes exposed. Then we will try something else." Yolanda sat in the recliner and talked about wound management. Position the patient for pressure relief. Reapply skin protectant and change the bandage as often as needed. Good nutrition is essential to healing. Elsa could feel the information draining from her head. She tried to look like she understood.

Yolanda stuffed paraphernalia into her bag. "Do you think you can handle showing your mom how to do this? I mean, I assume that she tends to Midge sometimes too? I could come out again, but you'd have to pay for another visit."

"Mom does the evenings. I can show her." Elsa looked out the window.

Yolanda stood up, shouldering her bag. "Now, Elsa, your grandma really needs your help in the next couple of weeks."

"She always does."

"That pressure ulcer is going to get worse. They start from the inside, you know. From the bone. Because of her disease, Midge's tissue tolerance is pretty low. That makes it easy for wounds to worsen, hard for them to heal. Your job isn't easy. She does need your help."

A week after the nurse's visit Elsa was awakened by her grandmother's wheezy cries. Elsa picked her way through the mess in the living room, where she slept, to Grandma's room. The old woman lay on her back, the blanket peaked over her permanently bent knees. A cloying smell saturated the air. Elsa reluctantly pulled back the blanket; the sheets were wet and sour, and Grandma's nightgown was soggy with urine.

"Oh, Grandma," Elsa moaned. She embraced her grandmother, lifting her up to free the wet nightgown from under her bottom. Elsa was careful to turn her head away from Grandma when she did this—once, her moist lips had touched Grandma's neck accidentally and Grandma had squawked in surprise.

Elsa tugged the nightgown over Grandma's head and laid her back down, facing the wall. Grandma didn't usually have problems making it through the night without peeing. Elsa knew that a lot of people with her disease wore diapers, but Elsa's mom had said that Grandma had enough indignities to put up with already. Elsa pulled Grandma's underwear off, easing the fabric under her hip. The bandage stuck in the cloth and slid away with it.

Elsa inhaled sharply. The blister was gone. In its place was a red crater rimmed with white, mushy skin. It was the size of Elsa's palm, gelatinous, littered with gray muck. Elsa groaned in disgust. Beneath the musty sharpness of stale urine lurked the garbage smell of the wound.

Elsa grimaced and turned away. Over the past week she had fastidiously monitored the waterproofness of the skin protectant and changed the bandage when it became crumpled. She had even upped Grandma's exercise schedule, not because of any explicit instruction, but because it seemed like a helpful thing to do. She liked taking care of the blister: it was simple; it came with instructions.

"I can't fucking believe this," Elsa announced.

Grandma whined, and Elsa turned around. Grandma was stuck facing the wall, near-naked, her soiled underwear caught around her thighs, the wound glaring like a stoplight.

"Oh God, Grandma, don't worry. You're going to be fine." Elsa freed Grandma's legs from the underwear and tossed it towards the laundry basket. Then she hunched down at the foot of the bed and cried.

When her eyes were sore and her forearm braided with trails of snot she realized that she didn't know what to do next. She ran into the kitchen to call Yolanda.

Yolanda seemed unconcerned. "That blister cap is around somewhere. It just detached because the urine weakened the skin," she said, her voice echoing weirdly in the cell phone. She offered to come out the next day and have a look. Elsa turned off the phone. She would have to change the sheets. When she did, she would probably find the detached blister skin. She shuddered. She looked out at the bleak valley and tried to figure out how she could leave her grandmother's house, leave the desert behind.

The next day, Yolanda appeared. "Stage three," she proclaimed, when she saw the crater the blister had become. "That means deeper tissues are affected—some fat, some muscle." She calmly taught Elsa how to scrub the dead gray tissue without disturbing the glossy red. Yolanda's reassurance that it was not shoddy caregiving but low blood pressure and poor nutrition that kept the wound from improving did little to reassure Elsa. Elsa had tried to renounce her duties the night before, dramatically. "Come on, Elsa," Jan had said. "The computer will be here next week. It'll make everything easier. Don't be selfish." But Elsa dreaded the computer's arrival. She was afraid of what Grandma might say.

After Yolanda left, Elsa arranged Grandma in her wheelchair. She was fussy—first she wanted her feet propped up, then a pillow behind her back, her hands in her lap, on the armrest, at her side. "What's your problem?" Elsa hissed, guilt springing up as soon as the words exited her mouth. Grandma responded with a gargling moan. Elsa squinted in embarrassment, replaced Grandma's arm carefully on the armrest, got a glass of water and a magazine, and shut herself into her mom's bedroom.

When the computer came, she wouldn't be able to retreat, she thought. She imagined a long list detailing the things she had done wrong in her caregiving. Missed baths. Rough handling. Accidentally spilling milk on Grandma's chest. And the crown: the blister. Grandma must hate her. Elsa flipped magazine pages violently and wondered whether, when the time came to receive the scolding, she would hurl Grandma's spoon collection across the room.

The computer arrived a few days later. Jan and Elsa weren't sure how to install the fiber-optic eyepiece and other paraphernalia, so it sat on the hearth for a week until Jan could call the company's tech support. Once the computer was successfully mounted to the wheelchair, Grandma couldn't operate it. Elsa pointed the eyepiece at her own head to demonstrate, but Grandma just bleated with frustration. Her first typed words were gibberish. Finally, during a visit to Grandma's doctor, a nurse's aide showed them how to adjust the speed of the typing program, and there in the hospital Grandma wrote her first sentence: PDOSF HI HOW ARE SDF YOU. At home she wrote: NGD WANT WHISKY. Jan's hand flew up to her suddenly pale face and she said, "This is the first thing you say to us? Your liver doesn't hardly work! And all the drugs!"

ALREADY DYING, came the reply. So Jan made a face and gave her a sip of Jack Daniels.

Elsa continued to care for Grandma as before. She was hesitant to check the screen for messages, afraid that the next one would be a tirade of rebuke. One day she sat down to give Grandma her hourly ice chips. The screen said, GOT SOMETHING TO SAY.

Elsa slowly lowered the cup of ice chips to her knee and waited for Grandma to type the next sentence.

YOU HATE THE DESERT.

"Uh . . ." Elsa replied. "It's all right. You know, a little hot." She gripped the hem of her shorts.

YOU KNOW WHY IM HERE.

Elsa blinked. "Is that a question? I guess it's a question. We've got to figure out the punctuation on this thing. I'll look in the manual." She tapped the cup of ice against her leg, leaving a wet circle on her skin. "Mom never said."

Grandma wheezed, her eyes glinting as she blinked. WANT TO TELL YOU IF I WRITE WILL YOU READ.

"I'll read it. Of course I'll read it."

GOOD.

Elsa fed Grandma her ice chips, silent and wondering.

Two days later, Grandma instructed Elsa to print the missive she had prepared. Elsa pulled the pages from the printer and read.

MY FAMILY WAS FARMERS IN MINNESOTA SO WAS SVENS WE GOT MAR-RIED RIGHT OUT OF HIGH SCHOOL SVEN WAS IN THE ARMY HE GOT TB AND WAS DISCHARGED BECAUSE OF HIS TB WE HAD TO MOVE TO THE DESERT DRY HOT AIR SUPPOSED TO BE GOOD FOR HIS LUNGS BY THAT TIME ALL THE GOOD LAND NEAR TOWNS HAD BEEN CLAIMED WE LIVED IN A CANVAS TENT FOR ALMOST TWO YEARS WHILE WE BUILT THE HOUSE SVEN WAS AN ADVENTURER HE LIKED IT BUT I DIDNT LIKE IT HERE FOR A LONG TIME.

I HAD JAN IN 1952 WE HADNT PLANNED TO HAVE CHILDREN WE THOUGHT ABOUT MOVING CLOSER TO BARSTOW SO THAT JAN COULD GO TO SCHOOL BUT WE WERE LIVING JUST OFF OF SVENS PENSION FROM THE SERVICE SO WE COULDNT AFFORD TO WE HAD A GOOD GARDEN AND SOME LIVESTOCK BACK THEN SO WE WERE DOING OKAY AS LONG AS WE STAYED HERE I TAUGHT JAN AT HOME UNTIL HIGH SCHOOL.

SHE LEFT RIGHT AFTER GRADUATION RAN OFF WITH THIS NUMBSKULL TODD MOVED TO HEMET SHE GOT PREGNANT WITH YOU AND DUMPED TODD I DON'T KNOW WHY SHE WISED UP.

WE VISITED WHEN YOU WERE LITTLE BUT AFTER SVEN PASSED I WASNT MUCH FOR LONG CAR TRIPS HE LOVED IT OUT HERE SAID IT WAS CLEAN I THOUGHT THATS FUNNY CAUSE ITS ALL DIRT BUT I LIKE IT TOO SO WIDE OPEN TINY FLOWERS IN SPRING HAVE YOU SEEN THEM ID LIKE TO BE BURIED OUT HERE WITH SVEN I KNOW THAT JAN WILL TRY TO PUT ME IN FOREST LAWN YOU SHOULD STOP HER DONT SELL THE LAND.

When Elsa finished reading she stared at the veil of brown grit that coated the windowsill: particles of desert blown in through the screens. Elsa's heart felt like it had been folded into a tiny, creased package. "It's really good, Grandma." She didn't know what else to say. "I'm gonna do the dishes now."

Later, when she checked on Grandma, Elsa found a message on the screen. She stood beside Grandma and bent down to read it.

I HOPE I DIE SOON TIRED OF BEING A BURDEN TO YOU AND JAN I KNOW YOU WONT BE SAD WHEN I DIE DONT BLAME YOU THIS WORK IS TOO MUCH FOR YOU.

"I'm just trying to help." Elsa's hands drifted upwards as if it were a question. She watched the alphabet scroll across the screen, each letter highlighted in turn.

Grandma blinked. YOU DIDNT HAVE A CHOICE SORRY FOR THAT.

Elsa turned her head and squeezed her eyelids together and swallowed. She straightened up and started clearing junk mail and papers off the coffee table. "How's your butt feeling?" she asked. The wound remained; it hadn't healed, but it hadn't worsened either. Elsa returned to the computer.

OKAY IT ITCHES DONT WANT TO DIE WITH A BIG SORE ON MY REAR GLAD YOURE HELPING ME.

Elsa threw the junk mail onto the table. "But I'm not even doing a good job! You got that blister because of me, and it's not even going away!" Tears leapt from her eyes.

Grandma gave a small, high-pitched sigh. IM THE ONE FALLING APART.

Elsa shook her head. "It's okay, Grandma. You're going to be fine." Elsa studied the couch.

NO DYING SOON WISH IT WOULD HURRY UP I KNOW YOU HATE IT HERE.

"Jesus, Grandma, we weren't gonna leave you out here to rot." Elsa looked at her grandmother: her slack torso propped in the chair, her hands balanced carefully on the armrests, overgrown fingernails curving over the edge. The thin skin on her face hanging down, the contours of her skull shining through, her eyes radiant like boulders at sunset. Her hair stringy with sweat and stuck to her jaw. Elsa lifted it, brushed it behind her ear, and pressed the back of her fingers gently against Grandma's cheek.

# Sliver

JENNIE PANCHY

A splinter, invader, roots in my foot,
big as a matchstick, clubbed on one end,
snug in its furious journey.
Toes tipped upward, I can see
it's sunk in the arch, blue as milk
under a chunk of skin. I am on the porch
of the house that keeps my grandmother,
keeping watch over her fragile life, the dangers
that are stairs; afternoon naps that swell,
bruise, and will not wake; lungs flattening
like butterfly wings. She's hidden
from the heat in the corner room, breathing
cool air lumbering from the conditioner's sieve,
working to pull air into her body, thin
as a whisker, pained by the glass
that keeps her from the orange
poppies that she could not plant,
their mouths below her window,
inhaling summer. When I call upstairs
to find where a needle's kept, she opens the door.
*Hot water, salted,* she says, and takes
each stair with delicate purple feet, joints
cracking like twigs, the tube hanging
from her nose like a vein, pooling in coils, disappearing
around the door, its mouth buried in the tank,
blue bullet, that holds her air. We sit
at the kitchen table, my foot cooking in a salty crock
of water; she holds the needle by the eye
and tips its tongue into a match's lit head,
her glottal breath stitching the space
around us. I was prepared to do this

myself, but I see what she's become: the adult
helping the child, shaving off
the indignity of this twist of things; the woman
who laced her skirt pockets with tiny branches
pearled with new berries
broken from the gooseberry bush,
jay feathers, milkweed silk, stones chosen
because they were less beautiful than other stones;
who tied stray pieces of yarn to her buttonholes
because they were lovely and lost;
who carried a boat alone through the meadow
before dawn and paddled into the hours
when we woke and wondered where she'd gone.

# Pure and Predictable

## PATRICIA DUNN

When I think of Egypt I don't think pyramids, mummies, political unrest, the Nile. That exotic place that the goddesses descended from. I think mother-in-law. Egypt for me is Safi.

"My name means pure," she tells me every single time she pours herself a glass of water bottled by the local manufacturing company called Safi. Each time, I nod. If my mother-in-law is anything, she is pure. Pure in her predictability.

I know she will shout, in English, "hypocrite" to the young woman who walks by us wearing the hijab and a form-fitting shirt embossed with glittered red letters, "LIPSTICK." She does. It's guaranteed she will ask, in Arabic, the woman who stands in front of us in the cashier line wearing the full covering, "Do you know your Qur'an! Where does it say you must dress like that?" She does. I know she will complain to the cashier about something she finds wrong with the store, something not like in America where she lived for almost twenty years, the way she always complained in stores in America about things wrong, not like in Egypt. She does. She does.

If there is anything Safi is, it's predicable.

Usually, as I board the plane from New York to Cairo with a stop in between at whatever European country's airline offered the best deal, I am filled with cross-cultural clichéd daughter-in-law dread. Starting with the complimentary orange juice (or water if the deal we had gotten was really cheap) and continuing straight through the preparation for landing, I obsess over what my mother-in-law will find wrong with me. Buckle your seat belts . . . My hair is not cut right for my face . . . Lock your trays . . . My eyeglass frames are too dark for my coloring . . . Put your seats in their upright position . . . And why don't I just wear a little makeup. Then there are the "advices" as she calls them, directives, given in the plural, never in a single shot, on the ways I should better live my life. Translation: How I need to be a better wife. If only I made her son take Q10 and some other such vitamins, her son, perfect until he met me, wouldn't need to take the "evil" chemical stuff for his high blood pressure.

But nothing is predictable.

On New Year's Eve Safi called my husband and me in New York, where we were both watching Dick Clark's countdown and recovering from the flu, and said, "It's positive." She had breast cancer. This I never expected. Even when I had heard a week earlier that she had found a lump in her breast, I never thought it would be cancer.

I know the statistics here in the United States. According to the American Cancer Society, one in eight women will be diagnosed with breast cancer. I've read the World Health Organization statistics: more than 1.2 million people will be diagnosed with breast cancer this year worldwide. But the woman who is found every day at her local social club in Cairo playing tennis and swimming for hours or running for miles around the track while most members sit and talk ("gossip," Safi would say) can't be part of that 1.2 million. The woman who eats organic while others gorge on takeaway from Kentucky Fried Chicken and Pizza King can't be a statistic.

Safi is the healthy one. My father-in-law is the sick one, the one with the weak heart and with sugar, as he calls his diabetes. The one whose hobby, Safi says, is sleeping. The one I expected to one day have to fly urgently to Cairo to see. Not Safi.

Three days into the New Year Safi has a mastectomy, her left breast removed. We fly to Cairo. I don't obsess about what Safi will find wrong with me, but what the doctors will find wrong in her.

Two days of travel, two days after her surgery, we arrive in Cairo. In the taxi on the way to the hospital I try to prepare my four-year-old son. "Grandma Safi just had an operation so she may not be like she usually is." I forget that Ali was only two the last time he saw his grandmother. He has no frame of reference for "usual." He doesn't know his grandmother's modus operandi: combustible energy.

The private hospital reminds me of the two-star rundown hotel in my neighborhood where I grew up in the Bronx. I look into an unoccupied room. A hospital bed that has to be adjusted manually. No remote. Heavy, "Gone with the Wind" red velvet drapes. No blinds. Dusty rugs on the floor. No sterile bare tile. A television with a knob. No clicker.

"They fix things here. They don't throw them away," my husband says as he catches the disdainful look I flash the X-ray viewing machine, in the corner of the room, that looks to be the first of its kind, ever. It's something I imagine from the 1940s, though I have no real idea what the '40s were like here or in New York.

On the elevator up to Safi's room, I almost choke on all of the national and cultural bias I have always professed not to have. "Why didn't we make her have the operation in New York," I would scream to my husband if we were alone.

When we reach Safi's floor a nurse wearing a bright white hijab and even whiter long dress welcomes us to Egypt in English and Arabic. Safi's door is closed. The nurse slowly nudges it open. There's a scream. It's Safi. She's welcoming us to Egypt, her Egypt. My son Ali, with no frame of reference, runs the other way. My husband kisses his mother, who looks more combustible than ever and, as I look at the decorations the hospital staff has put up for her birthday, I realize this time, without saying a word, Safi had shown me wrong. It was good she had her operation here. She calls for my son to come to her. I hear the power in her voice, a power that must have been passed down to her from the goddesses, and I forget that she's just had surgery. I brace myself for what I predict is to come—a litany of my wrongs.

Safi grabs Ali, who's hiding behind her son, and looks at me. "Thank you," she says. "Allah will bless you for this." I'm reminded of how much faith she has.

I walk over to her. I kiss her. I'm grateful that nothing in life is always predictable. Safi means pure, I nod.

# In The Bosom of the Family:
# Reflections on Families and Breast Cancer

## Janet Reibstein

It is a warm, sunny June day, 1959; I am in sixth grade, and in two weeks I will go off to summer camp in New Hampshire for the first time. My mother and I are walking into the boutique that caters to the teeming colony of twelve-to-sixteen-year-old girls bred in Great Neck, the suburb of New York in which we live.

"Now, remember: I'm not happy about this. So one. Only one," my mother warns as we enter the small shop brimming with pants, blouses, dresses, skirts, tennis outfits, bathing suits, pajamas, and underwear, all in sizes seven to fifteen. Along the side, next to the colorful bathing suits pinned to the wall, is a free-standing counter stuffed with boxes stamped with images of girls beaming above their cleavage in demure white bras. I flip through the dividers till I find the one labeled "Lovable."

It's taken weeks to get my mother to agree to this expedition. "Ridiculous," she'd mutter when I'd bring it up. "Next you'll be asking me to buy you Modess when you haven't yet gotten your period." I am possibly the last girl in my class not to wear a bra. I have suffered the indignity of changing for gym in an undershirt; on sleepovers, of hiding in the bathroom while getting into my nightgown; and—much worse—at the boy-girl parties I've started to attend, the absolute mortification of boys running their hands along my back during slow dances and feeling nothing but uninterrupted fabric. I feel certain that this gossip will spread hotly and widely (and it does): Janet doesn't wear a bra! My mother has, till now, turned a deaf ear to my abject pleas for a bra. My position has become desperate: I will enter junior high pursued by whispers. That all my friends, endowed with bosoms or not, have ritually ditched undershirts for bras—even undershirt bras—has left her unmoved. Till today, when, finally, the ritual is mine.

I select a training bra: 28AA. Even I can't see the point of an undershirt bra, the step before the trainer. For I do, by then, have more than primitive breast buds, meriting marginally more than undershirts. A "training" bra is just the thing: I've got tender, extended nipples, with some rounded, soft area forming "commas" underneath. I've been anxiously inspecting my chest for the arrival of something to flesh out the tops and sides, pushing and pulling in a vain search for the emergence of fleshy bits beyond. But it's remained roughly in this same impoverished shape for about eighteen months. They will stay so for a good while longer, but I don't know that yet. I won't get my period till close to my fifteenth birthday, at which point breasts will sprout suddenly as if in one of those time-lapse photography films so typical in 1950's science classes. Soon after that, things having to do with breasts will become complicated, and I will not for a long time realize how pleasing and relatively generous mine have become. But that is getting ahead of my story.

I leave the store with my one bra triumphantly stuffed into a plastic bag. I haven't thought through how I will get through two months away at summer camp with only one bra. I've won this battle, though my mother is less than gracious about it: "Honestly," she is still grumbling, though with a grudging grin—the mom shepherding the (almost) teen daughter through a normal and necessary (if in the mom's view, premature) ritual—as we leave the store, "what next?"

When I was sixteen—only a bit over a year of living with womanly breasts—I watched my young and pretty mother be wheeled from her first breast cancer surgery, the first of her breasts now gone (the second would be cut off eleven years later). Her surgery came scarcely a decade after the first of her two older sisters died of breast cancer in her midthirties, leaving three teenage daughters. Roughly three years later her other sister, in her early fifties but still premenopausal, would die of the same disease. Three were diagnosed, and two died, within a dark age of breast cancer. In this long, dark period, silence, shame, and ignorance prevailed, and diagnosis foreshadowed an almost certain death sentence.

Two months after her surgery I was in my mother's bedroom with her while she threw clothes into two piles: "no longer possible" was one; the other, "can still wear." Into the first went halter necks and low-cut necklines. A third pile began to form: "not sure." Into that went tops that clung, tops that defined the outline of her chest. In time, most of these migrated back to the "can still wear" pile. My mother, like most women of her day when reconstruction was not an option, got used to her prosthesis. Bras come into their own again after mastectomy and prosthesis: like my training bra, the right one under clothes lends a semblance of "normality."

Without a word of explanation, she offered me the reject pile to sift through. I knew what had happened to her: that her breast had been removed; that she had "cancer." Cancer, we all knew, had killed my aunt. Yet I hardly attended, consciously, to my mother's bodily mutilation, nor to the fact that the very symbol of womanhood that had led to her irritability scant years earlier had been summarily removed from her just as mine was blooming. Her survival was my preoccupation, not feminine identity nor bodily integrity.

Breasts were dominant not just in my own emerging identity but also within a breast-fetishizing culture; this was, after all, only two years after Marilyn Monroe's death. Yet our family discourse about the actual loss of my mother's breast (whether during intimate conversations or clinical ones) occurred exclusively in terms of health rather than psychological or gender identity terms: removing her breast signified hope of her survival on the one hand and the portent of her death on the other. Beyond that, "breast cancer" was a closed-off subject and so an unknown experience. Even the sisters, loving and close and eerily all members of this secret, underground society of breast cancer victims, hadn't ready language to share, help, or guide each other. So it was that my mother lay in bed recuperating for a month postsurgery with half her chest gone and without a direct comment passing between us about this particular loss. Indeed, in my family, breasts, per se, were seldom named.

Handing me the "no longer possible" pile, my mother uttered her one observation about her changed body. "You don't feel like a woman," she murmured quietly and finally, the subject now closed. But as she spoke, I became aware of mine—that I had two breasts to her one. Briefly the notion that Whoa! Hey! I wasn't going to lose them too in some way distant future, was I? floated between us. The moment passed. And with it, for the rest of my mother's life, passed any possible easy discussion of our bodies. The summer of my first bra stands in memory as possibly the last time my mother and I had a "normal" and relatively transparent exchange about breasts, however cranky and irritating.

This story represents a single, tiny way breast cancer can starve off normal channels of motherhood. It shows the particular pathos of being a breast cancer mother to a young daughter.

"Is that what I shall be like?" I'd think as a ten-year-old, regarding her through a spray of Arpége as she got ready for a party, as she'd slip on, first, a silky black slip, then over it something either floating or sleek, then zip it swiftly up and over her slim and curving torso. That link vanished with her breast. I imagine her, in turn, wistfully catching a glimpse of the tiny dark pink buds emerging against my scrawny frame as I'd change into my yellow stretchy bathing suit at our neighbourhood pool. I doubt after breast cancer she gazed freely at my body again. A mother-daughter line had been broken—a legacy of breast cancer untold within the medical journals.

One of the ironies surrounding breast cancer is that it strikes women in what for most has been a gratifying center of their gender, their breasts: breasts that have fed their children and attracted and sustained pleasure with their partners. Another is that a woman's disease becomes, perforce, a family one. Increasingly breast cancer is moving down the life cycle, hitting women in their middle adulthood, like me: in my forties, in 1995, when having a preventative bilateral mastectomy, I discovered that I too had cancer, like my mother, my aunts, and one surviving but one-breasted cousin. We are often now women in the prime of family life, steering relationships with partners and children. Our families, like the one in which I grew up, will be cancer families as much as the individual women will be women with cancer. A vulnerable woman means a vulnerable family. By definition, a family is under siege when its wife, mother, or daughter is struck. And this poses a real conundrum: a family, to help the woman who is the primary patient and not become a patient itself, needs to be hardy. But how can it be when its center isn't strong?

But knowledge of any sort is power; and I and my current family, it has to be said, are far more empowered now than I and my then family were when my mother was ill. Knowledge was mostly hidden from me as a sixteen-year-old when my mother was first diagnosed. I knew neither when medical appointments were held nor what was said in them until months and sometimes years afterward. Some of that concealment was willful—my parents protecting me from terror—and some simply medical practice of the day. Doctors—mostly men then—held knowledge and dispersed it according to their own whims, something, though, that could be bent and shaped, in part, through the patient's level of knowledge and power. This meant that the more educated and privileged you were, the more you could prevail upon your doctor to share his knowledge with you, which meant that women on their own hardly had a voice during medical consultations. In the case of my own parents, the fact that they were both well educated and that my father accompanied my mother to consultations meant that they knew more than most.

I, however, was told little—and when told anything it was filtered through my father's language and his judgement of what I ought to know. But even I, being a girl, and so deemed to understand more about breasts and the mysterious female body, and by virtue of being the oldest and already in advanced adolescence, was told much more than my three small brothers.

When I decided to have a prophylactic bilateral mastectomy, I did as much research—some of it with my husband, who accompanied me on key consultations and helped think through key questions—as possible. And, mindful of how shocking, mysterious, and frightening it had been to me and my brothers watching our mother change in shape, in physical robustness, and in personality as she struggled with her supposed death sentence, my husband and I told our two young sons about my decision. And then, because my postsurgical cancer diagnosis meant that I needed both Tamoxifen and further surgery, we told them about my diagnosis and our understanding of what it meant.

That, in comparison to my parents' task, was relatively easy. The threat to my life was so tiny it was easy to allay their fears. It was only coping with their response to the label "cancer" that posed problems, and to the prospect of seeing me be a surgical patient once again. But over the course of surgeries and treatment, my sons have had to witness me as a "sick" mother. During that time it was clear they were shaky. Each pushed the boundaries of his own ways of coping, one more emotional than usual, the other more reserved. If I'd been more ill, with a more frightening prognosis, they, like my brothers and I, would have endured a more delicate time. A mother's disease is a child's as well.

The fact that I have sons also must matter: I only had to deliver to them a verdict on my own health, not on their own potential illness, though in time they will have to become more emotionally aware of the potential each of them has to hand down a genetic predisposition to their daughters—and, in probably a different way, their sons.

Most breast cancers are not legacies that mothers will actually hand to their children, though when you are damaged and weak it is hard to believe that you are not failing your children. You are showing them, you feel, by your own example, how frail fate and life itself can be. And if your child is a girl, you are showing her in grim, exquisite detail how it just *could* be so for her.

Even if I still had my original breasts, I wouldn't be talking freely about them to my sons—one's eighteen and the other twenty-two, and my breasts were removed while one was eleven and the other fifteen. Breast baring wouldn't be in order. I like to think, though, that if they were girls I would: that I'd show them my current prostheses, for example. I'm due for a new reconstructive surgery soon. I'd like to think that if I had daughters I'd be talking, as I have been with my friends, frankly and graphically about what my better-shaped, new breasts will be like. To a limited degree I've done so with my sons. I cannot imagine such a discussion ever taking place back in 1964 or even, again in 1975, between my mother and me.

It is knowledge—of genetics, so that I knew breast cancer could have killed me; of what breast cancer could wring upon me physically; of its emotional impact on me as a woman and what it might do to my family; of the involvement I'd need from my partner; and of what our children would need from us—more than anything that marks how far we've come from my mother's first diagnosis in January 1964. It is knowledge that has passed from me, the mother, to my sons, and me, the spouse, to my partner, helping us to knit together and get through a series of emotional tests. As important as that knowledge, though, is the wisdom that has grown from it, wisdom with a Russian-doll flavor: breast cancer lives inside the breast of a woman who lives, herself, inside the bosom of a family. It is her disease and their disease—and one that they all help, and need help in, defeating.

# Narratives of
# Professional Life
# and Illness

ℰ๑

CORTNEY DAVIS, a nurse-educator and editor of two volumes of writing by nurses, begins this section. In "Becoming Flora" she addresses the role of literature in representing suffering to health care providers. As a representation, such experiences are quite distinct from the embodied experience of illness—when the boundary between the healthy provider's and ill patient's bodies disappears; when providers stop reading about the experiences of the sick other and begin writing about the suffering of the self. "When we caregivers write about our own bodies and illness experiences," Davis writes, "we approach the quest for empathic sensitization—that light of understanding—not from the top down, from theory to experience, but from the bottom up, from experience to understanding." The health care providers in this section who write narratives about their personal illnesses are, as the title of Anne Webster's poem suggests, doppelgängers. They are both "member[s] of the club" who "no[d] / noting symptoms" and patients who suffer both from the symptoms of their illnesses and the dynamics of the health care system. In addition, illness often represents at least a loss of status, if not professional disaster. The fact that the "My Body, My Self" essay is published pseudonymously by medical student C. Sebastian speaks to the potential professional damage caused by illness. She writes that during the diagnosis of her multiple sclerosis, she had been "living a double life—ducking in and out of the Neurological Institute." Even though her narrative describes "outing" her MS to medical classmates, her decision to withhold her name speaks to the professional pressure that health care providers feel to be well and define themselves as other than their patients. Yet Cortney Davis's poem, "It Is August 24th," powerfully illustrates the potential futility of this impetus. After examining a pregnant woman who has endangered her pregnancy because of a cocaine binge, the provider in the poem thinks, "I'm better than her." Yet all it takes is a potentially threatening man following her as she leaves the clinic to remind her that "I am a woman / like any woman— / just skin and hair and that sharp primal cry." Similarly, in Kate Scannell's "Leave of Absence," she writes, "*I am on the other side now.* . . . I had spoken the word 'cancer' many times before to my patients and their loved ones. . . . Hearing my doctor's words capsize my own life, I felt myself being pulled into the collective." Rachel Naomi Remen's essay makes clear that any control felt by physicians over bodies and illness is illusory. As doubtful witness to the repair of her own body's ability to heal, she writes, "This great wound, in the slow, patient way of all natural things, gradually became a hairline scar. And I, a physician, was not in control of this."

# It Is August 24th

CORTNEY DAVIS

and at last I'm leaving the clinic
with its faded paint, its finally empty waiting room.
Good-bye to the women and their screaming children,
good-bye to the pregnant blonde whose water
broke early at twenty-five weeks
after a coke binge she finally confessed to.
I'm leaving that tone in my voice
as I probed her vagina and quoted statistics of loss,
her uterus foul with bacteria. *From what?*
I wanted to ask. *From an all night party, his oily fingers?*

Walking into the sun past "Women's Health,"
past the dried scum on the pavement
where they scuff out their smokes,
tear gum wrappers into a hundred paper swans—
*on my tax money,* I say later to friends, *on my tax money*—
my skin lets go of that blonde, the bloody water
that blasted apart her thighs and filled my shoes
as I opened, carefully, with one hand's fingers,
the bluish lips. I think about her as I pass a man
dressed in a no-color sweatshirt, his eyes
twin blue stones.
He says *Hi,* so low I almost turn.

I'm used to being polite
to every patient who looks into my eyes
as if they were my friend, so I answer
*Hi,* and walk on. There is the soft suck of gum soles
as he falls in behind me, the sound
like sticky amniotic fluid drying on the floor.
After her exam, the woman lay back

and drew up her knees. I'm better than her,
I thought, as I dropped the speculum
into the bucket, peeled off my latex gloves,
hands pale, knuckles without her jail-blue tattoos.
*I know this is hard,* I said,
in that way one woman has
when she turns away from another woman.

Suck, suck, our shadows walk,
light wavering around us like the fringe of flesh
that rings the vagina. What should I do?
Walk faster? Turn to stare? Run
to the alarm box, the security man, wondering
how *he* feels today,
how much better than me as I punch the buzzer
once, twice, over and over?
I see the woman in the clinic
turn toward me, eyeliner like thumbprints
under her eyes. I say *The baby*
*will probably not survive.*
*This is some fucking mess,* she says, my car
on the far side of the ramp, the man
right behind me, both of us knowing
that I am a woman
like any woman—
just skin and hair and that sharp primal cry.

# Becoming Flora:
## When the Illness Narrative Is Our Own

CORTNEY DAVIS

She was the last patient to arrive that August Friday, an urgent add-on at the end of the day. I picked up her chart and flipped through to the nurse's note. The nurse's words oozed condemnation—"Patient twenty-five-weeks pregnant, thinks her water broke a few nights ago but didn't bother to call"—an attitude I was all too ready to pick up and run with. It had been a long busy week in the women's clinic where I work as a nurse-practitioner, and I was tired. Tired of standing, tired of listening, tired of doing exams, tired of the noisy kids in the waiting room, and tired of pleading with those mothers who continued to smoke, drink, do drugs, or jeopardize their pregnancies in other ways.

I took a deep breath and closed my eyes for a second. Then I walked down the hall and knocked on the door of exam room three.

The woman (I'll call her Flora) sat at the end of the exam table, undressed and draped from the waist down—blonde, angular, jittery, nail bitten, and high. I stood over her, fully dressed and crisp in my white lab coat. My smile was automatic and superficial.

"Hello, Flora," I said. "I understand you think your water might have broken. Tell me what happened."

"I *know* my water broke," she said. "I mean it was like a *flood* or something. It was maybe a day or two ago. I don't know, maybe last weekend? I can't re-member."

I moved the rolling stool closer to the table and sat down. Flora's legs were thin and veiny. Her feet were bare, half moons of dirt under the toenails; thick yellow calluses hardened her soles. I remember thinking that those calluses might be an apt metaphor for Flora's life.

"Is the baby moving?" I asked.

"I guess," she said. "Maybe not so much today."

"Are you having contractions?"

Flora shrugged and scratched her nose with her index finger. She had tattoos on her knuckles, the do-it-yourself kind made with a cork, a needle, and some blue ink. One tattoo was a heart with an arrow through it. The other was a heart torn in two, its jagged edges no longer approximated. She caught me staring.

"Oh, these. I did some time in Hanover," she explained, referring to a women's prison a few hours away.

"Broken hearts," I said, feeling a glimmer of empathy. "I guess we've all been there."

"No shit," Flora said, laughing and throwing her head back. I could see her teeth, small and uneven but brilliantly white. She was almost pretty. When I pulled the stirrups out of the exam table and motioned her into position, she apologized for her unshaven legs. I placed the sterile speculum into her vagina and a pool of foul, greenish amniotic fluid spilled down the speculum handle.

"Uh oh," I said, looking over the sheet to see her face. "It seems your water has broken. And I think you've got an infection. What's been going on?" In my mind's eye I pictured her at an all-night party. I conjured her man, his grimy fingers inside her. I began to feel remarkably clean, conveniently forgetting the seamier details of my own past.

After finishing the exam, I pushed back from the table, dropped the speculum into a bucket of disinfectant, and stripped off my gloves. My fingers were moist and wrinkled. My gold wedding band sparkled under the exam light.

"We'll have to get you right up to Labor and Delivery," I said. "It looks like your water's been ruptured for a few days—"

"Good," she interrupted. "I'm way ready to have this baby." After a pause, she added, "The baby'll be okay, right?"

"When your water breaks prematurely because of an infection, and when that infection's had a few days to take hold . . ." I searched for the right words then decided to give it to her straight. "This is serious, Flora. You're barely twenty-five-weeks pregnant. There's a chance the baby might not survive."

Tears welled up in Flora's eyes and streaked down her cheeks in thin single lines. She wiped her face, smudging her thick eyeliner into two black blotches under her eyes.

She looked at me. "I just did a little coke, not much. I mean, we had this party going on last weekend and everything. And then my water started coming out but the baby was moving a lot, so I thought everything was okay. I just came in today because the baby hasn't moved much since last night." She shrugged and smiled as if to say, *You know how it is.*

I placed my hand on her arm, the way I've placed my hand a hundred times on other patients' arms.

"I know how difficult this is," I said. I felt disingenuous, cold. I felt that my body was safe, and hers was in danger; that my body was whole, and hers was broken. I sent Flora upstairs to deliver the baby who, it turned out, would not survive. Finally, when it was almost dusk, I left the clinic.

On my way to the parking garage, I saw, from the corner of my eye, a man lounging against the brick building. As I passed, he scuffed out his smoke and fell into step behind me. We were alone on that side of the hospital. I heard the soft, squishy sound of his footfall, his steps echoing mine. Nervous, I walked faster then started to jog. When he picked up his pace, trailing me. I began to run.

Every time I open an exam room door and see a patient waiting inside—sometimes sitting in a chair, sometimes perched on the exam table—I wonder who she is, how we are different, and, most of all, how we are alike. Because I work in women's health, I have a professional advantage: I too live in a woman's body and so am subject to that body's strange and wonderful whims. Like many of my patients, I've given birth; I've offered my breasts, laden with milk; I've bled too much and too long; I've had lumps in my breast and surgery to remove them; I've felt the sudden sharp pelvic pains, like a knife in the vagina, that men will never experience. Because I am physically like my patients, I can empathize with them and better understand their stories and their symptoms. They believe that I am less likely to judge them. When I walk into a room, patients sometimes say, "Oh good, I was hoping I'd get a woman."

Still, there is always an invisible, ever-shifting boundary between a patient and her caregiver, a boundary constructed and maintained by both for the safety and well-being of both. Our women patients want us to be like them, yet they also want us to be strong when they are weak, healing when they are hurting, kind when they are overwhelmed, and knowledgeable when they are questioning. As caregivers, we want the same things—and more. Secretly, down deep inside, we want that line between the state of being a "patient" and the state of being "well" to be firmly drawn. Patients exist in bodies that are, for whatever reason, no longer cooperating. Caregivers exist in bodies that are functioning smoothly, allowing us to hum along in our daily tasks. Knowing well the wages of illness, we caregivers want to be the ones forever on the outside looking in, peering into patients' ears and eyes and throats, listening to their hearts, palpating their ovaries; we want to be the ones in control, who diagnose and then step back, returning safely home to our normal lives.

But what happens when that boundary, that elusive line, disappears, and we are magically changed, the essence of what is *us* suddenly transformed from the body of a healthy caregiver to the body of a suffering patient? How does being a patient who is also a caregiver, with pockets full of insider information about disease and healing, alter the way we experience our own illnesses, our physical and mental lapses? What if the converse happens and that line between patient and caregiver becomes a barrier, too deep, too thick, too wide to cross, and so instead of acknowledging our similarities, we harden our hearts to our patients' suffering and deny our own? What happens if we caregivers dare to write about our own illness experiences? Would this writing benefit us, our patients, or our readers?

In the 1970s, educators and caregivers (first physicians and later nurses) became intrigued with the idea of using fiction and poetry written about illness as a vehicle to encourage students' empathic connection to real patients. By reading about the experience of disease, by deconstructing plot and character and point of view, health care students might be better able to appreciate a patient's case history as a multilayered narrative, replete with metaphor, symbol, simile, and a main character who experiences the world and responds to sickness in a unique way. Maybe, through reading literature, students could be sensitized to envision patients in what John Updike calls "the light of understanding"—the ability to be empathetic, primed by the "identification, sympathy and pity" that resulted from their immersion in the lives of characters who, through fiction or poetry, became "real" to them.[1] By reading *about* illness experiences, students and even seasoned practitioners might appreciate the ways in which they were more like than unlike their patients.

This idea caught on, and soon literature courses were either offered or mandated in a third of medical education programs in the United States. Poems were being read at grand rounds; interns were asked to read Camus's *The Plague* before beginning their infectious disease rotations; pioneers in the field of literature and medicine penned textbooks about how to use stories and poems in health care education. These pioneers saw different functions for the literary arts. Some championed literature's ability to promote empathy, while others believed that by studying how moral dilemmas were resolved in novels, caregivers might learn the subtleties of ethical decision making in real-life patient-care situations. Today, the study of literature and medicine has become almost a mainstay, if not of actual medical and nursing education programs then certainly in discussions about such programs. After thirty years of mingling the clinical with the literary, theories abound. And in some ways, the question of how illness narratives might benefit caregivers and their patients has come full circle.

In a recent issue of *Literature and Medicine,* editors Maura Spiegel and Rita Charon wrote in their preface, "We are getting down to fundamentals, primary causes, asking again, with the benefit of all we have learned, the big questions: Why do stories matter? How is empathy bound up with narrative? What is a workable, ethical, legitimate, or *bearable* relation to suffering, that of others and our own?"[2]

Indeed, why do stories matter? Can we ever truly witness another's suffering? Does reading literature *about* illness sensitize our response to our patients—not just touch us in the moment of reading but grab us and shake us and change our lives? As a nurse, I have watched, monitored, recorded, discussed, and charted hundreds of bedside scenarios. As a poet, I've written about some of those same encounters, believing that, in the retelling, my interactions with patients and my observations about them might become accessible to readers, both laypersons and professionals, whose hearts and minds might then open more fully to the experiences of those who suffer. But when I or any other writer put our words *about patients* on the page, no matter how talented we are, how accomplished in imagery and metaphor, we can only represent the original event—the patient's reality—from a distance. Students and providers might be encouraged through literature to see their patients in the "light of understanding," and we women caregivers might be physically similar to our female patients, but in the end, we are *not* our patients. I don't know how other caregiver-writers feel, but I know that, for myself, the only events and emotions I can honestly and accurately witness are my own: what it's like when I'm the patient; what it's like to be a caregiver bending over the dying; how my body feels when it's invaded by instruments, illness, or the examining hands of my own physician.

When we caregivers write about our own bodies and illness experiences, we approach the quest for empathic sensitization—that light of understanding—not from the top down, from theory to experience, but from the bottom up, from experience to understanding. By revealing our own illnesses in poems and stories and then sharing our writing, we move from self to other, from the personal to the universal. When we write about our own emotions when confronted with a patient's suffering, or our own reactions to cutting cadavers in anatomy class, or our own feelings of inadequacy in the face of disease, or our own illnesses, something wonderful happens: the barrier between caregiver and patient becomes transparent. When we let our diseases or disabilities become the central narrative, we toss a metaphoric stone into the water. The ripples of our personal revelation spread both out and in, circle by circle, into the world and into our own souls, informing and changing the way we experience the greater, universal enterprise of caregiving and care receiving.

Writing about our own bodies and their failings, however, isn't so easy. We feel much safer, much less exposed, when we keep our hands in our lab coat pockets and our minds on X-ray results and what time the next patient is scheduled to walk through the door. It's less threatening to read or write about our patients' bodies than to write about our own—after all, their bodies are undressed and exposed routinely; ours are uniformly veiled and beyond scrutiny. Writing about ourselves is a two-edged sword. If we reveal our diseased bodies and minds, we fear others might lose faith in us. If we're patients, how can we be strong enough to cure other patients or to work alongside clinical colleagues? Yet if we don't dare name our own illnesses and examine them, we miss the one sure connection we have to witnessing our patients' suffering and to bearing our own. We are most like our patients when we risk speaking of being patients ourselves.

The writers represented in this chapter—doctors, nurses, therapists, and medical students—are women who have accepted this risk. By sharing their stories, they expose themselves, some for the first time, to their patients and coworkers. They admit to weaknesses, to doubts, to keeping secret their own illnesses. Some speak of becoming immune to their patients' suffering and in that admission speak of their own fragility and terror. Others speak of the burden of "knowing" too much about disease, especially when the disease is suddenly their own. All speak of separation and unity—the internal separation of being both patient and professional within one body; of women's body connections to other women even as they struggle, as professionals, to separate themselves from those for whom they care; of the shifting qualities of strength and vulnerability; and of the flimsy barriers between our multiple selves.

In my poem in this chapter, "It Is August 24th," I stand outside my patients' experiences, peering in at her from behind that invisible boundary that separates us—at least at first. I speak of how short the distance is between a nurse and her patient; how quickly we travel that passageway between being "outside" and "inside" illness. Anne Webster, in her poem, "Doppelgänger," also exists on both sides of that line, alternately in the body of the knowledgeable nurse and the body of the short-of-breath patient. As patient, she fears she might die; as nurse, she dials up radiology to listen to her own chest X-ray report. In this poem, Webster splits herself first into two, then into three: nurse, patient, and writer. Fern Cohen examines another aspect of the "doppelgänger" vision in her essay, "The Particulars." A psychoanalyst, she moves into the realm of the subconscious as she reveals her own reaction to a diagnosis of breast cancer. Her illness becomes the stuff of transference and countertransference, and her story weaves between the physicality of illness and the workings of the mind. Forging ahead with her analytic practice in spite of surgery, radiation, and fatigue, she observes her patients observing—or failing to observe—her situation. She relies on her accustomed, low-key responses to physical threat to help her survive. But can a caregiver, when experiencing illness, wall off not the patient but the suffering self? Cohen considers this "mind/body split," turning it over and over like a multifaceted gem.

Angelee Deodhar contributes a haibun, a form best described as poetry, often haiku, interwoven with prose. One important element in haibun is the writer's representation of the passage of time, and indeed Deodhar's poem examines what happened to her during eight hours, the length of one hospital shift. From behind her oxygen mask, the poet recalls that in medical school "they never taught us how to break bad news." Now, both doctor and patient, she writes, "Needing more oxygen / I break the bad news / to myself." Another element often found in haibun is allusion to the writer's travels. Deodhar uses the Himalayas as her trope, mountains impossible to climb, both physically and mentally. This author's images and metaphors allow us, as readers, to *feel* what it's like to be inside her body as she, now fully vulnerable, looks up at her physician with new insight, gained not in medical school but in her experience of being the patient.

In a pseudonymously submitted essay, C. Sebastian, a medical student, has MS, a diagnosis that fractured her life in two. In the hospital, functioning as a medical student, she assumes her professional self; she takes her "regular self," her patient self, to MS support groups. From the caregiver's vantage, she writes, "*Multiple sclerosis was the mechanism though which I would become an outstanding physician,*" but from the patient's point of view, "*Multiple sclerosis was random. It was a mistake, an error, a sham, a trick*" (Sebastian's italics). We often urge our patients to accept or challenge their illnesses, to change their points of view, to fight or to give in. This author suggests that we caregivers must, at some point, merge our professional and patient selves. As she struggles to find the point of integration, the acceptance of palliation, she realizes that her MS "*is a chronic progressive neurodegenerative disease. It is without cure. It is mine*" (Sebastian's italics). Yet her avoidance of identifying herself reminds us that we as caregivers are not allowed to be one with our own illnesses. The dark image of a doppelgänger duality still dominates our professional and personal identities.

And so, even when we are the caregivers, the professionals, the ones with medical and nursing tricks up our sleeves, our bodies can betray us. When they betray us—perhaps most of all when they betray us—we must claim them and celebrate them as *ours*. Even if we think we are somehow different from our patients, when we write about our own illnesses and our own responses to illness, we learn that we are not. In writing about our own illnesses, we caregivers initiate an important conversation: we view the patient and her illness from the converse side of the dialogue. We become open to new beliefs. We change. Which brings me back to that Friday in August, the day I thought my patient, Flora, was in danger, and I was safe.

I had parked my car that morning on the far side of the parking garage. Suddenly terribly afraid of the man who was following me, I began to run. He ran too, his shoes hitting the pavement in time with mine, a twinned *bam bam* that rang sharp and tinny under the garage's huge dome. Although only a few moments had passed, time slowed and I saw Flora's face, how in the clinic she had turned toward me seeking solace, forgiveness, *something* that I did not give her. Considering her as she sat in the exam room, I couldn't imagine myself in her situation. I couldn't imagine my body dirty, invaded, infected. I'd planted myself safely on the caregiver side of that invisible boundary that separated us, and I bricked up the wall so my patient couldn't reach me, and I couldn't reach her.

But running from that man, a man so close I could smell his sweat, I learned how suddenly we can cross that invisible boundary into another body; how we, who give care to others, can, in a split second, become women who need help and caring ourselves. Heart pounding, mouth dry, body vulnerable and trembling, on that August day, I became Flora.

## NOTES

1. "Testing the Limits of What I Know and Feel," *This I Believe*, All Things Considered, read by John Updike, NPR, April 18, 2005 <http://www.thisibelieve.org/>.

2. Maura Spiegel and Rita Charon, eds. and preface, *Literature and Medicine* 23 (2004): vii.

# Doppelgänger

ANNE WEBSTER


I'm here to tell you it's not that easy being
two people at once. The nurse that I am nods,
noting symptoms. Yes, bone marrow suppression,
pneumonia, left ventricular hypertrophy
indicate a poor prognosis. As the patient,
short of breath, head split by bolts of pain,
I push the call button, count minutes until
a frazzled woman with a clipboard rushes in,
only to wait again for the pill, the relief.
The other nurses, the doctors, know I'm
a member of the club. We talk critical
platelet counts, rocketing hypertension.
Alone, I dial the automated report number.
*Webster, Anne: today's chest film shows*
*increased infiltrates of pneumonia.*
Pus boils in needle sticks; my fever spikes.
Is this the fatal infection? I've seen it all
too many times to think I should be spared.
Yet the woman that is me weeps for the man
she would leave, the shining years left, for
grandchildren who will grow up without her,
even as the nurse in me notes vital signs, tallies
figures in the chart, numbers in the red zone.

# The Particulars

### Fern W. Cohen

About eight years ago, I discovered a small lump in my breast that turned out, alas, to be malignant. Fortunately it was contained and since a six-week course of daily radiation was the only further treatment following a lumpectomy, I decided to keep as much as possible to my regular schedule, at least when it came to seeing my psychoanalytic patients. I had been assured by my physicians that there was no reason not to work—although I should definitely expect to feel tired, especially toward the end of treatment.

And that I did, my late-treatment weariness compounded by the low-level exhaustion that had set in when the initial anxiety about the unknown extent of the cancer had turned me into an instant insomniac. Moreover, for the sake of continuity, I had largely maintained my patient schedule throughout the various medical and surgical procedures, a trade-off that I only later realized contributed significantly to my overall depleted state. To keep working was how I tended to handle illness in general, an identification with my father of which I was well aware and that usually stood me in good stead.

Several years earlier, it had been the way I dealt with a torn tendon in my rotator cuff when the necessity of shoulder surgery had come as an unpleasant late-winter surprise. As a tennis player, I wanted the surgery and the ensuing physical therapy out of the way since my surgeon had promised that, if I acted quickly, I could be back on the court by June, albeit my serve lagging behind. That timing was uppermost in my decision-making process (such as it was); scheduling the surgery on short notice, I canceled my Thursday and Friday patients without telling them why and was back at work the following Monday, arm in a sling.* Indeed, once I dealt with the various transference responses, the arduous regime of physical therapy both at the hospital and home did not seem to intrude on my work (although it certainly took over the rest of my life).

On the contrary, the experience reinforced the familiar analytic adage that everything is grist for the mill. One patient was immediately and quietly furious

---

* Since many patients can be profoundly affected by the separation and/or interruption, most analysts try hard to stay with the established schedule and routine; hence it is customary to give as much notice as possible before canceling a regular session or taking a vacation.

at me: she had been in treatment with me for a long time and had developed a sense of closeness and so felt excluded by my not having told her in advance. Our explorations around her fury at being "left out" became pivotal, at least to the extent that she was able to express her hurt and anger openly for the first time. To a fragile and quite paranoid patient who paled when he saw my arm in a sling, I explained the situation immediately, acutely aware of his tenuous equilibrium and the obsessive mechanisms with which he struggled to maintain control. He had been prompted to come into treatment by a fantasy of killing his wife with the camping ax they kept in the back of their car and was still quite terrified of the damage he might do: after an uncharacteristically long pause in the session, I decided to remind him that *he* had not caused the damage to my arm, whereupon he was able to pick up where he had left off. Another patient did not even notice my arm was in a sling until the next day!

Feeling upbeat, I spontaneously described some of these reactions in my peer supervision group and was taken aback by the unexpected counterpoint that ensued; several colleagues were surprised I had not alerted my patients: had I been too orthodox (classical) about not disclosing anything personal, lest the transference be contaminated, as it were? Nevertheless, I was persuaded otherwise, especially by the patient who had become so furious at me, since seeing my arm in a sling had also tapped into her deeper anxieties about losing me. Had I modulated her experience by informing her, her short-term comfort might have been a therapeutic opportunity lost. Thus, in the case of my having breast cancer, I hoped I could manage similarly, although clearly it was life threatening, whereas surgery to the shoulder was not. Being stalwart about medical procedures was quite characteristic of me.

Somewhat in self-defense, I should add that once I started to deal with the practical aspects of having cancer, with the exception of my patient hours, I had cut my schedule to the bone. Ironically, this dovetailed with a limit-setting enterprise that had already grown out of my struggle to differentiate myself from my father, for whom work had been all (he had worked vigorously until three months before he died at eighty-six). Accordingly, I had already created a midday break of several hours (for writing, grandchildren, and so forth), and I hoped it could provide a built-in structure for what lay ahead. If I had no choice about having radiation, I hoped to avoid drastically rearranging my patient hours. Moreover, I already knew that my schedule was about to become lighter: one analysand would be away for two weeks and another was due to give birth. Had that not been the case I might have planned differently, and while I sometimes found myself fantasizing that my patients were unconsciously accommodating me, it seemed to me, when the radiation was scheduled to begin, that everything could fit together without my having to miss too many beats.

It certainly had not felt that way when the diagnosis (in situ ductal carcinoma) was first confirmed, although typically I had not felt particularly alarmed in the six weeks following my discovery of the lump. Over twenty-five years earlier I had discovered a pea-sized lump on the outskirts of my right breast that had turned out to be a benign cyst, and I had been living with it quite happily for years. Admittedly, this new lump on the underside of my left breast felt softer, but riding on prior experience, I felt only mildly concerned; and although my internist offered to see me immediately, I felt calm enough to wait, especially since I had already just scheduled my regular checkup for the first mutually available time in four weeks. Still, a lump is a lump is a lump, and it was notable enough for me to have mentioned it "by the way" to my analyst, similarly to how I had told my husband.

I certainly do not want to give the impression that I thought myself immune to cancer—in the month of waiting I often found myself wondering why, in the heat of such a potentially alarming event, I tended to become a "cool cat." Identification yet again with my father, who for me tends to figure largely in matters of mind over body—with a large mix of denial thrown in. Another component, I later realized, had to do with my not wanting to be like my mother, who had chronically fallen prey to an assortment of maladies, some major but most minor, yet all of which disrupted the flow of her life. It was a dynamic I was vigilant about warding off, and it tended to make me push myself to work when I might have been better served by letting up. Overreactions were anathema to me.

Naturally, one does not choose one's defenses, and it wasn't long after the diagnosis of cancer that I found myself on the other side—confronting full-blown anxiety and gloom. Nevertheless, I must admit a preference for, even a degree of pride in, my initial composure and absence of anxiety, although it can turn out to be the calm before the storm. And in this instance, it did. The downside is that the seeming containment or mind/body split that gets me through the actual experience can catch me off guard afterwards, a kind of cold-sweat backlash. In between, there were even humorous phases, such as the times I found myself humming the Beatles' familiar tune, "I Want to Hold Your Hand." It was an inversion of course—what I wanted was someone to hold mine.

Perhaps I should mention that once I knew that the lump was malignant, I did not throw myself into research but relied instead on knowledgeable people whom I trusted, starting with my internist. Although my actual knowledge of breast cancer was quite limited, I had a general sense of what might be entailed and was immediately thankful that the days of automatic mastectomy were long-since past. No woman in my family had had breast cancer that I knew of, although much more immediate was the fact that my father *had* had breast cancer, with a consequent mastectomy, in his midsixties.

A stunning surprise to us all at that time, no one, including his physicians, seemed to think it had the same implications for me or my sister that my mother's having breast cancer would have held. And while I remember visiting my father in the hospital, it was scarcely discussed, typical of the extreme privacy with which he lived his life. In similar fashion, over twenty years later, when he was diagnosed with a slow-growing, inoperable malignancy from which he eventually died, he told no one about it but my mother, my sister, and me. It wasn't a secret, but given my sense of angry distance created by his dedication to his work, it also added to the sense of disconnect between his breast cancer and mine. Admittedly, at odd moments I did find myself wondering whether mine was on the same side as his, but neither my sister nor I were sure; at even odder moments, I thought it might be carrying identification with him a bit far. If I *was* going to resemble him, I wanted to emulate what I admired: to continue to work.

Naturally, one confronts mortality in one's own way, but for me, following the implosion of anxious gloom that set in when I learned that I had breast cancer, the critical watershed was the discovery that my lymph nodes were not involved. Despite the bad-news/good-news phrase with which my physicians all reassured, "It's malignant but small. You discovered it early, and you can be cured," the tortured waiting to learn the outcome of each of the various tests became a purgatory with little shelter from the black cloud that had settled around and within me. But as I progressed to congratulations that the lymph nodes had not been involved, treatment began to seem a necessary chore that I could fit into my life. Until then, my anxiety had spiked frequently with images of my family scattering my ashes in the country on my favorite meadow nestled within stone fences and rolling hills. While I did not plan my funeral, I did wonder who would attend and who might have been affected by my presence in their life.

Closer to home, as my husband and I began to contemplate the gravity of our situation, my having cancer seemed to intensify our closeness. With age, an increased sense of mortality had already crept into our lives, mostly in the form of banter about the aches and complaints that came with trying to cover the tennis court well. Now it hovered in a much more actual way. For me, it was localized in an unbearable anticipation of separation from him, from our children, and from our (then) only grandson, with whom I was totally smitten. While I realized the experience of loss would be theirs, I hated the thought of missing out, another constant of my emotional life.

In those abysmal early days, I noticed it was easier to wonder how my illness or dying might affect my patients, with whom, relatively speaking, I was less involved. Work had always been vital to my sense of self, but at least I was separated by the boundaries of the therapeutic frame, and if telltale chemotherapy were not entailed, my patients would not need to know. On the simplest level (I told myself)

I did not want to burden them. But really, as I contemplated the more extreme alternatives in the sleepless early morning hours of heightened vulnerability and fear, sorting the intersection of my patients' reactions from mine seemed daunting beyond anything I could handle. And although I did try to reassure myself that I could and would cope with the varied range of reactions the news of my having cancer would evoke, I realized when I was most bleakly honest that I was afraid my patients might abandon me out of fear or dread of loss.

But while I was spared that awful task, I was left with other quandaries, including whether or whom to tell. There was no question about our children, although my husband and I had agreed·during the tortured wait for the results of the needle aspiration that we would hold off until we knew more specifically what I faced. Thus, by the time I did tell them, I was able to be relatively positive rather than overwhelm them with the distressing uncertainty we had just gone through. And although I continued to have fantasies of the cancer going amok in my body, being able to talk about the limited nature of what it was that I would have to deal with was a lot easier, given the alternatives of which we were all too aware.

For instance, once I learned that the lymph nodes were negative, I began to feel sanguine about my progress, and as I headed toward the radiation, I began to worry primarily about the invasion of six weeks of daily treatments on my life, if only (I rationalized) on my time. Some of this was reality based, but much more was a displacement of my anger that included a number of meltdowns along the way. Nevertheless, once the treatments were underway, their set course helped mute my anxiety about dying at the same time that preparing for them allowed me to be distracted by logistical dilemmas that loomed disproportionately large, including another round of whether, and if so, whom else to tell.

Indeed, that question precipitated a rare argument between my husband and me, prompted by his remark that he wasn't even sure he would tell me if the roles were reversed. Because he is an extremely private person and a tease, I couldn't tell whether he meant it, but lacking all humor in the heat of those early days, I became furious at the thought of his excluding me—a seeming betrayal compounded by my awareness of how much I needed him. (And ever competitive, I hated the indignity of his not needing me in the same way that I needed him.)*

Although openness about cancer has become a prevailing cultural norm, my first reaction was to keep it completely private professionally since I did not want my patients to find out: as a therapist, I did not feel it was appropriate for my reality to intrude on their experience, putting me instead of them at the center

---

* Not hypothetical at all! Several years later, I discovered that my husband had been diagnosed with a form of cancer for which no treatment was yet required, and since he was asymptomatic, he decided not to tell me so as not to worry me.

of their concerns. Then too, and perhaps not so unrealistically, I worried about their abandoning me, just as I worried about the impact on future referrals should my colleagues learn of my cancer: I knew only too well how small the psychoanalytic community could be and how readily the word might get out.

Beyond that, I was also reluctant to tell friends. Although I am ordinarily fairly open about most things, I knew the knowledge would precipitate concern and I hated the prospect (always had) of having to deal with their solicitous phone calls. On the other hand, if I did let people in, clearly they would be entitled to ask. Thus while my ideal would have been to keep the knowledge of my having breast cancer solely within my family, I found myself changing ground rules frequently, and it soon became clear that any consistent formula would be hard to enforce. (Oh, how I longed to maintain my father's abstinent ideal.)

Every decision seemed to embody some conflict or ambivalence. For instance, should I tell the members of my long-term peer supervision group or my more recently formed Freud reading group? We were all both colleagues and friends. If I was able to talk about my worst mistakes and blunders with a high degree of comfort, how could I exclude them from something that was so central to me and consequently undermine their trust? I rarely missed either group's meetings, except to have the lumpectomy, for which I had offered a dental excuse; and although I could concoct a story, I was terrible at it, in contrast to my husband, who had a remarkable capacity to pull people convincingly into a tall tale and keep them there, a capacity I definitely envied when it came to the business of whether or not to tell.

Other wrinkles ranged from the mildly perplexing to the grandiose. For instance, two close women friends were in treatment with senior colleagues, and I did not want these senior colleagues to know; while I knew that confidentiality would provide some protection, could I ask my friends not to bring up whatever my having breast cancer would stir up for them? Surely, if the roles had been reversed, I would have wanted to bring up the subject with my own analyst. To make matters worse, I began to obsess about telling my analyst's wife. She too was an analyst and someone with whom I had worked on various projects; we were friendly enough, if guarded, given the awkwardness of my being in treatment with her husband. While I believed they maintained the boundaries of privacy regarding me, I didn't want him to be burdened with having to keep a secret from her, especially one that she might inadvertently hear about. Moreover, while I had mostly managed, as his analysand, to keep my competitive feelings with her on hold, it began to seem that I wanted them both, in loco parentis, to be concerned about me. So was I obsessing for his sake or for mine? Similarly, I wanted to tell a former supervisor why I would not be attending the study group we had just organized. Should I then allow him to share the news with his wife, an analyst whom I knew less well? It seemed that my having breast cancer continued to produce tremors long after the actual seismic event.

Ultimately, practicality won out as I relinquished my abstinent ideal in favor of a case-by-case approach, starting with a close friend and colleague at a conference one morning when we hugged hello and she asked how I was. Her shock when I told her prompted her stunned response that she had always thought of me as "invulnerable," but she quickly regrouped and sprang to action by encouraging me to contact another analyst friend who had just finished treatment for breast cancer and was up on the latest research. Continuing in an anecdotal vein, she mentioned that her friend's analyst had responded most humanly with "oh shit" when he first heard her news, and then she went on to ask how my analyst had been. "Just great," I said, plummeting into comparison mode, aware of the unmistakable stirrings of envy because *my* analyst had not lost his cool enough to swear on my behalf. It seemed that even my having cancer didn't guarantee immunity from rivalry or envy, though it definitely increased my tendency to compete. Of course, my analyst had been comforting and responsive throughout—but in his own style, including his inimitable brand of humor that at some point entailed his making a bet with me about the outcome of one of my tests, which he lost—and which I loved. In truth, my having cancer seemed to make me vulnerable to wanting comfort in any form or shape.

# Eight Hours*

## ANGELEE DEODHAR

At medical school, they never taught us how to break bad news. Comfort the patient, stay calm, do not fear, pain is only in the mind, or in that phantom limb. You're better says the physician, and with a Dracula smile orders more tests—blood samples, X-rays, echoes, referrals. If better, why all these investigations? You tire easily, so you must take more oxygen, at least eight hours a day. Tied to the oxygen cylinder, an umbilical cord to survival dream, of snow in the mountains and the ski slopes where we christied. Snowbound inside the white expanse of quilt, my knees tenting it into mountains over which only my fingers climb, play chess against myself remembering Cecil Day Lewis's quote:

Those Himalayas of the mind are not so easily possessed.
There's many a precipice and storm between you and your Everest.

Even the cicadas are silent, the hiss of the oxygen, the ticking clock, his gentle snore, the cocker whimpering in her dreams—moon glow intrudes. Earlier in the evening we'd watched a comet. With its flamboyant tail it whisked across the sky leaving other stars staring. In my mask, I am that comet, that space traveler racing past galaxies to keep a tryst with eternity.

needing more oxygen
I break the bad news
to myself

* A haibun: A combination of brief prose and embedded haiku, usually recording a scene or special moment.

# My Body, My Self

## C. Sebastian

In June, somewhere on the Iberian peninsula, the sensation began. Strange. Like nothing I had felt before. On neck flexion, a peculiar electrical surge ran down my lower back and into my legs and arms to my feet and hands.

*Disease devoured me. It swept in on silent, sour wings, and sniffed me out. The naive and hopeful scent of the healthy me wafted through the air and was too much to resist. Swells of sunscreen and sweat and laughter drifted up from striped canopies, rocky shores, and Botticelli's* Birth of Venus. *No one could see the bloodthirsty beast that robbed me day by day of my carefree life. For years, disease had waged its private war against me, attacking my most valuable parts, those to be protected at all costs, and I was (blissfully) oblivious.*

I would later learn to name this sensation; it was not unique to me, or my body. Others had felt it, and a French neurologist had lent his name to the phenomenon: Lhermitte's sign. After traipsing through nine countries in ten weeks with a backpack and a Eurail pass, I returned to New York to begin my second year of medical school. I promptly made an appointment with an orthopedic surgeon, thinking I had pulled something in my back and should have it checked out. This electrical feeling wasn't going away—in fact, it was becoming stronger and more persistent. After a perfunctory exam, the orthopedic surgeon declared me free of any orthopedic problems and directed me to see a neurologist. A neurologist? Why in the world should I see a neurologist? What could possibly be the problem? A laundry list of unsavory diagnoses spilled out of the doctor, including Lyme disease, lupus, and others, followed by, "But I think it's nothing. Just go see a neurologist."

*Disease poisoned me from the inside. One day, it pierced through my thin skin and I became it; it was all that was left of me. It could no longer be ignored. That day, I clutched a yellow and pink slip in a sweaty palm as I left the neurologist's office for the first of many times. Sunlight dazzled; wind threatened to topple that me who walked out onto the street that day, September 18. Unsteady, unsure, afraid. The slip read, "Mechanical irritation of cord, disc? demyelinating disease. MRI brain and c-spine, lumbar puncture."*

An MRI, an LP, an SSEP, a hospital stay, many neurological exams, and more than a few sleepless nights later, I received my diagnosis. Like the new convertible on a game show, my key turned in the ignition and disease roared to life. I carry a diagnosis of multiple sclerosis. I was in the middle of the first exacerbation of a chronic progressive neurodegenerative disease, the course of which is unknown, the only certainty being that I will live with it for the rest of my life.

*First, multiple sclerosis was the punishment for a crime I hadn't committed. What had I done to deserve this?*

Having never been a person particularly invested in hidden meanings behind daily events, I was nonetheless impressed that my diagnosis with an autoimmune disease came midway through our immunology block, and that I walked straight from my neurologist's office, where I learned my diagnosis, to our clinical-practice lecture on breaking bad news.

For a month I had been living a double life—ducking in and out of the Neurological Institute, avoiding questions about why I had stopped going out socially, why I was missing class, or how I fell down and skinned my knee. Even benign interactions with friends and acquaintances seemed disingenuous. It was the only thing I could think about and the one thing I couldn't say. One day, out of a combination of being utterly exhausted with dishonesty and intrigued by the coincidence of it all, I shared my diagnosis with a small group of classmates. This, the "outing" of my MS, was therapeutic for me at the time and spoke also of the safe environment of our group. People were supportive and confidential and I felt proud of them, of myself, of us. Maybe things would be okay. I was more comfortable after telling that group of people, more able to face the reality of my disease and its implications.

*Then, multiple sclerosis was the punishment for a crime of which I was entirely guilty. I perseverated on this karmic calculus, trying to pinpoint where I had gone so wrong, but found no satisfactory answers.*

There were days when I wanted to tell everyone I saw about my MS, and other days when I wished that no one knew. Sometimes, when I told a friend or family member about my disease, I felt like I was physically hurting them, as though I was doing this to them. I would watch as their faces fell, their eyes filled up with tears, and then it was my turn to act strong and console them, tell them I was going to be fine. I would be self-effacing or make a joke and they would say I was really something. I knew that it was only because of their care and concern for me that they were hurting, but it was still devastating. My situation, my condition, written on the faces and voices of my loved ones, was ghastly. I could hardly bring myself to watch, to bear witness to my own experience.

*Disease devoured me, consumed me, left me clinging to the threads an identity that I thought could not be rent. But I was one of the lucky ones. Like Geppetto from the mouth of the whale, I emerged a reconstituted me, a different me but still the same, with a taste for little things I thought were lost and instead remained, fearing the (un)known, mourning the only things I had lost for certain—my naïveté and my health.*

In the weeks following my diagnosis, I had wondered about other people with MS. Every blessed person who sought to console me spoke of their neighbor's hairdresser or their sweet little aunt who had MS and "really did well for a while; of course . . . you know, she can't really walk now . . . but she did keep on with her knitting, which she really enjoys," or some such meandering description of the declining condition of the mysterious disease of multiple sclerosis. But I still hadn't spoken with a single person who, like me, actually had MS. Call it denial if you will, but it was more a dearth of opportunity. We don't wear armbands or have a secret handshake. There is no demyelination salute or autoimmune swagger. I scanned for foot drop on the sidewalk, nystagmus on the train, and intention tremor in the produce department, but my detective efforts bore no fruit.

So my MS debut was important. I sat and listened to the panelist, absorbing the scene in the downtown hotel meeting room at an event hosted by the National MS Society. Scooters zipped and canes clunked and I felt alone in the crowd again. Two friends had accompanied me and I wondered strangely, obsessively, if people thought that they had MS and not me. The moderator was a prototype for the MS Barbie—blonde and bouncy, cheerleader-prom queen-marathon runner—"Isn't it a great time to have MS, ladies!?!" she effervesced as new therapeutic options were discussed by the physician panelists. The back of the room rumbled and so did my gut. (No—this is NOT a good time to have MS. It is a miserable time, thank you very much.) I asked a question about professional disclosure, damned the quaking of my voice, and retreated to the coffee, fruit, and conversation waiting in the back of the room.

I found, or rather was found by, a couple of the reactive rumblers lurking in the back and making snide remarks. They came at me with an index card that read "Professional Women's MS Support Group" with dates and times. One said, "We want you. The only rules of the group are that you have to be relapsing-remitting and be on therapy. No whiney people who are afraid of needles, no cheerleaders. We are a bunch of women with MS and we are pretty pissed off about it. You have to have kind of a bad attitude, and we think you would fit right in."

I never so appreciated the merits of my bad attitude.

The women in my group taught me, more than any book or pamphlet or physician, about life with MS. Strong personalities and fierce ideas about treatment options and survival strategies are traded like marbles on the schoolyard, and meetings are always intense. I feel cared for and connected and no longer alone. For all the love and support my friends and family have given me, I am most sustained by my every-other-Wednesday sojourn to the east side where I visit my community. We are businesswomen, bankers, attorneys, and journalists; we design gardens and program computers. We are medical students. We are a bunch of women with MS and we are pretty pissed off about it.

In physical diagnosis class, Dr. A. introduced the video on giving a pelvic exam by saying that it was the last time the ten-year-old film would be used. Made while she was a second-year medical student, the woman who produced the film had been diagnosed with multiple sclerosis shortly thereafter and had died this year of complications from the disease. *What!?!* Until that day, I had not considered that MS might dramatically shorten my life. I was constantly reshaping my ideas of what this disease could be.

*I struggled for hours and days and weeks over why this was happening to me. Causality was less appealing as the days brought thousands of new ideas for the source of my diagnosis. Multiple sclerosis was the mechanism through which I would become an outstanding physician. Multiple sclerosis was random. It was a mistake, an error, a sham, a trick. Pain and disability and urgent survival instincts to maintain my way of life came and inked out desire for reason or causality, and for now multiple sclerosis just is. It is a chronic progressive neurodegenerative disease. It is without cure. It is mine.*

Intellectually and emotionally, I was making solid strides. Unfortunately, my body was not. Vision through my right eye was declining and prompted a visit to my doctor. When I was admitted to the hospital directly from my neurologist's office, I didn't really know what to do with myself. Though I had considered being admitted for steroid treatment as a possibility, I still somehow believed that it wouldn't happen to me. My neurologist kept me off-service so I wouldn't be followed by other medical students or residents, and my friends kept a veritable vigil so that I wouldn't be alone.

The first morning in the hospital I woke up with a strange sensation in my hands and feet. By the time I was discharged, the sensation had spread to my lower back and abdomen. For months, the sensation persisted. It was as though someone had covered every surface with a layer of invisible sandpaper, or as though every object, even my own body, were burning me deeply on contact. This prickly, searing sensation also has a name: dysesthesia. It is not entirely uncommon in MS and would most likely go away as the flare subsided. Like everything else in MS, however, there are no guarantees, and cases have been documented in which dysesthesias have persisted over years.

*I'm worried about my body. I'm afraid my body has fallen in with the wrong crowd. My body slinks in after curfew and smells of cigarettes and wine coolers and the groping of inexperienced fingers. My body tells of traffic and a flat tire on the expressway, but I know the words are spun with forked tongue. Lies. Stuff and nonsense.*

This sensation, and the stiffness in the joints of my fingers, was nothing less than excruciating. The dysesthesia eliminated physical intimacy for me. Touch, except on rigidly circumscribed areas—face, arms, shoulders, legs—was unbearable. I endeavored to relearn what objects felt like because my previous understanding of touch was no longer valid. The dysesthesia effectively robbed me of any enjoyment I previously found in physical interaction with the environment. Simple tasks that I used to take pleasure in, like a hot shower or folding crisp, clean laundry still warm from the dryer—all these things I viewed anew, as challenges to be overcome. Can I make myself fold this sheet? Can I type this whole sentence without stopping? When I am introduced to someone, can I shake hands without wincing? Intellectually, I knew these things were not really "hurting" me, but what is pain? I am often asked if I am in pain and I say no, not really. I experience pain but it is phantom, like the embittered stabbings of an amputee's limb—the misleading, ill-advised firings of renegade neurons.

*My body is an unreliable source of information about the world. Innocent-looking sidewalks send waves of scintillating electricity up my legs. The finest cashmere is sandpaper to my skin. This is no decade-late teenage rebellion. It's a bona fide condition. My body is a pathological liar and I want to stop listening.*

Manipulating my previously nonthreatening environment was a test of willpower; some daily tasks were rendered all but impossible. Writing, a staple of student life, was extremely difficult due to muscle stiffness and the focal pressure it placed on my hands. My script was childlike, labored, humiliating. The tasks of physical diagnosis—palpation, percussion, and the like—are not well served by a lack of normal feeling in one's hands. My position as a medical student was in jeopardy and this reality was sobering. It flew in the face of logic that I could have made it this far only to have my career snatched right out of my traitorous hands. I was not resigned to this at all. Rather, I believed that one of the medications would start to work, and that soon my exacerbation would subside. I was hopeful.

*I put my body on restriction, grounding my body the fraud and its accomplices, the nerves. I dope up my body and tell it, behave! Now my body is quiet; if it says anything at all it is nasty. I know my body is simmering, angry over the punishment of sedation. But my vengeance is relentless.*

Palliation is a strange idea for a twenty-three-year-old medical student. That I may require medication for the rest of my life to make touch bearable is an idea I have worked myself around for the last several months. This was not without struggle, and even now I taste anger, metallic and foreign, under my tongue when I think of my many trips to the pharmacy, my copays, and most of all the side effects—drowsiness, confusion, photophobia, memory deficits that come off as thoughtlessness. I juggle different doses of various meds like prizes on "Let's Make a Deal"—bargaining, gambling, taking risks one moment and playing it safe the next. There are no guarantees, only probabilities.

The medication that I inject daily to actually treat my disease process is somehow infinitely more palatable. Preparing and administering a 1.1 cc injection of my anti-MS elixir of choice is oddly empowering, perhaps more so than swallowing a pill. The idea that a good cure should hurt a little persists.

When I began writing this account, I was thinking of my illness as the defining event of my medical education, or at least of this, my second year. I don't doubt this is true. There have been fabulous doctors and rotten ones, many examples from which to choose models for my own career. There have been myriad perspectives: cranky residents and kind nurses and medical fellows who just want to go home. But as a patient, I urge every doctor to try to place him or herself in the patient's shoes. Don't stand by the foot of the bed and tower over your patient—she feels small already—take a minute, sit down, listen. Particularly as a patient coping with the murky realm of neuropathic pain, I offer to the medical reader this small piece of advice embedded in a very personal and meandering tale: try to understand. Realize that you will never understand. Try anyway.

*MS slammed me back into the body I always thought I could rise above. Although initially I felt distanced from my alien-invaded body, I have become decidedly located within this erratic, unpredictable form, particularly now as my life has begun to "normalize" after my diagnosis. I can't check my MS at the door with my coat; no babysitter will watch my disease so I can have a night on the town. Though right now I have no visible disability, my myriad sensory deficits remind me constantly of my deficiencies and my traitorous body.*

As for my voice, I have not found it missing. I have tried on different ways of presenting, describing, revealing my MS. Like pairs of shoes, some are more comfortable than others, some pinch and I can't wait to get them off. My guess is that, with time, one or two will become my favorite, old, wear-around-the-house ways of talking about MS. Some will be more suited for the professional community. Others will be for special occasions, or for first (third? fifth?) dates. Some days I'll go barefoot, but you can't do that for too long.

# A Front-Row Seat

RACHEL NAOMI REMEN

It is hard to trust something you cannot see. Even after seven major surgeries, I have had, at times, difficulty in trusting my healing. In 1981, I developed peritonitis and sepsis when the sutures holding my intestines together gave way a few days after a six-hour abdominal surgery. By the time this was correctly diagnosed, I had become gravely ill. I was rushed back to the operating room where further surgery probably saved my life. I remember being pushed down a corridor at a dead run, the lights overhead flashing by, my surgeon, who was also my friend, running alongside my gurney. Medical culture being what it is, he was talking to me about my case as if we were two physicians lunching in the doctors' dining room, talking about a mutual patient. "You know," he said conversationally, "because of the infection we will have to close by primary intention." Filled with drugs and very ill, I remember thinking, "Primary intention. I used to know what that means." Then events accelerated and I lost track of it all.

Several hours later, I awoke in the recovery room giddy with the realization that I had once again survived. Barely conscious, I explored my abdomen with a fingertip. There was the big, soft bandage just as before. Comforted by the familiar, I drifted off.

The next day a nurse appeared to change my dressings. Chatting comfortably, she pulled back the bandages and I looked down expecting to see the usual fourteen-inch incision with its neat row of a hundred or more stitches. Instead, there was a great gaping wound, as open as any I'd ever seen while assisting in the operating room. My surgeon's words came back to me in a rush—primary intention—and today I knew what this meant. In the presence of infection there would be no sutures. The peritoneum and fascia would be closed and then the wound would be left open to heal on its own.

Deeply shocked, I looked down at the ruin of my abdomen. Surely this was a mortal wound. I remember thinking, "There is no way that such a thing can heal." The nurse chatted on cheerfully, unaware of my reaction. Taping the dressing back in place, she left the room. The next morning she was back to change the dressing again. This time I turned my head aside and wouldn't look. She spoke to me pleasantly while she performed her task. I didn't answer. I was in despair.

For several mornings, we went through this same routine, she pulling back the bandage, murmuring encouragement, I, head averted, awaiting the end. After a week or so, it occurred to me that against all probability, I was still here. Perhaps I would not die of this wound after all but would have to live with it. This raised a completely different set of concerns and obsessions. How would I live with this great hole in my front? Perhaps after many years it might fill in and become flat—a scar fourteen inches long and several inches wide. Until then no tight jeans or bathing suits. Could I wear extra-large clothes? Or fill the deep trench in my belly with cotton and tape so it would not show?

After a few days of such musings, it became obvious that if I was going to live with it, I would need to see it. So that day, when the nurse pulled back the dressing, I forced myself to look again, expecting to see the gaping wound of ten days before. But it was not the same. Astounded, I saw that it had begun closing in at the bottom and was distinctly narrower. And then an extraordinary thing began to happen. Day after day, she would pull back the dressing and I would watch as this great wound, in the slow, patient way of all natural things, gradually became a hairline scar. And I, a physician, was not in control of this. It was humbling. Yet I certainly had a front-row seat at the healing process. It was only much later that I realized that I had been occupying this same front-row seat since the moment I had entered medical school. The life force I had witnessed in myself was a birthright common to us all.

# Leave of Absence

## KATE A. SCANNELL

When I discovered that I had cancer one hour and forty minutes before leaving for Paris, I was transported into an eerie seam between thought and feeling. In this wordless void, I groped for understanding and emotion—the usual evidence of my existence. The shock of my disembodiment unmoored me from physical time, and I drifted chaotically through future, past, and present. When thoughts and feelings did stir, they seemed to belong to someone else, to some body that I had inhabited. It was as though I were watching them projected onto a screen from an archival recollection of my being.

Pressing against me in the void were the words the pathologist articulated through the phone: "cancer," "surgery," and, several times, "uncertainty." These words tried to penetrate me and locate meaning and emotional resonance. But I was not there in the usual ways to receive them.

While the pathologist spoke, I stared at my desk clock. The first thought that stirred was, "How long does 10:20 last?" At 10:19 I had been a healthy, forty-three-year-old physician embarking on a year's sabbatical from work. Suddenly, I became someone who might be as old as she would ever be, someone with a midlife journey violently foreshortened. Within seconds, I traveled through decades in a wormhole that delivered me closer to my death.

The airport taxi would arrive at noon. As I clutched the airline tickets, a strange logic supplanted my medical mind, which knew that disease did not heed human desire. But I am leaving for Paris, I told myself. I begin my sabbatical today. I can't possibly have cancer now.

"Would you repeat everything you said?" I asked the pathologist. I needed her words to charge at me again. I wanted them to pierce me and register an emotional or intellectual reality. She repeated "cancer." But my numbness only grew denser. Everything inside me stilled, melded to the moment before the pathologist spoke, and resisted forward time.

Seconds earlier I was poised to fly into my future. For months I had orchestrated two celebratory weeks in Paris to inaugurate my exploration of time, my philosopause. Weary from working sixteen years as a physician, I had secured a year's leave of absence to discover what might happen in my life were it not always weighted under the psychic toll of so many other lives and the grueling physical demands of my job. What would I think about if the suffering of hundreds of patients were not a constant backdrop to my psyche? What if the fears of missing a diagnosis or deciding a wrong therapy did not cycle through my head with disruptive regularity? What if my days were not fragmented into fifteen-minute segments in which my mind turnstiled into the world of yet another patient? What would I do if twelve-hour workdays vanished? How would I feel if rested, physically active, nourished by noninstant food? What would I write about?

I had not simply imagined my sabbatical time as an open space, but I had planned vigorously for it to be so. In the weeks preceding my trip to Paris, I had finally conferred with a financial advisor and a life insurance representative, written a will, procured new eyeglasses, and obtained a mammogram. I had launched my departure from long-term depth psychotherapy. Days earlier, I completed the work on my research grant. And, hell-bent to enter my sabbatical with a completely clear slate, I wrote through the nights to finish a book manuscript that I ceremoniously mailed to my literary agent in New York at 8:30 in the morning, precisely three and one-half hours before leaving for Paris. When I returned home from the post office, I unplugged my alarm clock: the luminosity of "8:55 A.M." faded away.

Only two remaining items nagged on my list of things to do: a phone call to the insurance representative to confirm my decision to purchase a life insurance policy, and another to my gynecologist to obtain my biopsy results.

Twice during the preceding week I was unable to reach my gynecologist by phone. At 9 A.M. I left another phone message, reminding her that I was leaving for Paris in three hours. I packed several more novels into my suitcase, overwatered my vegetable garden, and ate breakfast. I could just begin to feel time uncoiling. Beneath my skull. Around my eyes. In the knot at the base of my neck.

At 10:15 I tried to reach my doctor again. Unsuccessful, I phoned the pathology department directly for my results. The clerk recognized my name and assumed that, as was usual, I was requesting a pathology report for one of my own patients.

"No," I explained, "it's for me."

The clerk responded cheerily and placed me on hold. The sedating elixir of phone Muzak paradoxically intensified the disturbance I felt waiting: its attempts to manipulate my experience of time irritated me. Time—my time—was moving fast despite the slowed, dampened rhythm of an old rock tune.

Finally, the clerk returned and asked in a clearly directive manner, "Doctor Scannell, would you like to speak with one of the pathologists?" In this very moment, I was first aware of time bending. It bowed like a long bone about to snap. Instantly, I stood within the bending itself. Past and future dutifully flanked either side of me.

"Yes," I replied, already understanding what the clerk tried not to convey.

Immediately, one of the pathologists was on the phone. She relayed how sad she had felt when she realized that the specimen was my own. She said, "I look at tissue samples all day, and I rarely know the person to whom they belong."

"Do I have cancer?" I asked.

She was stunned. She had assumed that I had heard.

Two weeks earlier, in my quest to tie up all the loose ends of my life before commencing my sabbatical, I told my gynecologist that I was concerned about a short-lived symptom that we both knew to be common in healthy premenopausal women. But I had dreamed three consecutive dreams in which I harbored both uterine and ovarian cancers; the dreams disturbed me, my partner, and my therapist. I voiced embarrassment that these dreams would compel me, a physician, to seek my gynecologist's evaluation. Still, my gynecologist willingly obliged my concerns.

A piece of my uterus then traveled for two weeks from one microscope to another, failing to inspire a consensus of opinion from specialists in the department who remained evenly divided as to whether or not it showed cancer. The pathologist explained that, finally, it had been placed into an envelope and couriered across the San Francisco Bay to Stanford University where, just hours earlier, it was deemed benign. "But," the pathologist said, "I personally think it's malignant. I'm sending it to UCSF for another opinion."

I knew about "medical opinions." I formulated them every day as a rheumatologist. I knitted opinions from unclear science about mysterious diseases and uncertain remedies as a daily practice. Opinions were as solid as the prevailing winds and as clear as the practitioner's view. Opinions were constantly reformulated by facts that could change if yet another study were funded. I realized that even if the new pathologist sided with malignancy, I'd still be floundering in a murky gap between health and life-threatening disease. Reasoned opinions and medical facts could not orient me comfortably within this gap.

The clock on my desk was literally ticking. This comforted me in a strange way. It reassured me that there was some order to experience, that I would not be stuck forever in this moment, this bend in time in which I felt increasingly disoriented and numb.

I thanked the pathologist and apologized for putting her on the spot. I stared at the plane tickets in my hand as proof that I would be moving soon, at jet speed, into open skies, across the distances between me and my unlived personal life.

At 10:25 I hung up the phone, and it rang immediately. My gynecologist spoke, explaining that she had been waiting for better clarity of my biopsy report before calling me the prior week. After the explanations, she said, "We're still uncertain if it's cancer. And, if it is, we can't know if it's metastasized before surgery."

Hearing these words from her, my doctor, I felt the bend in time strain further. I felt my life organizing into a sharply divided "before" and "after," with "cancer" cleaving the middle.

*I am on the other side now,* I thought. I had spoken the word "cancer" many times before to my patients and their loved ones. I watched their lives capsize from the force of this single word. I tended to hold my experiences of these moments as one large and sad memory, monolithic in its universality, yet so fragile that, under certain circumstances, it shattered into individual parts. Hearing my doctor's words capsize my own life, I felt myself being pulled into the collective memory.

All the while I spoke on the phone with my gynecologist, my partner remained at my side, encouraging me to cancel our trip to Paris. The time would be tainted by worry, by separation from friends and colleagues, by alienation in a foreign country. Besides, now there were pressing practical matters to attend. In one ear were my gynecologist's words erasing the certitude of my future; in my other ear sounded my partner's voice urging me to abandon plans of my past. These sharp distinctions of past and future literally spoke to me, pressed against my life like a vise. My sense of my self as continuous through time began to fracture.

I desperately craved the continuity of my past and future self. I wanted to believe that the awful immediate moment could move on a spectrum, that it could yield to other moments. My gynecologist repeated things as often as I needed to hear them. My partner slipped me a note—*Air France would give us credit for a future flight.*

I hung up the phone. I turned to my partner and said, "If I have cancer, we will have gone to Paris."

Within the next ninety minutes, I made sixteen phone calls. I arranged preop evaluations for the day of my return, surgery the week following, cancellation of my sabbatical to provide me the potential for disability claims should I have metastatic cancer. I asked a friend to phone me in Paris with the UCSF pathologist's opinion. I called my therapist and told her that I probably had cancer, "as in my dream," and that I was leaving for Paris in this new, uncharted way.

I did not call the life insurance agent.

In the taxi en route to the San Francisco International Airport, time bent several more degrees until it cleanly snapped into a "before" and an "after" that fell away from the present in which I was stranded. Having failed dismally to plan my life, to structure time around it, I felt completely powerless in the insistent present. My mind and heart could not translate my experience, and I hovered in the seam between thought and feeling. In silence I rode the taxi to the airport, and soon I was suspended thirty thousand feet in the air, crossing time lines, entering a foreign country.

*Narratives of Advocacy:*
*From the Personal*
*to the Political*
ℰ

THIS SECTION EXPLORES what it means to utilize personal narratives to enact change. These contributions revisit each of the preceding sections, yet these are narratives through which the personal experience is made political. The first essay in this section is written by Carol Levine, whose work as an advocate for family caregivers has been discussed earlier in this book. Levine not only describes her personal experience as caregiver for her disabled husband but contextualizes this experience in familial, communal, and national policy contexts. Her narrative regards the translation of personal experience into a lifetime of advocacy for family caregivers. In her words, "As difficult as it is for me, I tell my story to open the eyes of professionals and policy makers to the realities of caregiving in today's complex medical and economic environment. What I did not expect, and what happens time and again, is that their hearts are opened as well. That is how real change must start—one mind, one heart at a time."

Marja Morskeift and Judith Nadell revisit the experience of illness—Morskeift's narrative describes her experience with multiple sclerosis to advocate for disability services, understanding, and access, while Nadell's essay echoes many themes from Susan Sontag's classic "Illness as Metaphor." She uses her own frustrations with mind-body self-help literature, debunking the popular myths of cancer to conclude "Sometimes Cancer Just Happens." Sucheng Chan's letter to her mother's physicians regards the relationship of the ill to the medical establishment—but her anger at physicians' culturally inappropriate care makes this a narrative of direct interpersonal advocacy. Sunita Puri's essay could belong to either the section on social constructions of womanhood or the illness experiences of health care professionals. She is a medical student and community activist who locates and critiques her struggle with eating disorders and body image in her experience as a sexual abuse survivor. "One major way I have tried to heal myself," she writes, "is by using my experience to raise awareness of how common sexual abuse is . . . I write and speak about my experiences to medical school classes, to members of the South Asian community, and to community health workers . . . Every word written, every phrase spoken, and every ear that listens are all crucial components of my healing." Puri's words make clear that the personal to political connections of illness narratives are both socially critical and individually empowering.

# Night Shift

CAROL LEVINE

Henry James haunts me. Not the ghostly apparitions in *The Turn of the Screw*. Not betrayed and dying Milly Theale in *The Wings of the Dove*. But the anonymous, obsessed narrator of *The Aspern Papers*.

One fateful January morning in 1990, my husband Howard and I were driving along a rural parkway and listening to a recording of James's novella. Suddenly, the car spun on an icy patch, hit a guardrail, and flipped over. I was not hurt but Howard was near death from a severe brain-stem injury. I remember ejecting the rented tape from the totaled auto and taking it with me in the ambulance to the nearest hospital. People do strange things in shock.

It would be four months before Howard slowly emerged from a coma and many more months before he uttered coherent phrases. Today, he is totally disabled, essentially quadriplegic. He has no memory of the accident and only fragmentary recollections of its aftermath. He can recall games he watched as a sports publicist years ago but not some important events in our life together.

He has been home for more than nine years and requires round-the-clock care. An attendant looks after him during the day; I am the night nurse. Trying to hold on to one of the few remnants of our preaccident life, we still listen to books on tape. Not long ago I played *The Aspern Papers* again. Maybe, just maybe, I thought, hearing it will restore lost memories. After all, this is the stuff of television dramas.

When the tape ended, I looked at Howard expectantly.

"Good story," he said. "What's on TV?"

Life is not a television drama. My husband will never recover his memory, his amputated forearm, or his old personality. Some things cannot be changed. But the indignities and irrationalities of the U.S. health care system, which add an unnecessary level of burden and stress to family caregivers like me, must be changed.

Caregivers in this nation are 25-million strong and provide nearly $200 billion a year in unpaid labor. We are also 25-million isolated individuals, our economic contribution taken for granted and our potential political power largely untapped.

I have spent twenty years as a professional in medical ethics analyzing thorny health policy problems. Yet I naively believed that the system would work for me when I needed it. And it did—in the beginning. Despite a winter storm and a widespread telephone outage, I could still make connections. Within hours of the accident, I arranged for Howard to be transferred to a major medical center. Trauma teams went into action. His life was saved.

But then his devastating and permanent disabilities became apparent. The system's previously attentive agents and agencies disappeared into the maze of voice mail. He became a "custodial" case—a losing proposition for profit-seeking insurers and a black hole for spending-averse policymakers. I was no longer able to be myself, a loving but grieving wife. I was unceremoniously transformed into a "caregiver." In this new job I had total responsibility but no voice or power.

To my chagrin, I was also back in a world dominated by gender stereotypes. As a graduate student in the 1950s, I had faced academic committees that frankly told me that they would not consider me for a fellowship because I might get married and pregnant. And so I did, but I still wanted to work. (I did eventually get a Ford Fellowship when the chosen recipient, a man, backed out.) As a young mother of three small children in the '60s and '70s, I had faced the nonexistence, never mind unaffordability, of daycare in the suburbs. It did not make much difference, however, since no one would hire me—and told me so—because I had young children. Without years of work experience and lacking a mentor, I pieced together freelance writing and editing assignments until one led me to the rewarding career I now have. I even received a MacArthur Fellowship in 1993. My two daughters had a greater world open to them. My son shares childcare equally with his wife. As far as my personal life was concerned, sexism was a thing of the past.

And then I became a caregiver. Not only are women the traditional caregivers, they are expected to do more of it, quietly and obediently, without special training. We are assumed to be hardwired for wound dressing, feeding tube calibration, and wheelchair manipulation. Perhaps my professional experience working with AIDS advocates, mostly gay men, had skewed my sense of reality. In this world men took care of each other through illness and death, albeit with a lot of help from the gay and lesbian communities. They challenged the system to provide what they needed, and the system responded. Outside this special sphere, however, old paradigms rule.

In the prosaic world of chronic illness, it is wives, daughters, sisters, aunts, and female friends who constitute the bulk of the caregiving workforce. Depending on the population surveyed, up to three-quarters of caregivers are women, most of them in their forties and fifties. To be sure, many men take on daunting responsibilities, but on the whole, women do more caregiving, provide the most intimate forms of care, and stay for the long haul. As a survey published in the *New England Journal of Medicine* reported, women provide most of the care for terminally ill people, without help from paid workers or volunteers.[1] Women also get less social support; a man can usually count on women to help out and to praise his efforts. For women, it's lonely duty as usual.

Often there is more than one person in a family who needs or may need help. I have an eighty-eight-year-old mother who lives five hundred miles away; she is fortunately in excellent health. For now, all we do is worry about each other. And I have one granddaughter who has serious physical disabilities; I am as involved in her life and as supportive of her parents as I can be but wish I could do more. At critical times I have rushed between two hospitals. I sometimes feel as though I am Caregiver Central.

When my husband's prognosis became clear and the long future stretched ahead of us, I looked for help. None was forthcoming. Even more appalling, the most judgmental responses came from other women—nurses and social workers. Some nurses, admittedly overworked, were so resentful of my continuing to work and failing to relieve them of their duties that I had to hire a "companion" to be with my husband in the rehab center until I arrived each day at 4 P.M. to feed him. When he screamed for help (regularly) or was uncooperative (even more frequently), I was blamed.

No matter what I did, it was never enough. That was not the case for the spouse of another patient with approximately the same level of disability. This patient was a woman, and her husband visited with great fanfare and flowers every few evenings. He also arranged for round-the-clock private nurses. The nurses rushed to greet him and to tell him how wonderful he was. When I noted the discrepancy, a nurse said, "You don't realize how rare it is for men to stay involved."

In long-term caregiving, all too often women are pitted against women. Nurses' aides and home health aides are generally women, and generally underpaid and poorly trained. Drawn from a largely immigrant or minority population, these women have jobs that are among the most demanding and stressful in the health care field, but they have little security and very few opportunities for advancement. They often feel—and sometimes are—exploited by the families of their patients. And yet the family caregivers are burdened by their own caregiving, worried about their relatives, and untrained in care management.

I no longer have conflicts with other women over my husband's care. Since the early days, I have hired male attendants, a decision on which my husband insisted and that I respect. But there are relatively few men who are in this category, and not surprisingly, the most skilled are better paid than women.

Of all the professionals involved in my husband's care over the years, only a few have ever expressed concern for me. Two were male physicians. One was a female nurse, who spoke to me surreptitiously, perhaps fearful that she was breaking the code. She said, "You don't have to do this. It's going to be incredibly hard. You can find a good nursing home." Despite her (accurate) prediction of what lay ahead, I could not then consider nursing home placement, nor can I now.

A social worker told me I was selfish when I refused to take Howard home from the rehab center without having home care services in place. His insurance company refused to pay. "Is there any assistance available?" I asked. "Yes," she said. "Quit your job and spend down your assets. Once you're poor, Medicaid will pay for a nursing home." Here was an offer I could refuse.

Even some of my friends and colleagues assumed that I would quit my job. That was never an option, financially or psychologically. I had worked too hard for too long to give up my work. Certainly it is hard to balance work and caregiving, but in retrospect, work has been my salvation. I am not alone. More than half of all caregivers are employed full time; others work part time. One study found that women employed full time were less stressed from caregiving than part-time workers because they spent more time away from their responsibilities and received greater financial, psychological, and social rewards from work. There is a difference, of course, between taking a leave of absence to be with a dying parent, where there is an expected closure, and quitting a job to take on long-term caregiving.

The Family and Medical Leave Act was supposed to help with some of these problems, but it only covers companies with more than fifty employees. Over half of all employees in the United States are ineligible, many of them women who work in the service sector. Currently, leaves are unpaid, a major drawback for caregivers. The prime beneficiaries of the law are new parents who can plan financially for time off. Although the National Partnership for Women and Families inaugurated a campaign to encourage states to use their unemployment insurance funds to pay new parents who take leave, this improvement would not help family caregivers of ill or disabled adults. California is the only state with a paid leave act.

Like many caregivers, I pay a heavy financial price for keeping my husband at home. Many essentials—home aides, costly disposable supplies, physical therapy, and appropriate wheelchairs—are not covered by private insurance. Medicare does not cover long-term care, and its benefits for rehabilitation are extremely limited. Medical costs in general are responsible for tremendous financial hardship. A survey of bankruptcy filings in 1999 estimated that nearly half were caused by expenses from either illness or substantial medical debt. Women heads of households and the elderly were particularly hard hit by these costs, even though they had medical insurance.

And this is to say nothing of the physical and emotional toll. Last year my managed care company paid more for my stress-related medical problems than for my husband's medical care. And what do I have to look forward to? A study of elderly caregivers who experienced stress found a 63 percent higher rate of death than occurred among their noncaregiving peers or among caregivers who did not experience stress. This only confirms the many stories I hear of caregivers who die before their supposedly more fragile family members.

Managing care can be exhausting, frustrating, and mind bending, whether one deals with the private sector, as I do, or with government bureaucracies. I recently spent more than three months trying to find a way to have Howard's blood drawn for a routine checkup. The approved lab within "pushing" distance is not wheelchair accessible. The only accommodation the lab would make was to offer to draw my husband's blood in the street! Finally, it turned out there was a solution that the managed care company did not even know about: the lab provided home services, and for less money.

If Henry James haunts me, Kafka captures the irrationalities of my caregiver's universe. Professional caregivers, who should be compassionate, are uncaring; management experts, who should be efficient, waste time and money; and information providers, presumably the experts, know less than the people asking for help.

And perhaps there's a bit of Beckett too. Each day I say to myself, "I can't go on." And then I say, "I must go on." I am not a hero or a martyr, even if these seem to be the standards that the system expects. But neither am I stoic, meekly accepting the status quo. For now, I am able to provide Howard a tolerably good quality of life. My children and grandchildren impress, delight, and stimulate me. My project at the United Hospital Fund, a research and grant-making organization in New York City, focuses on improving policies and practices that affect family caregivers. Among other responsibilities, I supervise grants for several pioneering hospital programs that could change the caregiver's environment.

There are some other promising signs: there is bipartisan support for legislation providing a tax credit of three thousand dollars a year for caregivers and caregiver support grants for states, although its enactment is being held hostage by politics. These would be very modest steps, but a beginning to what Mona Harrington envisions in her book *Care and Equality: The Establishment of Care as a National Value.*[2]

Implementing such a vision is a challenge both to liberals, often suspicious of inserting family needs into anything but an antipoverty or a "women's" agenda, and to conservatives, traditionally suspicious of anything nontraditional. Caregiving is certainly a women's issue, but it is more deeply a human issue. Either as a provider or a recipient of care, everyone will be in the caregiving lifeboat at some point, looking for rescue.

Some caregivers say their lives are enriched; others find spiritual solace. I respect their feelings, and sometimes I envy them. Nevertheless, I steadfastly refuse to find this experience ennobling. I will not be a poster wife for caregiving. As difficult as it is for me, I tell my story to open the eyes of professionals and policymakers to the realities of caregiving in today's complex medical and economic environment. What I did not expect, and what happens time and again, is that their hearts are opened as well.

That is how real change must start—one mind, one heart at a time.

## Notes

1. E. J. Emanuel, D. L. Fairclough, J. Slutsman, H. Alpert, D. Baldwin, and L. L. Emanuel, "Assistance from Family Members, Friends, Paid Caregivers, and Volunteers in the Care of Terminally Ill Patients," *New England Journal of Medicine* 341 (1999): 956–63.

2. Mona Harrington, *Care and Equality: The Establishment of Care as a National Value* (New York: Knopf, 1999).

# Sometimes Cancer Just Happens

JUDITH NADELL

In the last decade, I had cancer twice: breast cancer in 1992 and thyroid cancer in 1998. Today, I feel healthy and strong—and expect to remain so for a good long while. But I didn't always feel so confident. Let me tell you why.

I was devastated by my breast cancer diagnosis. Seeking information to help me cope, I came across articles, books, and TV shows on the mind-body (or holistic) model of illness, which says that mind, body, and spirit are interconnected and profoundly influence one another. Won over by attention-grabbing titles like "Let Your Mind Heal Your Body" and "Think Your Way to Health," I initially embraced the model wholeheartedly.

Parts of the mind-body approach were helpful to me. I can't imagine how I would have gotten through some pretty dark days without the mind-body techniques of meditation and visualization. But gradually I came to feel that many holistic health proponents distort the mind-body connection. How? Oversimplifying the connection, they argue that the wrong kinds of thoughts and feelings create illness and that it's only by changing these that we get well. This explanation of why we get sick and how we recover made my bouts with cancer much more difficult than they otherwise would have been. Three myths or false assumptions are, I believe, at the heart of this oversimplified concept of illness.

## THE INNER-DEFECT MYTH

The first myth, which I call the Inner-Defect Myth, asserts that illness is a sign that something is awry in our inner lives. For starters, listen to what Dr. Bernie Siegel asserts in his book *Love, Medicine, and Miracles: Lessons Learned about Self-Healing from a Surgeon's Experience with Exceptional Patients:* "The simple truth is, happy people generally don't get sick."[1] Believing that cancer usually fulfills a psychological need, he goes on to argue that traumatic loss typically precedes a cancer diagnosis and, if that loss isn't "properly dealt with," the body often responds by developing a "malignant growth."[2]

So ... how did I respond to the idea that something out of balance at my core led to my breast cancer? Frankly, it sparked deep feelings of guilt and self-blame.

And I'm not alone in having those feelings. As Dr. Jimmie Holland explains in her book *The Human Side of Cancer: Living with Hope, Coping with Uncertainty,* a medical diagnosis often shakes the very basis of one's identity, making even the most psychologically sound among us feel guilty, ashamed, and defective. These feelings of self-blame are especially powerful, Dr. Holland argues, when the illness is cancer.[3]

Absolutely. During my life, I've had run-ins with several serious medical conditions. But none of them delivered the psychological wallop of cancer. One minute I was fine; the next minute—pow—I was someone who gets cancer. And since, for most people, cancer evokes distressing images of misshapen, diseased cells spreading throughout the body, it's not surprising that I felt almost ashamed of my illness.

These awful feelings were multiplied many times over by my initial acceptance of the popular notion that there's something called the "cancer personality." According to several mind-body proponents, we cancer patients fit a particular profile. In the book *Getting Well Again,* Dr. O. Carl Simonton and the four other authors write that cancer patients tend to be emotionally repressed and pessimistic; they feel unloved and unappreciated; their lives lack meaning and purpose.[4] To my dismay, more than a few people seemed to accept this blame-the-patient view of my illness. When I had thyroid cancer, an acquaintance looked at me soulfully and asked, "Why do you think you got cancer again?"—her assumption being that I got cancer a second time because something was still out of kilter in my inner life.

It's understandable if we cancer patients blame ourselves for getting sick. Being ill makes us feel helpless; blaming ourselves may be less anxiety producing than accepting the fact that sometimes there seems to be no reason at all why we get cancer. But isn't it an oversimplification to view the health of the body as a reflection of psychological or spiritual health? Does an infant with leukemia have unresolved personal issues? What about the role of heredity, diet, environmental exposure, even random chance?

Plus there isn't a whole lot of evidence to support the cancer-personality theory. Look at the traits typically associated with the so-called cancer personality—emotional repression, childhood pain, dissatisfaction with life, you name it. Do you know anyone who couldn't lay claim to some of these characteristics? Conversely, don't we all know someone who radiates psychological health but has been diagnosed with cancer?

This brings me to my first message. If you feel burdened, as I did, by an essentially blame-the-patient interpretation of your illness: please take yourself off the hook. Doesn't it make more sense to view the myth as defective, not the person who's ill?

## The Mandated Cheerfulness Myth

If the first myth makes us responsible for getting cancer, the second makes us responsible for recovering from cancer. This Mandated Cheerfulness Myth argues that maintaining a positive attitude is essential to getting well. Indeed, Dr. Siegel goes so far as to claim that "attitude . . . is [get this] the single most important factor" in getting better.[5] In similar fashion, Dr. Lawrence LeShan asserts in his otherwise quite wonderful book *Cancer as a Turning Point: A Handbook for People with Cancer, Their Families, and Health Professionals* that our immune systems can fight cancer only when we turn our supposedly inherent negativity into positive, upbeat energy.[6]

Clearly, dealing with cancer is much easier if we're optimistic and hopeful. But this be-positive-at-all-costs edict threw me for a loop when I had breast cancer. I felt anxious about feeling anxious, fearing any emotion that smacked of negativity would do me in.

Insisting on a positive frame of mind leaves those of us with cancer little room to respond authentically. Shortly after my second cancer diagnosis, a well-intentioned friend called to see how I was doing and kept assuring me, "Don't worry. Don't worry. You'll be fine, just fine. And aren't you lucky you caught the cancer early!" Her maddeningly chipper comments left no space for me to say, "Hey, you know what? I don't feel fine. I don't feel lucky. I feel angry and scared."

Experiencing enormous anxiety after the phone call, I turned to my journal to sort out what I was feeling. Once I started writing, I couldn't stop, until finally, with tears streaming down my face, I jabbed my pen into the paper, scribbling over and over, "This is no small thing. This is no small thing. I've got cancer again. Shit." And guess what? As soon as I gave myself permission to stop pretending that everything was hunky-dory, my anxiety lifted.

So here's the second bit of advice I'd like to pass along: if you've received a ticket from the Attitude Police because you've had the gall to feel depressed, angry, or terrified about having cancer, I hope you'll take the ticket and tear it up. Yes, attitudes and emotions affect the immune system, but, Dr. Holland emphasizes, we don't know whether "the[se] blips in hormone levels have any connection" to the onset of cancer or to recovery.[7] The reality is, the upbeat don't always survive cancer while plenty of scared, angry folk do.

## The Transformation Myth

The Transformation Myth says that if we really want to get well, we must fix the painful personal issues that led to illness in the first place. Arguing (incredibly enough) that "there are no incurable illnesses, only incurable people,"[8] Dr. Siegel contends that once a patient repairs what's askew, the body "can eliminate the disease because it's not part of the new self."[9]

During my first bout with cancer, this idea that I'd get better if I transformed what needed repair gave me a much-needed sense of control—at first. But soon I crashed with a loud thud. My breast cancer diagnosis had shaken me with volcanic force. Every loss, regret, and fear I had ever had exploded to the surface. Beliefs about myself, my relationships, my priorities—all underwent deep seismic shifts. My life seemed riddled with fault lines threatening to give way at any moment. The transformation myth made me feel that I had to resolve these complex issues quickly. What if I didn't fix things fast enough or if, heaven forbid, I fixed the wrong things? After a while, my cancer began to feel like a test I had to pass. If I flunked (that is, if I died), it would be—much of the holistic health literature seemed to suggest—my own darn fault.

Nowadays I consider heartless the notion that death may be a sign that perhaps, just perhaps, someone didn't do the inner work needed to live. Nowadays I know that lots of people survive cancer without resolving deep inner conflict—just as lots of people survive without experiencing any major turmoil at all. Everyone's experience is different.

No, I don't believe we get ill because there's something deep inside that needs fixing. Yet I have to acknowledge that, for me, cancer did serve as a catalyst for healing emotional wounds and awakening the spirit. Let me explain.

Back in the fall of 1992, reeling from the impact of my breast cancer diagnosis, I signed up for a series of biofeedback sessions, hoping they'd help me manage my anxiety. Skeptical that they were doing any good, I went to my third session and dutifully tried to slow my breathing and relax my muscles—but succeeded only in feeling more anxious than ever. Tension at an all-time high, I was suddenly flooded—absolutely flooded—by a golden, honey-colored light. And then I began to cry, and cry, and cry. But they were wonderful tears. My fear gone, I felt a profound sense of peace and joy.

By nature an analytic, linear type of person, I wanted a rational explanation for what had happened and kept asking myself, "What *was* that?"—feeling a bit like folks in the old westerns who'd ask, "Who *was* that masked man?" as the Lone Ranger rode off into the sunset.

In spite of myself, my encounter with the golden, honey-colored light set me off in a spiritual direction—so much so that several months later, I woke up one Friday morning, singing "Rocking My Soul in the Bosom of Abraham." "This is strange. Why in the world am I singing this?" I wondered. "What could it possibly mean?" Then I heard myself answer, "Go to synagogue tonight"—a surprising response from someone who had rejected religion decades earlier.

That evening I did go to synagogue and, on the way in, I picked up some literature outside the sanctuary. One of the items was the synagogue newsletter called (how perfect is this?) *The LIGHT!* Chuckling at the coincidence of it all, I entered the sanctuary, sensing deep down that I—a card-carrying skeptic—had somehow stumbled upon a kind of faith.

Cancer can bring about other changes too. If we're lucky, we emerge with a greater appreciation of our own inner strength. I, for one, now sense within myself a bedrock strength I hadn't known was there.

But I have to admit that, in some ways, I also feel more anxious than I used to. Sometimes a twinge in my little finger can be enough to make me think I've contracted that dread disease, pinkie carcinoma. At first, I berated myself for this heightened anxiety. Having faced a life-threatening illness, I thought that from now on I should be staunchly fearless. With time, I came to see that we cancer patients may leave our cancer behind but not our fear about getting ill again. That fear comes with the territory.

Cancer shatters the myth of invulnerability; it teaches us that we're going to die, that we're not going to be here forever. Painful as it may be, this deepened awareness of mortality reminds us how precious life is, how important it is to make the most of the time we *do* have. A final story illustrates my point.

When I had breast cancer, I mentioned to a friend that I was thinking about becoming a literacy volunteer after I finished treatment—something I had intended for years but had never gotten around to doing. As I spoke, an image flashed in my mind of me and a student sitting side by side, exchanging triumphant smiles, as the student finished the first book she had ever read. So powerful was the image that my eyes filled with tears and I had to stop speaking. In that moment, I knew I couldn't put off becoming a literacy volunteer; it was something I *had* to do. Soon afterwards, I starting volunteering and, since that time, have worked with undereducated adults and at-risk children, helping them learn to read—work that's brought great joy and a sense of purpose to my life.

Many mind-body proponents believe that we get cancer exactly for this reason: to teach us how to live fuller, more realized lives. This brings me to my final message: I don't believe we're meant to get cancer. Yes, some of us may emerge from cancer transformed, but I don't think that's why we got ill. And there's no guarantee that transformation—if it even occurs—will bring health. We may resolve personal pain; we may visualize ourselves well and happy; we may discover a spiritual foundation; we may commit ourselves to doing meaningful work. These are wonderful strategies for living well, and taking such steps helps us feel we're playing an active role in getting better. But such measures don't—much as we'd like—necessarily banish cancer from our lives.

Sometimes cancer just happens.

NOTES

1. Bernie S. Siegel, *Love, Medicine, and Miracles: Lessons Learned about Self-Healing from a Surgeon's Experience with Exceptional Patients* (New York: Harper, 1990) 76.

2. Siegel 124.

3. Jimmie Holland and Sheldon Lewis, *The Human Side of Cancer: Living with Hope, Coping with Uncertainty* (New York: Harper, 2001).

4. O. Carl Simonton, Stephanie Matthews-Simonton, and James L. Creighton, *Getting Well Again: A Step-by-Step Self-Help Guide to Overcoming Cancer for Patients and Their Families* (New York: Bantam, 1992).

5. Siegel 76.

6. Lawrence LeShan, *Cancer As a Turning Point: A Handbook for People with Cancer, Their Families, and Health Professionals* (New York: Plume, 1994).

7. Holland and Lewis 19.

8. Siegel 99.

9. Siegel 124.

# A Case of Exhaustion

MARJA MORSKIEFT*

One Saturday morning, fifteen years ago now, I got up early, brimming with plans for the weekend ahead. I would take the bike and go to the market to store up on some plants for our still-vacant garden then sing some songs to my eleven-month-old son, his absolutely favorite pastime. I would record his first words: "moo" and "meow." The weekend cleaning was also still waiting to be done. I had been out late the night before, saying goodbye to a student to whom I had given a crash course in Portuguese.

Halfway through my bike trip I noticed that I could hardly get the pedals moving. I was crossing the bridge over the canal but I was crawling! Must be tired, I thought; I'd better turn in early tonight. I was leading a busy life and enjoying every minute of it. "A woman's hand and a horse's mouth should never be idle" is what my mother had taught me. Finishing my master's thesis in remedial education, finding a part time job, weaning our almost one-year-old son, giving crash courses in Portuguese because I was hooked on the language—no wonder I was feeling tired.

Having finally reached town, which seemed to have moved to China, I felt I needed to get back home soon. Everything was fuzzy; I was seeing through a gray haze. Something was definitely wrong. The journey home, in stages, took me forever. Several times I even had to sit down beside my bike to get my strength back. As soon as I got home, I crashed.

That was when my expedition through the jungle of medicine started, a world I had earlier gotten to know through small problems—appendicitis, a sprained knee—all easily remedied, and that would be the case here too; I was convinced of that.

I was turned inside out and the doctors found nothing alarming, which was a good thing, even though my fatigue persisted. "Fatigue" was a euphemism for sure. A debilitating exhaustion held me in a vicelike grip. My body seemed to be made of lead, and the air around me felt like molasses. All kinds of weird phenomena came and went. My vision was blurred and I couldn't focus properly. I

* English translation by Hanneke Meulenbroek

had tingling sensations in my fingers and rubbery legs. My hands and feet weren't responding and kept failing to reach or step where I wanted them to. My digestive system was suddenly doing overtime, making me get skinnier every day. I had burning muscle pains, and an ever-present, dreadful, all-consuming sense of nausea.

I felt so tired that at times I thought I would drop through the floor any minute, chair and all. My senses apparently did their own thing. After what I called a lapse—I clearly had good and bad spells—everything looked crooked and I tended to veer to the right when I moved.

I could hardly find the words to describe all the things that were happening to me. I did try, but even to me it all sounded ridiculous. I saw the incredulity, the pitying looks. I tried to ignore the condescending or ridiculing remarks of the medical examiner, the home care manager, and even some of the consulting specialists ("I feel tired sometimes too, you know, but you give in too easily"), the judgmental comments of outsiders ("Still suffering from that postnatal depression then?"), the well-intended advice of acquaintances ("Perhaps you should have your chakras healed!"), and the indifference of some of my extended family ("Well, at least it isn't a broken leg"). After all, there was nothing wrong with me, was there? My blood, constantly being tested, was fine each time. I didn't have cancer or diabetes or rheumatoid arthritis, so what was I going on about? I should take a good rest, take a break, go on holiday, get therapy. In the meantime I was doing everything in my power to get better, to feel better. I was to blame for feeling so exhausted: "Aren't you overdoing it a little, my dear lady, what with going to college, holding down a job, and taking care of an infant?"

It's all in your mind, everyone said after a while, and so did I. I started shopping around in the alternative health circuit. Everyone who wished me well knew of some miracle doctor, usually someone far off and expensive. I kept strict diets, got to know my chakras, and had my past life as a witch in Scotland healed; I imbibed, injected, and inhaled—losing all my savings in the process.

When I was told, "The reason why you're so unsteady on your legs is that you as a person are not grounded; you'd better start working on that," I suddenly saw the light. That didn't make any sense! I'd been making important decisions ever since I was twelve years old; I'd been living on my own since I was eighteen. There simply had to be something else wrong with my legs—I was walking like a drunk by now. There definitely had to be something the matter with me.

It became clear that my pituitary gland was not functioning as it should. At least it was clear that my hormones were acting up. With renewed energy I embarked on various hormone treatments, antihormone therapies, and implants, all of which literally made me sick to the stomach but were covered by my medical insurance. And yet, what was happening to me remained difficult to explain to the outside world. How could hormones make you feel so tired? It *must* be postnatal depression (four years after my last delivery?). A woman's complaint then, not to be taken seriously. But that didn't explain why I walked the way I did.

I kept being labeled a malingering drama queen and hypochondriac, which, consequently, did not qualify me for any medical aids or domestic care. Sometimes, after one of my so-called lapses, I had a range of a mere fifty yards for weeks on end, although I did manage to double the distance when I was pushing the stroller. Fortunately, my kids loved riding in their buggy, and no one pays any attention to a waddling, lopsided mother with two frolicking toddlers. Still, even before reaching the local convenience store, I was completely drained. No energy, no coordination, my legs gone, my sense of balance gone.

Nonetheless, I did learn to cope, to get along with my exhaustion, and I managed to devise my own strategies and survival techniques. I adopted a strict regime and carefully planned my activities. I went to bed in the afternoon, even when it meant having to find someone to look after my two boys. I bought as many time-saving devices as I could to recover from those days when I had been burning the candle at both ends.

The overpowering exhaustion gradually changed to extreme fatigue to fatigue. Thanks to these self-devised, self-imposed confines, the good spells that made life bearable were increasingly prolonged and became more frequent.

And then finally, after five and a half years, a godsend—but also as the Sword of Damocles—I was diagnosed with a genuine, socially accepted disease: multiple sclerosis (MS). I was very much aware that this label would make my life a whole lot easier. I now had a passport to domestic care, medical aids, and home-care devices. This would wipe those disdainful, disapproving looks from people's faces and change them into commiserating ones.

How wonderful it was to have a "really-horrible-oh-how-dreadful" kind of an illness! Still, my elation soon faded after the bulk of home-care devices had been made and installed—quite an undertaking, I can tell you. Lovely, when you're already low on energy. My relief was displaced by panic. Being possessed by a demon that is not ever going to go away is not something one looks forward to.

Yet, things have picked up for me since. I now allow myself to feel worn out, burnt out, washed out, like a wet rag. Whatever people may think, I simply go to bed during the day. I know my body and its limitations fairly well by now and manage to fit my daily routines around my fatigue. I adhere to a strict schedule (rest—activity—rest) and when I don't (this is too much fun to miss out on) I resign myself to the consequences—the pain, the being out cold—or pour out my troubles to a friend, a woman well acquainted with the whole shebang (a good bout of moaning always works wonders), or tell her the things I should have done to prevent it all. Managing a chronic condition that is typically erratic and running its own rugged course is a craft I keep refining. When I least expect it, a relapse ruins my carefully planned schedule, heralding that dreadful exhaustion that, in turn, inevitably triggers the panic. I haggle and plead (please, not my eyes; rather the fatigue than never being able to read again), chuck my principles overboard (frozen dinners), ask my GP for help (that he can't give). Finally, I resign myself to my fate and hope for the best. The world around me, however, never sees all this. When it's not going well, I retreat to my own little lair. When things are okay, nobody sees how much of my energy goes into "just" functioning normally.

For me, though, it's a real handicap.

Imagine having to access an inaccessible venue, like a theater foyer sporting an enormous staircase and no lift. Just try waiting for two hours for a wheelchair-adapted taxi to arrive after having attended an enervating training course that has already used up your energy resources for the entire day. Try and circumvent the medical arena unscathed, to survive multiple stays in the hospital, to get your home accessible enough to recruit adequate domestic help. Exhausting!

I'm just as tired as before, but by dealing with it shrewdly I also have lots of drive left for what really counts in life: raising my kids, loving and caring for all those who are dear to me, campaigning, teaching, studying, writing, and making music.

The fatigue often has the better of me, I have to admit. It's an opponent that is not to be underestimated. I wish the rest of the world would realize this. Think of how much energy it would save those of us with an ailment that tires you out.

# The Intersection of Illness, Personality, Culture, and Social Services

SUCHENG CHAN

*This essay is a slightly revised version of a letter I sent a social service agency during my mother's illness. There was little coordination among the various organizations that sent nurses and social workers to visit her, which meant that every time someone called me to discuss my mother's situation I had to start from scratch. This letter was an attempt to summarize the situation, but also to provide one account that could be shared among all of the people serving her. Three months after I wrote this letter, my mother's condition worsened. She had another stroke and passed away at age ninety on November 30, 2004.*

As a follow-up to our telephone conversation yesterday, I would like to give you a summary of what has been happening to my mother since she developed bleeding ulcers in June.

My mother grew up in a culture that draws a sharp line between family and nonfamily. Chinese people talk with family members about various private matters, but they refuse to talk to nonfamily members about such topics. In short, they think their mental health, sex life, medical history, and related matters are none of anybody's business. Therefore, even though you will ask a Chinese interpreter to assist you as you interview my mother, she will very likely be uncooperative because she thinks the questions you will be asking are inappropriate from her cultural perspective. Let me give you some examples.

After my mother's recent illness caused by bleeding ulcers, the doctor arranged for a nurse to check on her and take a blood sample. My mother, however, told the nurse that she did not want anyone to bother her. During earlier illnesses, my mother was never a good patient because she hated following other people's orders. In this instance, though, I gave the nurse permission to visit because I felt my mother's physical well-being trumped her mental well-being.

Meanwhile, I was also informed by my mother's HMO that a social worker needed to do a psychiatric evaluation of her because she had seemed so confused. I told them that the person visiting my mother must not mention the words "psychiatrist," "psychologist," or "mental illness" because older Asians like my mother perceive mental health and illness in a way that differs significantly from the views of Americans. I explained that Asian immigrants, especially older ones who had grown up in an Asian country, clam up or even become hostile and agitated whenever those words are mentioned. They think they are being told that they are crazy. Apparently, the message got through and the person who administered the questionnaire to my mother answered "I don't know," whenever my mother asked, "Why do you need this information?"

When my sister and nephew talked to my mother that evening, they found out that she was very angry about the evaluator's visit. She said the woman was stupid because she kept saying "I don't know" when my mother asked why she needed the information she was trying to extract. My mother had reacted in a similarly unfriendly way when another caseworker from her HMO visited her after she had a stroke in June 2002. When the woman asked my mother, "Do you ever get depressed?" my mother answered in a visibly defiant way, "No, I always try to be happy." When even more intrusive questions were asked, my mother refused to answer them. After the woman left, my mother said to me, "Americans are so rude: they think they can ask about the most intimate details of a person's life even though they are meeting you for the first time!"

It was during the weeks when my mother was losing blood and was therefore quite anemic that various people—nurses, social workers, psychologists—started calling and visiting her. So many people called her that she became very annoyed and refused to answer their questions. She was even more wary when strangers, such as the social worker from Adult Protective Services, showed up at her door without prior notice. Afterwards, my mother told me that she thought this man must be a scam artist out to get her money. She said she had learned to be extremely cautious because she had heard on TV and the radio, as well as read in the Chinese-language newspapers she subscribes to, that crimes against seniors were becoming more prevalent and that seniors should not allow strangers to enter their homes or sell them anything over the phone. What made her think that the social worker was a crook was that he asked her whether she knew what county she lived in. My mother said that if he did not even know what county her town was located in, he must not be from the area. The social worker, of course, was simply trying to test her mental acuity, but she interpreted his question in an entirely different way. This is a prime example of cultural misinterpretation: there is not only a language barrier but also a cultural one when health professionals and social workers deal with older immigrants like my mother.

When your Chinese American colleague called my mother and talked to her in Chinese, she was likewise wary of him. I asked her, "Since he can speak Chinese, why didn't you talk to him?" She said it was because many Chinese have entered the United States illegally in the last fifteen years or so—a fact she learned from the Chinese-language newspapers—and that they are desperate to earn money in whatever way possible, so why should she talk to them? In short, she does not trust a Chinese-speaking stranger, either. The point is this: whenever she appears to be confused—the favorite euphemism that health care professionals and social workers use to refer to what they think of as dementia—there are culturally appropriate reasons why she acts that way.

The stroke she had in 2002 damaged the area in her brain that enables human beings to make sense of the sounds they hear. She recovered her ability to communicate in Chinese much better than her ability to communicate in English, but there are occasions when she sounds garbled, regardless of what language she is speaking. Despite this, she *has* been able to communicate with people she trusts—her family doctor, her neighbors, me, my sister, our husbands, my nephew, and her younger brother—fairly clearly and coherently. Whenever she is angry or annoyed, however, she gets agitated and asks people to stop bothering her. What she means by bother is related to the fact that she is a very proud woman who does not like to appear stupid. When other people put her in a situation in which she may appear stupid because she can no longer speak clearly, she gets agitated and her speech indeed will sound like gibberish. She has said repeatedly and emphatically that it does not matter how many more years she lives; what she wants above all else is for everyone (family members, neighbors, doctors, nurses, social workers, *everyone*) to allow her to live in peace and quiet in her own house during the remaining years of her life.

She is so adamant about remaining in her own house because she believes, like many Chinese people, in feng shui (geomancy). She thinks she will die peacefully if she remains in her house because my father, who died in 1992, died quickly without any illness or prolonged suffering. As a devout Buddhist, my mother believes that a good death is as important as a good life. She keeps saying how lucky my father was to have left us without suffering any pain or debilitation. She fervently hopes to have the same good death as my father did. She believes that she will have one only if she continues to live in a house, such as hers, that has good feng shui.

I also want you to know that my mother still knows her mind and can communicate her wishes very emphatically to her family members. When she prepared her advance directive for health care, she made my sister and me promise her that we would never put her in an old-folks home or ask doctors to prolong her life by life support systems or any other extraordinary means. She reminds us that her older sister, who lived in China, died at age ninety-six after suffering from Alzheimer's disease for some fifteen years. My mother does not want to suffer the same fate. She says she has lived a full life and had a very happy ninetieth birthday celebration, so she is ready to go. She doesn't want anybody—and she means *anybody*—to attempt to prolong her life if she becomes a vegetable.

The fact that so many strangers visited her this past month really made her angry. She is especially upset that strangers continued to call her or show up at her front door even after she was discharged from her second hospital stay. She said the nurse at the hospital had told her she is now "off" their list because all her vital signs are good. I checked with the clinical supervisor at that hospital, who confirmed that they had indeed discharged her, not only from the hospital, but also from any posthospitalization care.

I regret to inform you that people like you, who mean well and who want to be helpful, are causing my mother continual distress. In other words, you are making the situation worse and any further visits you make will impede her recovery. You should have the wisdom and culturally sensitive professional understanding to leave her alone while she is recuperating. Not only is she getting better, but her family and neighbors are constantly monitoring how she is doing.

My sister was a caseworker for the Social Security Administration for many years. She understands fully why you, as well as people from other agencies or health care facilities, are required to call or visit my mother. But we cannot persuade our mother to answer your questions unless we are told ahead of time about these calls or visits. The nurse-practitioner who talked to me this morning insisted that my mother had been notified. What she does not understand is that speaking in English in a stern schoolmarmish way to a ninety-year-old woman whose native tongue is not English is not necessarily the most effective way to give prior notice.

Finally, I wish to emphasize to you that my sister and I are not negligent daughters. We are not ignorant children endangering our mother's well-being by letting her live in her own house. Let me assure you that my sister and I know what we are doing. We are determined to enable our mother to remain in her own home as long as possible. If you wonder why my mother has not moved in with either my sister or me, it is because she absolutely does not want to. She says that as she lives out her days, she wants to retain the freedom (a word said clearly in English) to do whatever she likes, whenever she likes. She says that when people hover over her all the time, they make her nervous and she feels as though she is an inmate in a prison or mental hospital ward or old-folks home. I can assure you that if she is not crazy now, such a move, forced on her against her will, will make her crazy faster than any illness or old age will.

The bottom line is this: you are dealing with a strong-willed and capable woman who will strenuously resist letting other people, particularly staff from government agencies, make decisions on her behalf with regard to where and how she lives. In order to carry out my mother's wishes, I have retained an attorney to explain to me the complexities of the law with regard to senior citizens. I expect the attorney to act as an advisor as we negotiate the labyrinth that forms America's health care system and mediate the interventionist social service systems that impinge on my mother's life.

# Happiness in Quotation Marks

## Sunita Puri

Mama is cooking *rajma* downstairs. I can hear the pressure cooker spewing out frightening bursts of air and emitting a garlicky, gingery smell throughout the house. It is a Wednesday, and the house is swollen with heat and heavy with humidity, even at night. I focus on the smells of dinner, on my mother quietly singing to herself, on the dampness of the bedsheets beneath me as I try desperately to forget who is on top of me and what he is doing. I feel myself leave my body and, hovering somewhere near the ceiling, I watch the scene externally, a feeling of detachment settling in as my twenty-year-old cousin finally stops, his breath hard and heavy on my face when he says, "Don't ever mention this to your parents."

Years pass with songs by Sheryl Crow, fat-free mint chocolate chip ice cream, a vision of tears in a high school hallway. Long nights with Algebra II books, of pacing back and forth across my room and cramming facts of world history into my head, of blocking out the nightmares with recitations of active and passive transport in mitochondrial membranes, of the long car rides to the nutritionist, the frenzied gulping of Diet Coke in order to mask the weight I had lost, of feeling and counting every rib before falling asleep at night.

I remember the beginning of high school in these fragments and glimpses that I otherwise try to bury. At the time, I thought that what I was doing was *good* for my body and mind, that the intense discipline of cutting down calories and cutting out snacks would somehow help me to stick to the rigid schedule of studying that I had developed for myself. My "happiness" was reduced to a number on a scale, and it has taken me years to realize that I should put this happiness in quotation marks. More importantly, it has taken me fifteen years to realize that, after my cousin left our home, I began to hate my body for the five years' worth of memories it lodged, for the loss of control these memories represented, for the guilt and shame over the choices I didn't have. And when you hate something that much, all you can do is try to destroy it. After all, my body was a very easy target.

As a chubby child who loved food, I was always chastised by the aunties in my community for eating too much—or at least more than their skinny little daughters did—and dressing poorly and generally not being what a young Indian girl should be. In my *kathak* dance classes, I was always asked to play the role of Krishna, a male Hindu god, because I was just not feminine enough to be a *gopi* or, certainly, Radha. The aunties would shamelessly speak of my fat, my big build, and my mother's inability to take the time to control my eating habits or change my style of dress. "*Chi, chi, chi,*" the aunties would whisper, "what good is her mother's education if she cannot even teach her child how to dress?"

Because I thought that my appearance embarrassed my family, I worked very hard in school to prove that there was *something* about me that could be a source of pride to them and to myself. The skinny little girls lagged behind me in school; I was always placed ahead in math, reading, and science, and the aunties changed their tune slightly: "Well, even though you are fat and ugly it's okay because you'll be educated and have a good job!"

Their cruelty only became more intense when I developed early and was so mortified by my out-of-place breasts that I actually quit *kathak* classes because I could not stand to hear the comments they would make. I worked extra hard in school to divert attention away from my appearance and towards my positive capabilities. School and "achievement" became the ultimate distractions; the more I achieved and the more positive attention I gleaned, the less I dealt with my feelings about myself and my body, and the less my parents asked about my emotional state. As long as I continued to perform at a certain level of academic achievement, they convinced themselves that there was nothing wrong with me. With grades as an emotional barometer, I could safely retreat from the complexities of feelings and real human experience.

In seventh grade, however, I made the decision to lose weight out of concern for my own health, although there was a small part of me that wanted to show my parents that I could look good *and* be an academic superstar. I worked out religiously at the gym and tried to eat better foods, although I never once felt the pressure to deny myself something that I wanted. I lost weight and maintained a healthy weight for my height for about three years, until I began high school.

The line between health and sickness blurred in my mind. As ninth grade progressed, I traded gummy bears for carrot sticks, thinking that I was trading bad eating habits for better health. I cut out all snacks, eating only three meals a day, in the name of rebelling against wasting money on unnecessary food and, in the process, being better to my body. Cutting snacks led to cutting breakfast: if I could do without snacks, maybe I could do without breakfast! And if I could do without breakfast, I could perhaps skip lunch as well. Physiologically, the less food I ate, the lighter and, surprisingly, more energetic I felt. I played on my high school softball team, was actively involved in our physical education class, and felt an emotional freedom that I had not felt in a long time. Psychologically, I felt an independence and a lack of attachment to anyone or anything besides my academic work. For the first time, it did not matter to me if my crush of the week did not notice me in class or say hello to me in the hall; as I lost more weight and I lost my period, I felt no joy over having a clear complexion and fitting into tiny clothes. These things, which earlier would have raised my hopes of guys noticing me, had no emotional resonance in my mind.

Slowly, better health became fewer calories, which became lower weight, which became numbness, which ultimately became anorexia, although I lashed out at anyone and everyone who associated that word with me. Surprisingly, there were very few people who actually did. At the height of my sickness, when I weighed eighty-five pounds (at five feet five inches), I ran into my Spanish teacher from the year before, who commented, "Wow! Sunita, you look great! How did you do it?" Whenever my parents, who were constantly panicked about whether I would last another day, expressed their anger and concern over my health, I simply retorted, "Well, my teacher thinks I look great!"

Despite my statements to the contrary, I was desperately unhappy. No amount of weight loss seemed to fill the enormous emptiness that I felt somewhere in my chest. And yet, what kept me going each day was the thought that when I stepped on my scale in the morning, I may have lost even more weight. My younger brother tried anything and everything to make me laugh, to make me relax and have a normal bowl of cereal with him in the mornings before school. My father became frustrated and gave up on any hope of my eating a normal meal. My mother cried, screamed, and began to fast on Mondays in hopes of God healing me quickly. I was oblivious, completely detached from it all. I lived as I did when my cousin harmed me: floating somewhere nearby, never wholly present, watching from outside my body as life happened to me, controlled despite my feelings of being in control.

To me, anorexia is the ultimate representation of psychosomatic illness, of how social experiences translate into bodily breakdown. Those who gape, aghast, at anorexic women believe their behavior to be voluntary; I call it an involuntary survival strategy. When you're in the throes of a sadness that you do not have the vocabulary to name, all you can think about is keeping your life on track by numbing yourself to the point where emotions are a foreign concept or a figurative four-letter word; reducing your entire life to the tiny things that are manageable actually makes sense. For me, that was food intake. For others, that is sexual promiscuity or abstinence or cutting or drinking or doing drugs or something else that has the potential to be *centering*. And, in my particular cultural context, food was so intertwined with family and with love; a rejection of both certainly was a rejection of a family that did not protect me and that did not allow me the space to ask for protection.

This narrative is less about my experience of one illness and much more about how experiences of violation have fundamentally altered my relationship with my body and therefore the choices I make about preserving or consciously not preserving its health. Painful events have lodged themselves in parts of my body, and I can actually *feel* the onset of memories viscerally before fragments of flashbacks smear their messy details across my mind. I can feel loneliness, anger, and fear in my breasts in particular. One of the "happiest" moments while I was sick was when, while in the shower, I looked down at a flat chest. My breasts had entirely disappeared, and despite how weak, emaciated, and hypoglycemic I was, my face lit up and I actually felt proud of myself for the first time in months. And what exactly was my accomplishment? Literally eliminating a part of my body, forcing a hotbed of memories to shrink out of existence. Despite months of my mind convincing me that I was heavy and needed to lose more weight, at that precise moment I actually felt *light,* as if something emotionally burdensome had simply been lifted from my *chest* in particular.

I did not starve myself to look like Kate Moss. I did not do it because I thought my thighs were too big or my ass was too fat. If I reread my diary entries from that time and think about the context of my starvation, it is totally clear to me that I just did not know of any other way to weave a life around my sexual abuse. How does one simply erase years of pain and abuse in one's own home? The rage that I felt but was unable to communicate or direct towards anyone who was actually responsible became a weapon I used against myself. Guilt, shame, anger, and self-hatred combined with an uneasy relationship with my body; a desire to please others and to strive for perfection proved disastrous. Abandoning a part of my life that I did not choose, erasing events that I did not want and did not have the voice or power to protest, necessarily involved getting rid of every physical and emotional reminder of what had happened. An androgynous body and an emotionally anesthetized mind were my keys to forgetting.

I have served as a domestic violence counselor for my community for years and am a very involved student activist, but there are times when I want to stop it all and give up simply because I am so disappointed by the dynamics within my South Asian American community. It is enormously difficult for me to write these words, especially as a woman in a community that has always tried to suppress the voices of women who have suffered at the hands of men—particularly male family members. I direct my anger, however, not just towards the men who abuse but also towards the women who participate in abuse by denying its existence or, alternatively, creating a context in which young girls such as myself make our bodies the outlet for our anger and pain stemming from abuse. I know that my relationship with my body, and my awareness of its deficits, would have been far different had I grown up in a community where the bodies of daughters were not treated as some sort of representation of good parenting. This treatment of women's bodies is certainly not restricted to the South Asian community, however; the all-American insistence on a certain type of body is problematic enough. But I have felt more watched, more physically evaluated, more judged in every way by women of my community than by white women, or women of any other community for that matter.

Another important component of South Asian immigrant community dynamics that has influenced my disordered eating is the constant preoccupation with what others think or say about one's family. Most of the women I have worked with who live in unbearably abusive families do not feel as though they can assert themselves, let alone leave, because they are so paralyzed by the fear of what other community members would say or think about their decision to leave an abusive marriage. A result of a persistent exposure to this particular community dynamic has resulted in my feeling that the opinions of *others* should structure my actions, thereby feeding my perfectionistic tendencies and my desire to please others. I am not trying to blame my community for my past preoccupation with what others think; but the fact that the opinions of others are so highly valued in South Asian immigrant communities adds to the potency and place it has had in my life.

My ethnicity and position as the daughter of immigrants has also made formal treatment so difficult to conceptualize and find. The dominant medical and psychological discourse on anorexia focuses almost exclusively on white upper-class girls as examples and case studies. And approaches to body image in different, loosely defined "ethnic groups" are often full of stereotypes and demeaning assumptions that actually lead to mistreatment and misdiagnosis of women of color suffering from eating disorders. For example, I often hear that eating disorders are rare in the black community because black women are part of a culture that values bigger women. I hear the same thing about Latina women, and I often hear that Asian American women are naturally thin, making it more likely that physicians or other providers would simply *expect* Asian women to be skinny and thus they overlook a woman possibly engaging in self-starvation or bulimia.

I hate these sweeping stereotypes because of the arrogance and ignorance they simultaneously display, but also because they underscore how invisible people who look like me are in America in general and in medical treatment facilities in particular. Nobody knows *what* the term "South Asian" refers to, let alone how to deal with the particular cultural dynamics that an anorexic Indian

American woman may be trying to negotiate. The ignorance and assumptions I encountered during treatment certainly made treatment much more alienating and difficult. There were at least three therapists who blamed my culture and "Indian family dynamics" for my anorexia. And a nutritionist I briefly visited asked me if I could stop eating Indian food while I was recovering because she had no idea how many starches and fats one serving of *daal* contained. While some of my relationship with my body had also to do with living as a brown girl in white America, the fact that therapists objectified and simplified my difference did not make me feel—or want to feel—any more comfortable in my skin.

I write this essay during the first weeks of medical school—an enormously exciting time when I am thinking intensely about combining the sociocultural and psychosomatic perspectives on health that my experience has afforded me with the biological and structural perspectives that I am learning through anatomy, physiology, and clinical correlates. But it is also a slippery time during which I have confronted my tendency to deal with stress in unhealthy ways.

I doubt that some illness narratives ever really end. I have often debated what defines the "end" of an illness such as anorexia. In fact, I wonder if anorexia is really the true illness of which I write: I tend to think of it much more as the syndrome that brought out the real afflictions that I tried so hard to bury and forget. Perhaps illnesses are mere awakenings—an attempt by the body to force the mind to heal, or to compromise life itself.

One major way I have tried to heal myself is by using my experience to raise awareness of how common sexual abuse is and to refuse to let experiences that I did not ask for or deserve limit my capability to do anything I want to do in this world. While it is difficult for me to do so, I write and speak about my experiences to medical school classes, to members of the South Asian community, and to community health workers so that they might be able to support a client, friend, or loved one who has endured such experiences. Every word written, every phrase spoken, and every ear that listens are all crucial components of my healing.

# Narratives of Advocacy: Activism, Education, and Political Change

℘

THIS SECTION ADDRESSES the use of narrative in public advocacy. It also highlights the role of illness narratives in giving voice to those who are traditionally voiceless and may not have access to public expression, including prisoners, impoverished women, and women with HIV. In this role, narrative facilitates a more public audience for the experience of often silent or silenced women. Narrating becomes a tool of advocacy in itself, a methodology by which otherwise marginalized voices can be heard. The first essay, "Narratives and Advocacy: A Gendered Connection," explores the use of illness narratives in policy making and the fine line between advocates using narrative as strategy and the risk of such narratives becoming co-opted by governmental and political forces, removed from the ill individual's experience, and reduced to anecdotes. The remaining contributions to this section in many ways revisit the problems of narrating illness discussed in section one; they are all based on oral interviews with women experiencing illness. Cheryl Harris Sharman's "Surviving but Not Quite Thriving: Women's Mental Health in East Harlem" is based on interviews with a woman not only struggling with mental illness but also with poverty, alcoholism, gender-based violence, and other physical ailments. This interview study is one in a series that was initiated to advocate for greater understanding of mental health in the inner city, as well as for Medicaid support of working-class women with mental illness. Similarly, Nancy Stoller's collection, "Prisoner Stories: Suffering and Death," chronicles stories gathered from reviewed files of women inmates in California. Although names and details have been changed to protect identity and confidentiality, these stories were utilized in a class-action lawsuit to illustrate the medical neglect that is rampant in the U.S. prison system. Kathy Boudin's narrative is also about the inmate experience; however, hers is a narrative of an insider. Boudin describes the importance of storytelling to her work as an AIDS activist and educator during her incarceration in a maximum security prison and the tricky negotiation of ill prisoners making themselves heard to prison authorities, the outside world, and one another. She also contextualizes within her essay the narrative of a woman who has since died from AIDS but whose voice carries on in her poignant words.

The last two essays of this collection similarly give voice—albeit from the perspective of two physicians—to women whose experiences might not have been heard otherwise. Laurie Rosenblatt's "Teaching about Care at the End of Life Using Creative Nonfiction Monologues" utilizes the oral history of one woman experiencing cancer to discuss the impact of such narratives upon health care trainees at Harvard Medical School. The advocacy of this duo of narratives—Rosenblatt's and her patient's—is in the transformation of future generations of physicians. The advocacy goal here is to "focus learners on their own responses as they begin to look at the personal and professional effects of witnessing suffering." Rita Charon, a physician, literary scholar, and one of the pioneers of American narrative medicine, ends our collection. Although most of the personal narratives in this anthology represent individuals taking the postmodern stance of moving away from physicians' narrative authority, Charon's essay perhaps represents a hopeful future for physician-patient relations. Indeed, her essay begins not with her seeing a patient in her own office, but with the line, "I wanted to see Mrs. Nelson at home, in her own bed." Charon initially "barges" into the room, all doctor, but is soon eased into a community of care around Mrs. Nelson. She utilizes literature and fiction to reflect upon Mrs. Nelson's story, which is also the story of the relationship between Mrs. Nelson and herself. "We can recognize," Charon writes, "with the help of these literary frameworks and fictional texts, that our communities of presence *matter* to ourselves and our patients, that they enact and embody some deep currents within our selves and our culture that yearn toward the genuine and the healing. Such work, perhaps not unlike testimony studies and oral history, gives voice to silenced accounts of suffering and also gives body to instances of care." In giving voice to Mrs. Nelson's otherwise untold story, Charon is simultaneously giving voice to her own story. Theirs is a reciprocal midwifery: illness narrative giving birth to caring narrative while caring narrative gives birth to illness narrative.

The nested stories within stories and voices within voices in this section create a model of connectivity—whereby advocacy and action emerge from the individual experience of suffering, the experience of the witnesses to suffering, and the relationships between them all. Each author in this, our final section, informs and is informed by the stories of other women to whose narratives she gives a platform and an audience.

# Narratives and Advocacy:
# A Gendered Connection

MARSHA HURST AND SAYANTANI DASGUPTA

As a writer, I understand the power of stories. Stories humanize policy, and offer the personal context in which policies and positions actually matter to people. . . . Properly told, stories have the power to move people, to change minds and hearts.

—Musa Mayer, 2005[1]

Musa Mayer, a writer and an advocate, has had metastatic breast cancer. Mayer's above quotation makes clear that advocacy is the connective tissue between illness experience and public change. Advocacy is fueled by life stories, stories that transform illness from an individual experience into a collective phenomenon.

Is making personal narrative publicly actionable a gendered act? Is there a connection between the moral voice of women in our society[2] and their use of that voice as agents of change? Indeed, the public voice that extends directly from the private story has become a characteristically female medium of advocacy, secondary to a collective social history that prohibited women from taking on most public roles. Certainly the feminists of the 1970s built a movement on reconstructing the personal as political. The personal oppression experienced by individual women modeled the oppression of the female sex, and giving individual voice to experience raised the political "consciousness" of the narrators and the listeners who connected to each others' stories. However, one need only look at gay men's activism in the AIDS crisis to realize that this construct of public advocacy, being based on private narrative, community action emerging from individual suffering, has been adopted by many other advocacy movements, particularly when those communities are marginalized and without access to dominant modes of public expression.

Narratives that empower advocacy are what Michael Bury has called "moral narratives." "Moral narratives introduce an evaluative dimension into the links between the personal and the social."[3] The moral narrative struggles with contextualizing the self and then reaching out of that context to accomplish a larger goal.

In the arena of public policy, however, there is an uneasy border between the moral voice of personal narratives and the purposeful construction of these narratives as a strategic tool. The effective narrative in a public policy arena is one that links compelling personal experience with the more abstract issues of value and morality. The most direct use of personal stories involves personal testimony at public, usually legislative, hearings. Personal stories motivate public policy; they can serve as a basis for knowing how to craft that policy; and they clearly empower the support needed to pass legislation. If successful, the story may come to embody a policy directive. However, there is also a potential for these stories to take on a life beyond that of the teller—a potential for them to be directly or indirectly co-opted. The personal-to-political strategies of the 1970's feminist movement had an obvious cultural impact on public life in the United States, in negative and positive ways. The strategy of using personal stories to have political impact was once uncommon, and perhaps revolutionary. In recent times, however, there is a social recognition of the importance of personal stories that arguably did not exist in the same form prior to the feminist movement. One need only look at modern presidential campaigns, with their hunger to incorporate the stories of "everyman" and "everywoman," to realize that even the most dominant cultural forums have now recognized the power of the personal story. This in no way negates the importance of personal storytelling, but it makes it more necessary than ever for us to listen to stories with a critical, discerning ear and to ask questions such as who is telling the story, whose agenda is the story serving, and of course, does this story enhance or obscure other voices and other stories?

Legislative testimonies are narratives with a political purpose. They are most effective when the stories are factually accurate, coherent, and connected to relevant and important values.[4] The clearest examples of personal stories that empower legislation are found in laws named for the teller or victim of the story. In these instances, the story connects a lived experience with a social issue, and consequently a person wronged with a public policy solution. In recent history, the stories of personal experience that have most successfully led to public action have been stories of children, particularly female children. Megan's Law, for example, the best-known state sex-offender law, requires notification if a known sex offender is released in the community. The law keeps the iconic image of the seven-year-old New Jersey girl, who in 1994 was "lured into her neighbor's home with the promise of a puppy and was brutally raped and murdered," in the public's awareness.[5] Megan's story raises some complex issues for both children's advocates and those who advocate for self-stories in general. It is clear that what happened to Megan is unspeakably atrocious, and that as a society we are interested in safeguarding all children from such occurrences. Yet children who are sexually assaulted are most likely to be assaulted by someone they know, and so laws like Megan's Law effectively obscure this aspect of the wider story of child sexual abuse by playing into parents' concerns regarding sexual abuse from strangers.

In addition, Megan's identity as not only a child but a female child may have much to do with both her personal story and the story of Megan's Law. Our cultural construction of the "vulnerable child"—whether male or female—is in fact heavily gendered. If the swooning nineteenth-century female invalid—set in stark contrast to the capable, intellectually powerful male physician—was the iconic passive victim of her time, then it can be argued that the child is her modern equivalent. Children embody a kind of voiceless vulnerability, and the child who suffers from illness has always been the most poignant embodiment of the "innocent victim," and thus of the moral compulsion to act. This action is most often in the paternalistic model, such that the narrative becomes one of passive (read female) vulnerability protected, rescued, and ultimately spoken for by dominant (read male) cultural institutions such as medicine, law enforcement, or government. This narrative helps legitimize the power of these institutions while contributing to their unimpeachability.

The Katie Beckett Act is familiar to almost every parent whose child has a severe long-term health condition. The act provides state-based Medicaid waivers so that children with special health care needs can be cared for at home. Katie Beckett's story, usually told by her mother, Julie, is almost an American allegory. The young child is very sick. Her loving family wants to take care of her at home and the doctors agree, but the family is middle class and made destitute by the child's illness; they cannot pay for care at home, and government insurance will only pay for care in the hospital. Katie's mother's story reaches a local representative, who corners the vice president on an airplane, and the vice president brings the story to the president's attention. President Reagan[6] had been looking for just such powerful examples of government "overregulation," and the Katie Beckett waiver for home care was born. In this story, one mother's narrative changes political history. The route from the personal to the political, from the family to the president, has a movie-perfect ending. Simultaneously, of course, Katie Beckett's story gains a life beyond Katie, her family, or even the Medicaid waiver with her name. Her narrative is utilized by a government with its own political agenda while in the broader sense it protects that government from critique. How can we criticize those who heroically help to protect the most innocent and vulnerable among us?[7]

Of course not all personal stories that become public campaigns are female stories, but the vulnerability suggested by a female narrative is clearly important to the frequent success of children's stories in compelling action. The Ryan White Act[8] is an oft-cited example of a story that was used to compel an unusually rapid organization of effective advocacy in health policy, funding, and legislation.[9] Ryan White, age sixteen (two years before he died), told his own story in testimony before the president's commission on AIDS, connecting his suffering from AIDS with suffering from the stigma of AIDS.[10] Yet even though Ryan White was able to quite literally speak on his own behalf, his narrative has suffered to a great extent the fate of many other "vulnerable victim" narratives: the story has been in many ways hijacked. Despite his own testimony urging recognition of AIDS-related stigma, Ryan White's story was, and perhaps is still, publicly constructed as the story of the "innocent" victim and is cited in stark contrast to the stories of "guilty" victims—those who acquired HIV through sex or drug use. Indeed, unlike Ryan White, most children are quite literally voiceless in that they do not have access to public forums of expression, and like White, they usually do not have the social power to either construct or contradict others' construction of their stories.

In policy making, the way the problem to be solved is defined is a function of how the "causal story" is constructed.[11] This means that a situation "comes to be seen as caused by human actions and amendable to human intervention." Causal stories "describe harms and difficulties, attribute them to actions of other individuals or organizations, and thereby claim the right to invoke government power to stop the harm."[12] The causal stories discussed here have moved occurrences from unintended to intentional: cancer is not a random occurrence but preventable by government action; we may not have intended a child to be so sick, but we can prevent her further suffering through legislation. The story that reframes an illness into an occurrence in which preventable harm is done often has a gendered core of caring and caregiving, no matter the sex of the narrator-advocate.

Paul Gelsinger tells a causal story about his son Jesse's death in a gene therapy trial at the University of Pennsylvania in September 1999. Jesse Gelsinger had barely turned eighteen, the age of medical consent, when he volunteered for a gene therapy trial. He had a mild form of the genetic disorder ornithine trans-carbamylase (OTC) deficiency syndrome, which was successfully managed; but, at the researchers' request, he volunteered for the trial, purely to help "newborns and other children." He died soon after enrolling in the trial.

Paul Gelsinger, who is now a public advocate for the protection of human subjects in research, tells Jesse's story frequently, connecting the story to moral values and public policy. The power of Paul's narrative is in the suffering of a parent, but also in the narrative construction of trust betrayed. It is a tale of intentionality—the researchers did not mean to kill Jesse, but they did knowingly put him at additional risk and intentionally hid that risk.[13]

Paul's testimony to the U.S. Senate explicitly constructs the causal story: "I have read that my son's death has been called by one of the leaders in this field as 'a pothole' on the road to gene therapy. His death was no pothole. It was an avoidable tragedy from which I will never recover." And by defining the problem as intentional deception, he has identified the public policy solution: government must be vigilant in its oversight of human subjects research so that "no more fathers lose their sons."[14] Only then will the government deserve our trust.

Testimony before policy-making bodies gives us the clearest example of how stories are constructed to influence policy. Causal-story testimony narrates a personal history, and the construction of that history is related to the type of policy it sets out to influence. It is typically a story of the innocent victim wronged by the failure of those charged with keeping the victim safe. There is a direct wrongdoer—the doctor, the attacker, the drunk driver—but the real cause of the tragedy is the failure of the government to protect the public. And the solution is the policy that would enhance that protection and prevent future tragedies.

Over a decade ago, Catherine Reissman asked the critical question about oral histories: "Why was the story told that way?"[15] Iconic stories that influence legislation or policy are told with an explicit purpose, and they are constructed to further that purpose. But sometimes stories take on a meaning that is detached from the body giving them voice. They are reconstructed and removed from the integrity of personal experience. And in this distancing there is risk of damage to the advocacy cause itself.

The Nelene Fox story is one such example. Fox, a thirty-nine-year-old mother of three, was diagnosed with breast cancer in 1991 and was soon found to have metastatic disease. Her insurer, Health Net, refused her request for autologous bone marrow transplant (ABMT), stating it did not cover "investigational" procedures. With the aid of seventeen hundred donors, the Fox family raised $210,000. Fox underwent the treatment in 1992 and died a few months later. Her husband and attorney brother sued Health Net for their refusal to pay, and the jury ruled in favor of the family. The award, $89.1 million, was the largest ever levied against an insurance company for refusing to provide health coverage benefits.[16]

The Nelene Fox story became an allegory: the evil insurance company denies coverage for a life-saving therapy and the victim dies; the story—and the AMBT-therapy bandwagon effect it was said to have caused—is blamed for the delay in obtaining clinical trial results that seven years later showed ABMT, a tortuous therapy to undergo, to be more costly and no more effective than conventional therapy. The story is believed to have prevented evidence-based scientific data from being collected and applied, and thus to have acted against the best interests of patients. Twenty thousand women underwent a bone marrow transplant for metastatic breast cancer before clinical trials results showed that ABMT therapy provided no additional treatment benefit.

The American advocacy community tells this story over and over as a warning about jumping on story-driven bandwagons. Interestingly, it is told as an admonition to women and to advocates, not to the physicians who treated these thousands of women with an unproven therapy. It is really a thrice-told tale: first told by Nelene Fox's family and friends to raise money and then to sue the insurance company; then told by women and their physicians to encourage use of an unproven therapy; and now told by advocates as a warning about the power of stories.

Stories also become detached from their moral voice when they become formulaic—in other words, no longer truly personal narratives. Barbara Ehrenreich, in "Welcome to Cancerland: A Mammogram Leads to a Cult of Pink Kitsch," confronts advocacy itself in her own personal story.[17] Her journey to "cancerland" begins with simultaneous exposure to a suspicious mammogram and a pink-ribboned teddy bear. At once she enters the world of breast cancer treatment, breast cancer culture, breast cancer advocacy, and the industry that feeds off of breast cancer itself. Ehrenreich's personal journey is also a devastating critique—of the science that chooses treatment over prevention, of the breast cancer organizations that feed on corporate support, of the "ultrafeminine" marketplace of breast cancer products (not the least of which are infantilizing teddy bears), of the thousands of Web-posted stories (mostly upbeat narratives with uplifting moral messages), and of breast cancer advocacy itself. Narratives used to raise money for advocacy organizations are the acceptable stories of the "redemptive powers of the disease." In this "seamless world of breast cancer culture . . . cheerfulness is more or less mandatory, dissent a kind of treason.[18] The stories Ehrenreich finds on breast cancer Web sites have lost their moral authority.

"The plural of anecdote is policy," says Daniel Fox, president of the Milbank Memorial Fund, a health-related foundation that publishes *The Millbank Quarterly.*[19] Fox's pejorative use of the term "anecdote" instead of "story" echoes a concern of some analysts, advocates, and even policymakers over the power of narrative, implying a juxtaposition of narrative knowledge with "scientific" knowledge. "Using narrative to make public policy," says former Massachusetts state legislator John McDonough, "requires the same standards of validity as those applied to case study. Lack of accountability is the bane of storytelling in the policy environment. A story needs to be true and presented in a context that does not distort its relevance to the policy choice at hand."[20]

Pierre Bourdieu suggests that "narratives about the most 'personal' difficulties, the apparently most strictly subjective tensions and constrictions, frequently articulate the deepest structures of the social world and their contradictions."[21] This is certainly true of narratives used in advocacy. There is a tension, however, between the power of a personal life story, power that resides in its experiential uniqueness and voice, and the purpose of advocacy, which is to construct meaning for a larger public. The power of one story is in its personal truth, while the power of collective public voice is in its commonality. In the world of advocacy, narrative knowledge is often expressed as a drive toward using the personal illness experience to engage the public, toward making the narrative actionable. The drive to make the personal public may inherently manipulate and even distort the personal truth.

Giving voice to our stories means giving structure to those stories, giving them form that will always be related to the purpose of their telling. And in advocacy, giving voice to a story is about the connection between the personal experience and the public purpose. The way we tell our stories will attribute cause, blame, responsibility—and point to a way to make the world better for someone else. And if in the process we give coherence to the story by telling it again and again, as Arthur Kleinman says,[22] we also may be giving the story a life—an embodiment of message and meaning—that departs from the body of the teller for a greater good. In order to maintain the advocacy power of women's narratives and to protect their stories from becoming anecdotes, advocates need to guard the integrity of these stories and monitor their uses. The important role women have played in empowering advocacy through narrative threatens to be lost, or perhaps overwhelmed, by the plethora of stories constructed or even solicited for a narrow purpose.

## NOTES

1. Mayer, Musa. "When Clinical Trials Are Compromised: A Perspective from a Patient Advocate," *PLoS Medicine* 2 (2005): 358.

2. See, for example, Carol Gilligan's seminal 1982 book, *In a Different Voice: Psychological Theory and Women's Development*, reissue edition (Cambridge, MA: Harvard UP, 1993).

3. Michael Bury, "Illness Narratives: Fact or Fiction?" *Sociology of Health and Illness* 23 (2001): accessed from Ebsco Host 6 Oct. 2004.

4. Walter R. Fisher, *Human Communication as Narration: Toward a Philosophy of Reason, Value, and Action* (Columbia: U of South Carolina P, 1987).

5. *Parents for Megan's Law*, 4 Feb. 2006 <http://www.parentsformeganslaw.com/html/questions.lasso>.

6. Reagan, perhaps not surprisingly for an actor, is often referred to as the president who started the incorporation of "story" into political voice.

7. Patricia Guthrie, "Waiver's Namesake Advocates for Kids," *Atlanta Journal-Constitution*, 15 Oct. 2005 <http://www.familyvoices.org/hcf/ma-kbw.htm>; Julie Beckett, "The Long Road Home," *Exceptional Parent* 26.6 (June 1996): 68–69.

Katie Beckett herself is now a founding and active member of an advocacy organization called Kids as Self Advocates (KASA), a part of the Family Voices project funded by government and private foundations. As a disability rights activist, she now lives the back story of successful child-health advocacy; see Katie Beckett, "The Katie Beckett Story, *KASA*, Family Voices, 4 Feb. 2006 <http://www.fvkasa.org/katie_story.asp>.

8. The full name of the act is the Ryan White Comprehensive AIDS Resources Emergency (CARE) Act.

9. C. C. Poindexter, "Promises in the Plague: Passage of the Ryan White Comprehensive AIDS Resources Emergency Act as a Case Study for Legislative Action," *Health and Social Work* 24 (1999).

10. Ryan White, "Ryan White's Testimony before the Presidential Commission on AIDS, 4 Feb. 2006 <http://www.geocities.com/SoHo/Exhibit/8222/rwtest.htm>.

11. Deborah Stone, "Causal Stories and the Formation of Policy Agendas," *Political Science Quarterly* 104 (1989): 281–300.

12. Stone 281–82.

13. Sheryl Gay Stolberg, "The Biotech Death of Jesse Gelsinger," 31 Oct. 2005 <http://www.frenchanderson.org/history/biotech.pdf>.

14. Paul Gelsinger, "Gene Therapy: Is There Oversight for Patient Safety?" hearing before the Subcommittee on Public Health of the Committee on Health, Education, Labor, and Pensions, U.S. Senate, 106th Congress, 2nd sess., 2 Feb. 2000 (Washington, DC: GPO, 2000) 106–447. (Y 4.L 11/4:S.HRG. 106–447.)

15. Catherine Kohler Riessman, *Narrative Analysis* (Newbury Park: Sage, 1993) 2.

16. H. Gilbert Welch and Juliana Mogielnicki, "Presumed Benefit: Lessons from the American Experience with Marrow Transplantation for Breast Cancer," *British Medical Journal* 324 (2002): 1088–92.

17. Barbara Ehrenreich, "Welcome to Cancerland: A Mammogram Leads to a Cult of Pink Kitsch," *Harper's* 303 (Nov. 2001): 43–53.

18. Ehrenreich 49, 50.

19. Fitzhugh Mullan "Me and the System: The Personal Essay and Health Policy," *Health Affairs* 18 (1999): accessed from Proquest Direct 4 Feb. 2006.

20. John E. McDonough, "Using and Misusing Anecdote in Policy Making," *Health Affairs* 20 (2001): accessed from Proquest Direct 4 Feb. 2006.

21. Pierre Bourdieu, "The Contradictions of Inheritance," *The Weight of the World: Social Suffering in Contemporary Society*, ed. Pierre Bourdieu et al. (Palo Alto, CA: Stanford UP, 1993) 511.

22. Arthur Kleinman, *The Illness Narratives: Suffering, Healing, and the Human Condition* (NewYork: Basic Books, 1988).

# Stories from the Inside

KATHY BOUDIN

In the prison that I inhabited for more than two decades, storytelling is a basic form of communication among the women: "grief stories" told in a family violence support group or on the shoulder of a friend in a cell; "war stories" about illegal acts where women got away or landed in prison; fantasy stories about the good life lived under conditions of poverty and abuse until this arrest broke it up; stories shared with children on visits to try and hold together the family that may or may not have existed before; and life stories, stories told and written with laughter and tears about the paths of our lives. Women tell and retell the stories of their own lives in order to piece together the meaning of their lives. It was therefore no surprise that narratives—both oral and written—ended up playing a critical role inside the prison population when the AIDS epidemic swept into the prison like a tornado and stayed instead of moving on.

In a 1988 blind study, close to 20 percent of the women coming into the prison tested HIV positive.[1] Families of women on the outside were disintegrating, and inside the prison, even as women in neighboring cells disappeared and died within weeks, the word "AIDS" was not said aloud. Fear, shame, and stigma kept us uneducated and quiet, no different from most of society. We all lived together, yet women died alone.

Telling stories was central to how we created a community inside the prison as the means of coping with the epidemic. After getting permission from the superintendent to organize around the crisis, thirty-five women sat around a table, each of us sharing what led us to want to do something about AIDS in the prison. One woman told the story of her sister dying of AIDS, her nephew left behind, eight years old and HIV positive. Another told a story of how women on her living unit were so afraid that certain people might be HIV positive that everyone was whispering about them and wouldn't sit near them on the couch. Another woman bravely said, "I am HIV positive" and told a story about how, when she left an open pack of cigarettes out on a table in the day room, in spite of how driven people were for cigarettes, no one would touch them. By telling our stories out loud, we broke a silence and began to transcend our isolated experiences of fear and suffering. The stories created a "we" from the "affected" and "infected" and were the basis for the community that helped us cope with the epidemic.

People use narratives to understand their own lives. Human beings rely on the narrative organization of experience as a way of both giving meaning individually and communicating.[2] In recent years, much has been written about the role of storytelling for individuals facing illness. Arthur Frank, in *The Wounded Storyteller: Body, Illness, and Ethics,* writes that for individuals to give voice to their illness is to no longer be defined by external definitions of their illness, including those of medicine. In reclaiming their stories, they reclaim themselves.[3] In prison, this notion is made more complex by the layers of definition imposed upon incarcerated individuals. Not just being ill, but the very definition of being a convict, a criminal, a prisoner, someone defined by a number living in a cell, strips the ill inmate of the power of self-definition. Storytelling is a way for women to assert their humanity in the face of illness and imprisonment. In *Intoxicated by My Illness: And Other Writings on Life and Death,* Anatole Broyard writes,

> The patient has to start by treating his illness not as a disaster, an occasion for depression or panic, but as a narrative, a story. Stories are antibodies against illness and pain. . . . I think that language, speech stories, or narratives are the most effective ways to keep our humanity alive. To remain silent is literally to close down the shop of one's humanity.[4]

In prison almost everyone had a story to tell about AIDS: those who were ill with HIV or AIDS, as well as those who were affected by the illness of family members and friends; those who were afraid because of behaviors that put them at risk or who were made afraid by their own fears or by living together so closely in prison. In prison, faced with the AIDS epidemic, we relied on narratives and stories to build a culture of survival, empathy, recognition, memory, and struggle for change.

Over the next months, we became educated about HIV and AIDS ourselves and then set out to change the awareness inside the prison. We divided ourselves into small groups to lead discussions, always with a woman who was HIV positive and willing to talk openly about it—a PWA (person with AIDS); that was the term being used at the time in the AIDS movement by those who were willing to be open about their status. We spoke to large numbers of women in the prison population, going to their living units and classrooms—telling stories and asking for their stories. The purpose was to build amongst ourselves a consciousness and an openness that would lead to empathy to replace stigma and fear. In some ways, this process was parallel to the 1970's feminist movement's reliance on personal narratives. Women told their personal stories of how the AIDS epidemic was affecting them because it helped them individually; at the same time, out of the stories came a collective consciousness and potential for collective change. This was the beginning stage of our organization that we called ACE, AIDS Counseling and Education, that went on to become a program in the prison through which prisoners could become educated, educate, counsel, and comfort each other. And out of this program women became advocates for one another both in the prison and when they went home.

We told stories not only to increase awareness, but in remembrance of those of us who died. When the inevitability of death hovered over us, we promised women that if they died, we would hold a memorial and their lives would be honored, the story of their lives told. And as woman after woman died, we held to the promise. The memorials were held in the presence of their quilt panels, painted by friends of the woman—drawings of her favorite song, food or cigarettes, and sayings that she was known by. Then friends would stand and tell a story, something about the woman who had died, something funny, something personal, something that continued her presence among us.

When we decided to write a book, *Breaking the Walls of Silence: AIDS and Women in a New York State Maximum Security Prison*,[5] it was clear that the book would be told as a narrative to convey how we, as women in prison, took on the challenge of the AIDS epidemic. The book would be made up of many voices, telling the stories by those who were part of the process—their memories of the early days when there were no medicines, little knowledge among the doctors and the fear that led people to die alone with no one around and no name for what they died from. The narratives would keep alive the history of the struggle that we went through as a community and hopefully inspire others.

Arthur Frank says that rarely is there a collective voice because of the privatization of medicine that isolates people.[6] Yet the women's health movement, the disability movement, and the AIDS movement are all exceptions, examples of people coming together and transcending the individual isolation of coping with illness.

When Katrina Haslip was preparing to leave prison at a time when there were no medicines other than AZT and Bactrim, the timing coincided with the beginning work on the book. Katrina had become a leading force in the ACE program, and she was an open PWA after years of silence. She was preparing to go home on parole and was committed to activism "in the street," as we referred to the broader society outside of prison. The book project became a vehicle for her to write about her personal development. Katrina wrote in the tradition of *testimonios*, a form of narrative bearing witness to a social urgency, usually by those who have been silenced, excluded, and marginalized by society.[7] She wrote the story of her own transformation for the community that had embraced her and given her the strength to break her silence to become an open leader in the struggle over HIV and AIDS.

I often ask myself how it is that I came to be open about my status. For me, AIDS had been one of my best-kept secrets. It took me approximately fifteen months to discuss this issue openly. I could not bring myself to say it out loud. As if not saying it would make it go away. I watched other people with AIDS who were much more open than I was at the time reveal to audiences their status and their vulnerability. I wanted to be a part of what they were building, what they were doing, their statement, "I am a person with AIDS," a "PWA," because I was.

Somewhere behind a prison wall in Bedford Hills a movement or community was being built. It was a diverse group of women teaming together to meet the needs and fears that had developed with this new epidemic, AIDS. These women believed that none of their peers should be discriminated against, isolated, or treated cruelly merely because they were ill. They believed that it was necessary for this prison to build an environment of support, comfort, education, and trust. I was a part of this process. In the center of its establishment I stood, struggling with my own personal issues of HIV infection.

While held in some sort of limbo, I felt as if the women of ACE had built a cocoon around me, for me. I felt warmed by them and so totally understood. These were the women who understood my silence and yet felt my need to be heard. They gave me comfort when I needed it and an ear when I needed a listener. They helped me to grow stronger with hopes that one day I would be able to stand alone and still feel as safe. Empowered! I took from them all that they were capable of putting out. I gave back to them what I was given. It was as if I mirrored back what they put out. I had never before noticed in my peers this ability to care so deeply. For I, too, had labeled them prisoners, cold and uncaring. Yet they had managed to build a community of women: black, white, Hispanic, learned, illiterate, robbers, murderers, forgers, rich, poor, Christian, Muslim, Jewish, bisexual, gay, heterosexual—all putting aside their differences and egos for a collective cause, to help themselves. I could not believe my eyes. Right before me lay a model of how we, as a whole, needed to combat all the issues AIDS brought, and we were building it from behind a wall, from prison. We were the community that no one thought would help itself. Social outcasts, because of our crimes against society, in spite of what society inflicted upon some of us.

We emerged from nothingness with a need to build consciousness and to save lives. We made a difference in our community behind the wall, and that difference has allowed me to survive and thrive as a person with AIDS. To my

peers in Bedford Hills Correctional Facility, you have truly made a difference.
I can now go anywhere, and stand openly, alone without the silence.
> Katrina Haslip, 1990[8]

When *Breaking the Walls of Silence* finally arrived in galley form we celebrated. Inmates who were part of the ACE organization, civilian staff, prison administrators, and guests gathered in the ACE office, while Katrina, with Carmen (another key PWA from early ACE years), both of whom had been paroled, came back into the prison to participate. Katrina was rolled into the office in a wheel chair, a smile spreading out from under the white gauze mask covering her face, and she was holding a copy of the book on her lap. Carmen walked with a cane; her thick hair that she had cherished was so thin that she looked like a different person. She moved with austere dignity. After eating and celebrating, we formed our traditional circle, and holding hands we sang our theme song—"Sister": "Lean on me, I am your sister, lean on me, I am your friend. . . ."[9] Katrina died one month later, and Carmen, three months later. Each of their narratives, along with all of the other women's stories in the book, continue as a living force. These narratives both reveal and contribute to the critical reciprocal relationship between the individual and the community in coping with the AIDS epidemic.

## NOTES

1. New York State Department of Health, *Focus on AIDS in New York State,* AIDS in Prison Project Fact Sheet 26 (Apr. 1994), newsletter ed. Miki Conn (Albany, NY: NYS Department of Health AIDS Institute, 1994).

2. Jerome Bruner, *Acts of Meaning* (Cambridge, MA: Harvard UP, 1990).

3. Arthur Frank, *The Wounded Storyteller: Body, Illness, and Ethics* (Chicago: U of Chicago P, 1995).

4. Anatole Broyard, *Intoxicated by My Illness: And Other Writings on Life and Death.* (New York: C. Potter, 1992) 20.

5. The Members of the ACE Program (AIDS Counseling and Education) of the Bedford Hills Correctional Facility, *Breaking the Walls of Silence: AIDS and Women in a New York State Maximum Security Prison* (New York: Overlook, 1998).

6. Frank 1–25.

7. W. G. Tierney, "Undaunted Courage: Life History and the Postmodern Challenge," *Handbook of Qualitative Research*, Norman K. Denzin and Yvonna S. Lincoln, eds. (Thousand Oaks, CA: Sage, 2000) 537–53.

8. Katrina Haslip, "Forward," *Breaking the Walls of Silence* 9–10.

9. Cris Williamson, "Sister," *The Changer and the Changed*, 1975; reissued 2005 by Wolf Moon Records.

# Prisoner Stories:
# Suffering and Death

## Nancy E. Stoller

In 1998, lawyers for plaintiffs in *Shumate v. Wilson,* a class-action lawsuit challenging women prisoners' lack of access to health care in three large California prisons, invited me to review several thousand pages of depositions to generate a statistical overview of the problems that these women were encountering.[1]

My research staff and I were deeply moved by the accounts that emerged from prisoners' letters and interviews. Reviewers would sometimes cry as they read through the files. During our project we constructed over one hundred narratives summarizing individual women's stories. The narratives demonstrate traumatic—and often futile—attempts to see a doctor or a nurse-practitioner. In them we could see detailed the process through which adequate health care was not provided, as well as the dire consequences.

Medical neglect is a prime theme that runs through the stories: medications are not handed out on time, treatment is delayed, and follow-up is missing. Women with HIV/AIDS, gynecological problems (including pregnancy), hypertension, asthma, orthopedic problems, injuries, and a wide array of other health problems report forbidding obstacles as they seek effective and humane treatment. Some delays are even years in length. In numerous cases, the pains of chronic disability and the final throes of illness are accentuated by institutional barriers and punitive discounting of human needs.

Of our many narratives, I have selected seven to give the reader a sense of what life can be like for a woman prisoner with a serious health problem. Details are changed when necessary to protect the confidentiality and identity of the prisoner. All names have been changed.

### "Heavenly Jones"

*A twelve-hour delay in treating a stroke*

At 6 A.M. Heavenly Jones woke her roommate by tapping on her bed. The roommate jumped down from her bunk to find Ms. Jones breathing with much difficulty, phlegm running from her mouth and her eyes glazed. One side of her body was paralyzed, and she was waving her other arm uncontrollably. She had also urinated on herself.

The roommate hit the emergency button and pounded on the window. A guard was the first to respond. She asked him to get the MTA (medical technical assistant, a person who functions simultaneously as a guard and nurse's aide). After being alerted by phone, the MTA called a prison nurse, who refused to come. The nurse told the guard "to see if it was really a stroke" and, if it was, to call the prison's in-house fire department. The guard reported to Ms. Jones's roommate that the MTA did not want to come unless it was an emergency. The roommate informed him that it *was* an emergency, so he phoned the fire department.

Soon the fire department arrived with two prisoners and the driver. The roommate does not know if any of them had medical training. They came with one oxygen tank that they did not use. By the time an outside ambulance arrived at approximately 7 P.M. (thirteen hours after Ms. Jones's stroke), she was paralyzed and unable to speak. She was transferred back from the local hospital to the prison infirmary about two weeks later, and the roommate is afraid Heavenly will not receive any physical or speech therapy.


## "Gloria Anthony"

*Twenty-three month delay in ordering treatment for a tumor*

One February, Gloria Anthony found a mass at the base of her neck. A prison doctor referred her to a surgeon.

Three months later, a sonogram and X-ray of the neck were ordered. A month after that, she said the mass was causing pain and headaches. The X-ray showed muscle spasm and disc narrowing, but no mass. Six weeks later, Gloria saw a surgeon, who advised removing the lump, but nothing was done.

Four and a half months later, she was again diagnosed with the mass, and an orthopedic reevaluation was ordered. Two weeks later a neurological consult was obtained, which found the lump and again advised surgery. Finally, after another month, the prison's medical review committee recommended removal of the mass by surgery. Almost a year later at the time of her last interview, the mass was still there.


## "Daphne Christian"

*Punitive treatment during end-stage disease*

At the time of her last interview, Daphne Christian had hepatitis B and C, advanced cirrhosis of the liver, and end-stage liver disease. She had ascites, a very swollen abdomen, difficulty eating and holding down food, pitting edema of entire lower extremities, severe, sharp pains in the area of her liver, and white or tan stools. Her liver medication had been discontinued, and when she asked why, she was told, "It won't do any good." She was told that she was on the list for a liver transplant but was not hopeful that she would get one. She feared dying in prison.

A doctor threatened that if she wouldn't accept assignment to the SNF (skilled nursing facility, also referred to as the infirmary by many patients) permanently, he would discontinue her meds. She didn't move because she didn't want to give up her job, her cell, and her "good time" (which she was generating daily by working). The doctor discontinued her potassium, Lasix, Lactulose, spironolactone, Tagamet, muscle relaxer, and pain medication, leaving her on only some psych meds. She and the doctor got into an argument and she called him an asshole, so he wrote her up and she lost some good time. As her legal adviser writes, "Her present punitive denial of care by the CMO (chief medical officer) puts her at risk for cirrhotic hepatic coma, peritonitis, pneumonia, renal failure, and essentially alienates her from her only source of medical care."

Her denture plate was seized by staff as contraband and thrown in the garbage. She needs her dentures to eat and cannot eat with prison-issue dentures, as she has major bone loss in her jaw. She waited weeks to get treated for bronchitis and was given aspirin, even though it's contraindicated for people with end-stage liver disease. She cannot get a special diet.

## "AUDRE CLIFTON"

*Eighteenth-month delay correcting an infected surgical pin*

Audre Clifton's leg was smashed in a severe automobile accident several years ago. Her leg and ankle were reconstructed with many pins and plates before her incarceration. While incarcerated, she began complaining of intense pain and visited sick call numerous times. Her skin began to be pierced by the hardware in her ankle, and the skin became red and filled with pus. The area became obviously infected and yet the prison continually ignored her repeated requests for surgery. She filed several formal complaints regarding the delayed surgery. The pain was so bad and the problem so clear that housing staff helped her request an emergency visit. After months of complaining of intense pain, she was scheduled for removal of the pin, but the outside appointment was canceled because she was not given a pass to see a doctor (no explanation for the cancellation was given). The surgery was not actually performed until nine months later—almost a full year after she began to request help.

## "Marie Compton"

*Grossly inadequate treatment after extensive burns*

Marie Compton suffered severe burns on over 50 percent of her body. When she was incarcerated, she had only one pair of custom-made pressure garments. Outside contacts attempted to send in other prescribed pressure garments, but these packages were refused and sent back. As a result, her burns began to show massive scarring. She was forced to wear the same one garment for months without washing it. This is completely unhygienic and dangerous to her condition—it is likened to wearing the same pair of underwear for months on end. She was also denied physical therapy at the prison. As a result, her muscles tightened up and she was unable to walk. She spent most of her time in a wheelchair that was unsafe and difficult to maneuver on her own. When she was finally able to stand up, she could only do so on the tips of her toes because the muscles were too short. She also had extreme difficulty getting the medications she needed. Pain meds and lotions to help the burns heal were prescribed by outside doctors, but often they were never ordered. She wasn't even able to get olive oil to help loosen the skin.

## "Rosa Prentice"

*Lack of follow-up care leads first to systemic infection and later to blindness in one eye*

Rosa Prentice has advanced sickle cell anemia. She has a lifeport that needs to be cleaned once a month. If someone does not clean it, she becomes dangerously susceptible to infections and severe illness. At one point, her lifeport had not been cleaned for six weeks. Because of this, Rosa developed a massive systemic infection and a severe case of pneumonia.

Rosa also has had severe complications with her eyes as a result of the sickle cell anemia. In August 2000 she went to her prison doctor and told him that the vision in her left eye was worsening. He said he didn't like the look of it but was not an ophthalmologist, so he decided to send her to the hospital that night. At the hospital, the doctor wouldn't tell her what was wrong, only that she needed surgery immediately. The next day, as she was going under for the surgery, the doctor told her that there was no guarantee that the operation would work. When she awoke, they told her a blood clot had formed and caused severe nerve damage. She had probably lost most of the vision in her eye permanently. She immediately went into a severe depression and sickle cell crisis and was given two units of blood and released to the prison five days after the surgery.

Four months later, the hospital ophthalmologist recommended another surgery to remove the cataract on the same eye to see if it would help her vision.

However, he had never worked with a sickle cell patient before, so Ms. Prentice wanted the opinion of a specialist before getting more eye surgery. This delayed her surgery an additional month.

## "Harriett Marcus"

*Inadequate care leads to a miscarriage*

Harriett Marcus was one month pregnant when she arrived at prison. There she received blood tests, vitamins, and calcium, and the baby's heartbeat was checked. She was transferred to another facility along with other pregnant women, supposedly because they would receive better care. At this facility Harriett began to have a thick brown discharge. A doctor gave her Monistat for a yeast infection, but the infection only became more irritated. Then Harriett felt the baby "balling up" inside her, but a nurse denied her permission to see a doctor.

Harriett was previously a nurse's aide and therefore she knows how to read blood pressures. Hers was often 140/100, which she knew was high. One night, she felt the baby continually "balling up and releasing." So she went to an MTA, who, after checking her, said that he couldn't detect a heartbeat. She went to a nurse who sent her to a doctor who finally sent her to the infirmary. At the infirmary, two MTAs argued in her presence about whether or not they should send her back to her unit because the ultrasound was unavailable. They finally called a doctor, who sent her to the hospital. At the hospital, the ultrasound confirmed that there was no heartbeat. Later, when she requested a copy of the autopsy and pathology report, she was told by the prison medical service there was nothing like this on file.

## Notes

1. For more information about this project, see Nancy Stoller, "Improving Access to Health Care for California's Women Prisoners" (California Policy Research Center, U of California, 2000) and Nancy Stoller, "Space, Place, and Movement as Aspects of Health Care in Three Women's Prisons, *Social Science and Medicine* 56 (2003): 2263–75.

# Surviving but Not Quite Thriving:
## Women's Mental Health in East Harlem

CHERYL HARRIS SHARMAN

*This essay employs an ethnographic approach to understanding women's health in East Harlem, New York. Studying mental health in the complex, changing environment of East Harlem was like peeling back the multiple layers of an onion. Toward that goal, I followed five women for five years as a freelance health journalist. There was no grant, no institution, no employer, just my residence in East Harlem and my growing concern for the lack of mental health care available to my neighbors. To grasp the totality of their minds, I had to examine the totality of their lives. I had to probe the disabilities of their physical selves, their physical spaces, and their relationships. One of the women I followed, Tara, embodied this complexity on a profound level. Peeling back the layer of her depression revealed depressing interactions with her environment—failed attempts to receive disability, a heart attack, depressed friends, routine poverty. Layers of heart disease, obesity, and problem pregnancies affected her life alongside the layers of her children's and husband's disabilities and illnesses, alongside layers of physical and sexual abuse. Each layer further weakened Tara's health. And yet Tara fought back, found the necessary treatment, functioned well. I began to see this as part of her illness narrative. Writing her story and advocating for her depends upon recognizing this; her story is complex and multifaceted, and it defies simple categorizations or diagnoses. In Tara's story, like the stories of many other impoverished women, illness, poverty, violence, personal resilience, motherhood, and community are all forces of risk and resilience that coexist side by side. Mental illness, like other illnesses, cannot be understood as it affects these women's lives without understanding the context of their lives in total. Tara, for me, is the beginning of such a journey of understanding.*

Bordered by Ninety-sixth Street to the south and Fifth Avenue to the west, East Harlem boasts over 100,000 residents—mostly Puerto Rican and African American—squeezed into two hundred square blocks. From the tops of the public housing projects, the largest concentration in New York City, locals with median incomes below the poverty line overlook the Upper East Side, one of the wealthiest neighborhoods in the United States. More than 36 percent of East Harlem receives federal income support. The infant mortality rate is nearly double that of the rest

*289*

of Manhattan. Asthma, diabetes, and cancer also ransack lives at higher levels than the rest of the borough. According to the last census, "Female householders with no husband present" account for almost one-third of families.

At first glance, East Harlem might to some people embody the stereotype that you must avoid this place, or die here. Yet only upon closer look do boundaries of race, ethnicity, sickness, and sanity reveal themselves to be the fluid, fragile borders they are. Only on closer examination does the role of gender move to the foreground. Only by even more intimate examination can we see beyond the immediate struggles to the invisible structures that threaten to sink women in East Harlem.

It took me five years to take this closer look. Intending to investigate mental health, I found five women willing to share their experiences with depression, postpartum depression, and schizophrenia. I found three of them on the same block. The first time I met Tara, in 2001, she was thirty years old and sat in a borrowed chair on the sidewalk in front of her building.

It was a beautiful day and everyone sat outside on the street. Her building is one in a row of brownstones that wear the architecture of the nineteenth century. They do not crumble, visibly, from the outside, but they are on a long walk toward total deterioration. Tara sat smoking in the black folding chair, the kind you'd take to a ballgame or the beach. Two of her children played in the crowded street and she bellowed out to them from time to time to mind the cars. In contrast to her two small children, who never made a sound, Tara commanded an audience with her every word. She didn't speak, she roared.

"Where do you live?" she asked me, preempting my questions with one of her own. I was startled by her bluntness but soon realized that Tara knew everyone who passed in front of her chair. If she didn't know you, and on that first day she didn't know me, she demanded to be introduced. That day, and every other day that I've seen her, Tara wore her long blond hair in a frayed knot at the nape of her neck, never fussed with fancy clothes, and never wore makeup.

"Oh, I know those houses," Tara responded when I gave my address. She lifted her hand above her head and said, "They're a good thing. They go to people who make less than this much and," she lowered her hand to her full chest, "more than this much." Tara was the street sage, the sidewalk her stage. She sat in that chair all day, every day, playing cards, watching the children—hers and everyone else's—gathering and giving information. Over a span of three years, Tara came to my apartment once and I came to hers once. Other than that, we met on her street where she's more comfortable than anywhere.

From the first day we met, Tara was open about her depression. "I couldn't do anything," she said, adding, "I was like this." She slumped her ample frame down in the chair, fixing her piercing blue eyes in a catatonic stare. "I was in [the public hospital] for sixty days. If anyone was to say to me, 'Have you ever been in prison?' I would say, 'Yes, I have. At [the public hospital].'" She shrugged her shoulders and raised her brow. Tara told a story with the deadpan of a native New Yorker and the dramatic pauses of a thespian.

Tara was sixteen during that psychiatric hospital stay. It was the early 1980s. Crack cocaine had moved into East Harlem as the factories shut down. Tara's grandmother had cancer. Despondent, Tara's mother tried crack. Addiction followed quickly. Her father too succumbed. Her biological parents lived on the streets.

Tara's stepfather, the father of her two brothers, took good care of his boys, Tara, and her two older sisters; but his diabetes and heart problems eventually made it impossible for him to care for them. Their grandmother could not care for them either. Tara had no supervision and routinely skipped school. Her grandmother died. One afternoon she ran into a friend of her grandmother's in an East Harlem park. He raped her.

Strung out on crack, her mother admonished her, "You should'a been in school."

Her oldest sister had a baby and, after a cesarean delivery, a bottle of codeine pills. Tara saw the pills as her way out, taking over forty of them in an attempted suicide. Her sister found her. The public hospital admitted her to the psychiatric ward.

Medicaid covered Tara's stay in a shared room with four or five other women. She felt held against her will, acted out, and often found herself in solitary confinement.

"That makes you more angry," Tara said. "You're like, 'I was angry when I came in here. I'm more angry now lookin' at these padded walls.' That's why now if I feel, like, down and depressed or something. I try not to go to a hospital because it's not nice at all. I find that city hospitals are the worst for a psych problem. It felt like prison."

Tara returned home from the mental hospital depressed. If people were rude, she cried or grew agitated. The medications prescribed by her doctor made her tired. She stayed home every day and slept. Then she began to accompany a friend's mother to a free support group twice a week on the Upper East Side.

The support group showed Tara how to avoid unhealthy patterns. "Try to change things around," they told her, "get out more, to make sure life isn't so gloomy." Tara benefited from hearing others share their strategies for fighting depression's powerful grip. "That helped me more [than medications]," Tara said, "other people, coming out and speaking about their depression and how you could overcome it. That's what helped me overcome it. I felt so much better. I felt great. I was active again, able to do things."

Tara finished high school and started college, even though she and her siblings lived in and out of foster care for the next four years. One younger brother suffered sexual abuse in a foster care home. Her two younger sisters were adopted by foster parents in Queens. The brother developed paranoid schizophrenia.

Tara's mother stopped smoking crack. "She said one day she just woke up and," Tara paused for effect, "that was it. She never did it again. She just wanted her kids back. She cleaned up off of drugs and fought for us." Her father stopped, relapsed, went through treatment, attends AA meetings, and remains clean today. Her mother never needed a treatment program. "She don't need nothing," Tara said proudly. "She wanted her kids," Tara said, adding, "a woman has more of the willpower."

Tara completed two years toward an accounting degree, married a wealthy man, and had a baby boy. But her husband beat her and she couldn't bring herself to leave him. When she nursed her son, Tara explained, her husband would "take my baby off my breast, throw him in the crib, and force me to have sex with him." One day she refused. His beating put her in the hospital. The hospital photographed her wounds and he went to prison for six years.

Tara now lives with another man whom she calls her husband. They have three children together, the youngest born in February 2004. His disabilities prevent him from working or caring for the children.

Tara's oldest son, now a teenager, has diabetes. By four, he had meningitis, asthma, and such poor motor skills that the hospital urged Tara to get him to attend a muscular dystrophy school downtown. She secured disability for him, after applying four times, and the subsequent review process proved too complex and overwhelming for her to continue the fight.

The middle two children, a boy and girl both under the age of ten, have kidney disease. At three, the girl had her kidney removed. Without health insurance, Tara maintains complex charts to monitor which doctor or hospital last treated which child so she knows where to go the next time.

In 2002, Tara decided to combine her knack for math with her knowledge of medicine to become an EMT. Days before starting the program, she suffered a heart attack. She was thirty-one years old. Her doctor ordered her to collect disability and never work again. She didn't qualify. "What do you need disability for? You're young," they told Tara. "You discriminate?" she responded with her usual fire. "I didn't know you had to be an old person to be on disability," she told me. "Maybe it was because, you know, because I'm white."

Despite these setbacks, Tara is still a fighter. For instance, reunited by her mother's sobriety, Tara, during the years of my research, invested extraordinary energy in their relationship. She walked a dozen blocks each way to see her mother twice a week or more, said wonderful things about her mother's care for the brother with schizophrenia, and spoke of her mother's past addiction with pain but without anger. "She'll say," Tara quoted her mother, "'I never stole from no one, never owed nobody nothing, never stole from my children, never sold my body, never robbed anybody,' which is very true."

The man Tara lives with now refused to come to the hospital for the emergency birth of Tara's last high-risk pregnancy. I helped her bring bags upstairs the day she came home, so I met him or, more accurately, saw him. He didn't speak to me and stayed in bed. Tara thanked me for my help, hugged me, and closed the door. "Now come here," I heard her tell him, "and meet your fucking daughter." It was an uncomfortable end, but not a surprising one, to what should have been a joyful day. Tara perseveres—perhaps even thrives—in the midst of chaos and conflict. This is all she's known her entire life.

Tara endured rape, physical and sexual abuse, a suicide attempt, her parents' addictions, and foster care. She has had a husband beat her, multiple miscarriages, and heart attacks. She battles obesity and the myriad health problems of her four children. She and the other women I met in East Harlem have health histories and lives that defy easy answers. But such women are nonetheless real, nonetheless hurt. Every day they get out of bed. Every day they do it all over again.

They are mothers and sisters, daughters and lovers, wives and friends. They may make your copies at the local copy shop, ring up your coffee at the corner store, wash your hair at the midtown beauty salon, serve as the security guard at your job. They are real women who force us to find real answers to abstract questions: What is our responsibility to the mental health care of disadvantaged women and children? How does gender affect access to health care and the distribution of benefits? Questions like these concern researchers and politicians, but women like Tara are more concerned with finding next month's rent, feeding their children, and fighting for their lives. Advocating for women like Tara requires us to see the world through this lens of survival, to recognize that her story, like every story, defies simple solutions and demands complex and multifaceted answers.

# Teaching about Care at the End of Life
# Using Creative Nonfiction Monologues

## Laurie Rosenblatt

By telling stories, people organize and understand experience. Narrative positioning or the point of view from which a story is told influences the listener's
distance from the protagonist. Medical stories often feature patients but use
the care provider's "objective" viewpoint as a way of focusing attention on the
disease rather than on the patient. Such stories allow care providers to stay on
task and shift away from patients to a distance that protects them while they
provide treatments and perform procedures that cause pain to the patient. In
the nineteenth century, the case history became the foundation for the development of medical theories of disease. Therefore, in considering how the
different rhetoric of monologue affects its use in teaching care providers, I'd
like to compare it to a case description written in 1895.

> At the end of the year 1892 a colleague of my acquaintance referred a young
> lady to me who was being treated by him for chronically recurrent suppurative
> rhinitis. It subsequently turned out that the obstinate persistence of her trouble
> was due to caries of the ethmoid bone. Latterly she had complained of some new
> symptoms which the well-informed physician was no longer able to attribute to
> a local affection. She had entirely lost her sense of smell and was almost continu-
> ously pursued by one or two subjective olfactory sensations. She found these most
> distressing. She was, moreover, in low spirits and fatigued, and she complained
> of heaviness in the head, diminished appetite and loss of efficiency.
>
>      The young lady, who was living as a governess in the house of the managing
> director of a factory in Outer Vienna, came to visit me from time to time in my
> consulting hours. She was an Englishwoman. She had a delicate constitution, with
> a poor pigmentation, but was in good health apart from her nasal affection.[1]

This 1895 case of Sigmund Freud is told in the voice of the physician who
approaches the patient as Sherlock Homes might approach a crime—a style
that persists in medical case histories: something's wrong with the machinery
of the body/mind and if the disturbance can be found, it can be fixed and the
patient may go on her way, cured. There is considerable evidence that Freud

in fact did not treat his patients in such a detached manner, but in this report he stands outside of the patient's experience and describes the story of her symptoms with technical language and surgical detachment.

In contrast, something I call the case study monologue shifts the locus of understanding from the doctor's observations to the patient's experience. By "hearing" the patient's voice, we gather a sense of her values and the physical, practical, and existential challenges she faces, as this contemporary case study monologue shows.*

Case Study Monologue: There's Only So Many Things You Can Make a Joke About—Then You Stop.

I was 29 years old when I was diagnosed with stage III inflammatory breast cancer. It's the worst kind. I had surgery, then high-dose chemotherapy, a bone marrow transplant, and finally radiation.

After that I was okay, in remission, until four years later. One day, I felt like I couldn't breathe and I thought I had pneumonia; it turns out I had fluid in my left lung and around my heart. I had a mass on my hip as well. So I had several operations to get the fluid out of my lung and my pericardium. And then I did another round of chemotherapy with Taxotere, which really kicked my ass. For me, it was worse than the bone marrow transplant. It was horrible—hor-ri-ble! It caught me by surprise because I never got sick from Adriamycin. Everybody was amazed about that. It just didn't make me sick that way. I felt shitty, of course, but I think the thing that really made the Taxotere much worse was that I'm allergic to it, so they had to pump me full of steroids before they could even get it into me. The worst part—and this sounds really shallow—was that I gained fifty pounds. So I was fat and I was bald and I knew it.

When I got the recurrence, all my friends were going to graduate school and starting to have families—and what am I doing? Chemotherapy! That was hard. I felt like I was really falling off the road. I felt that at the beginning, but I thought, "Well, it will be one year, no big deal. It won't change my life." And it did.

I'm not saying that I'm glad it happened, but there were positive things that came out of the first time around. It just got really difficult the second time. A lot of it was emotional. You know you don't get cancer exclusive to the rest of your life. You go into it with all your shit; everything comes with you. I remember thinking when I was a kid, I just couldn't wait 'til I grew up. When I grew up,

* This case study monologue is constructed from an interview with a forty-year-old woman living with advanced breast cancer. The study from which this interview came was approved by the Dana-Farber IRB. Permission to use the interview and story was obtained from the subject and her surviving partner.

everything would be magically okay; I would have a great life and I would have happy relationships. I've realized by having cancer that you never really grow up. You just get older. It all stays the same, it's just older. How disappointing. That's the hardest thing about having this illness—it doesn't go away. It's like my past, this crazy, dysfunctional thing that won't leave me alone. It's very cruel.

The third time it ended up recurring in my right breast. I started radiation. And in the middle of the radiation the tumor in my lung started growing. I haven't been in remission for very long at any stage. This is my sixth recurrence.

I meant to say, when I got sick the first time, I didn't realize—everything happened so fast—I didn't realize that I was going to be sterile afterwards. Not that I wanted a kid then, anyway, but it's nice to have the option. And lately—it's not an issue, it's just a very sad thing—right before I recurred this time, my partner and I were considering adoption, considering parenthood. I felt that I was in a place where I could actually be a decent parent. So we were really excited. And for a while after I recurred she would still talk about it, would say, "Oh, well, whenever this treatment's over." And I'm thinking, "I'm going to be dead." Or, "How can you talk about having a kid when all bets are off now?" I mean, as far as I was concerned, and am concerned, once you recur you are in a whole different category of cancer patient. It's going to kill you, sooner or later. It might be later, but it's still going to. This is going to be how I die. So having a child is not a part of what I can do now. And every time the cancer recurs, I think, "There goes another part of my life." I remember my therapist from the mind-body clinic saying you have to have a long-term goal if you're going to survive. So, I'm like, "Shit, I've got to get a long-term goal." I don't know what it's going to be. Right now it's just "stay alive until September."

What I do now, if I can work, is design housing for community development corporations, low-income people, people with AIDS, whatever. I always had a hard time with private client architecture because I just feel I'm too much of a social justice person. The housing I designed was different from any other public housing to that point so I felt good about it. And then I got sick again, so somebody else took over that job and basically finished it because I was out of work for over a year.

I guess the housing project seems even more important to me now that I know what it's like to get Medicaid. Nothing says disrespect like Medicaid. I have never been so insulted in my life as I have been at the pharmacy whenever I whip out my card. It's amazing. Everything changes. You know, I've never had food stamps, but I have become more aware of how people treat you when you have public assistance. When somebody whips out food stamps in the grocery aisle, all of a sudden the cashier has this superior attitude. It's humiliating. I have been in the pharmacy and taken out my Medicaid card, and they'll yell, "This woman here has welfare," or "This is a welfare prescription," and I'm thinking, "Shut up." I don't know why they have to announce it like that. They don't announce, "This person has Blue Cross"; they don't do that. I think it's about punishment. I think it's about being punished for being poor. I'm feeling when I'm in line and this is happening that I somehow have to explain myself: "No, no, no, I've been to college"; "I'm a professional person and I just had a bad string of luck." Why am I explaining this to the person at the counter? It's none of their goddamned business.

When you have a chronic illness you feel isolated for so many reasons. People just don't get it, and they get sick of it, I mean, I swear to God my friends sometimes think, "Would you die already!" I mean, not really, but in some ways it's like, "Shit, are you sick again?" When I first got sick, everybody was there, and I understand that people can only sustain that for a period of time, then they've got to go to work and live their lives, "I'm sorry, you're sick, but see you around." So it's interesting and frustrating how people react; and cancer is not like diabetes or lupus or any other chronic illness because there is nothing that strikes terror into people like cancer. The only thing more frightening is AIDS. There's a stigma about having cancer—even among my peers—there's fear, especially from women my own age. They want to know what I did wrong because they don't want to do that. So they ask, "Did you smoke?" "Were you not a vegetarian?" trying to find reasons to explain why this happened to me.

I understand that, but I also feel isolated because life isn't going to wait for me. I was actually lucky when I got sick; I didn't have any health insurance and it turns out that that was a good thing. If I had health insurance, I would have nothing because I would have had to pay 20 percent of half a million dollars—that's more money than I can come up with, and that's what the bone marrow transplant cost.

On the one hand, I wanted things to be normal. On the other hand I realized I had fundamentally changed. I was not the person I was before. Not in any way. In fact, I didn't really want to be the person I was before because it turns out I wasn't a very nice person. See, I was very much attached to my past before I got sick. And was still in that drama, or trauma, whatever. Being angry. I couldn't come to terms with crap that had gone on twenty years before. And I didn't want to. I didn't want to stop being angry. I didn't want to let go of it. And then I got sick and at some point I had an epiphany: "Why am I wasting all this time on that?" And letting go made a huge difference in my ability to empathize with other people or even sympathize or see other people as human beings instead of "that's a man and they're this type of thing." I was very scared of life. After I came out of that experience of being so sick and almost dying, the real possibility of death, and living large for a long time, I realized that I am not that person anymore. And now I probably have too much sympathy, but I think that's still better than being cold hearted.

In a brief span we learn where this young woman's vulnerabilities reside. Yet the subjective quality is also an illusion. I constructed this "telling" by taking sixty-two pages of transcribed interview and reconstituting a story in the patient's "own words." Construction (or reconstruction) of the patient's narrative in this way is as much mine as Freud's construction was his. However, the monologic construction has a different teaching agenda. Focusing attention on the woman's sense of self and her experience of her illness complements the more detached, technical understanding of her disease. Positioning myself within the patient's experience allows me a greater understanding of the interface between the patient's life and the illness. Reconstructing the patient's narrative mitigated my suffering as I cared for and ultimately lost this patient. Thus the constructed monologue also serves as a memorial, a remembering and working through of the provider's sense of loss. I use monologues like the one discussed here to teach students with different levels of clinical experience—from nurses and physicians in practice for many years honing their skills in palliative care to first-year Harvard Medical students in a course called "Living with Life-Threatening Illness." We attempt to close the gap between the patient's perspective and that of the student's self-protective distancing and encourage discussion about how, as care providers, we handle and use the information provided by a patient's story.

Patient monologues introduce first-year medical students to the experiences, issues, and feelings they will confront when they meet their patients. Reflection and discussion in small group meetings gives students a chance to think about their emotional reactions to painful material and strategize about upcoming interviews with their assigned patient-teachers. When reading monologues of younger people, they talk about how frightening it is to hear cancer spoken of in their own style of speech and in the context of their own concerns about careers and relationships.

Working with more experienced clinicians, we read monologues aloud, each member of the nine-member group taking a turn for a paragraph or two. Speaking the story makes it much more emotionally immediate. Hearing it in different voices makes the feelings and events seem closely shared, almost universal. By the end of the reading, several of these seasoned clinicians are usually crying. The discussion leads to personal memories of loss in their own lives and to the relationship between those losses and the challenges and rewards of a practice in which we try to alleviate suffering in people who are dying.

NOTES

1. Sigmund Freud, "Miss Lucy R. Aged 30," *The Standard Edition of the Complete Psychological Works of Sigmund Freud*, vol. 2, ed. and trans. James Strachey (1915; London: Hogarth Press, 1958) 106–24.

# Narrative House Calls and Cultural Memory: Communities of Women, Communities of Presence

RITA CHARON

I wanted to see Mrs. Nelson at home, in her own bed. She had been in the hospital and nursing homes so many times, in so many strange beds. Even seeing her in my office was not enough—I wanted to see her at home. So I met her niece Dorothy on the corner of 7th Avenue and West 151st Street, and she escorted me through the maze of a public housing project to Mrs. Nelson's door. We started in the kitchen, sorting through the pill bottles that covered the table; I wrote up new prescriptions and reviewed the blood test reports left by the visiting nurse and the requests sent by the physical therapist. Everything in the house spoke of sickness—a wheelchair in the kitchen, a hospital bed I could just see through the door into the bedroom, a large Hoyer lift to transfer a heavy body. Dorothy told me that she supervised home care not only for her aunt but also for her mother and an elderly cousin. She seemed worn out, in need of relief, not sure why she was the one to be burdened with all this work. And yet she also seemed unconditionally committed to her aunt, and I wondered what role my patient had played in this niece's life.

Rose, the home attendant, was in the room with Mrs. Nelson, giving her a bed bath. My impatience made me barge into the room, assuring Rose that it was fine if she wasn't yet done. I had come to her house for this. There was Mrs. Nelson, robed in a colorful wrap, gray and thinning hair sparkling, skin well lotioned. "Dr. Charon," she says, "they told me you were coming." We were smiling at one another, laughing out loud in our delight. My hands caressed her shoulders as she leaned toward me from her bed. "Here you are," I kept saying. "Look at you, here you are." She looked great—not only were her lungs clear to bases bilaterally and her heart rate regular, her abdomen soft and nontender, her legs not swollen, and her feet pink and warm, but she was in command in her own home, gazing out her windows to her stretch of Seventh Avenue and gathering around her those she wanted to be with.

As we spoke together, the visiting nurse arrived. About five minutes later, the physical therapist joined us. Dorothy's cousin Vicky popped in. By now, there were five of us with Mrs. Nelson in her room, each with appointed tasks in her care, magnetically drawn to the life force of this eighty-nine-year-old minister, church choir singer, sister who, although ailing in many ways, was the undeniable heroine of this scene. It was much easier for us all to do our work when together by her bed instead of on individual phone calls to my busy office. But there was more. Here we all were, a community of women (it didn't seem to matter that I alone was white), affiliated by virtue of our mutual care of Mrs. Nelson, enriched by one another's expertise, buoyed up by one another's presence. Dorothy's burdens felt lifted, I feel sure, when she saw how not alone she was. The visiting nurse and physical therapist, unused to doctors making house calls, must have felt a surge of new commitment to the care of this patient. We were all together in this community of presence, and weren't we going to make it work?

It is unusual for me to make house calls. (It is rare for any doctors in New York City to make house calls, except for those assigned to units specifically set up to do them. Ordinary doctors almost never leave the office or the hospital.) Why did I take the unreimbursable time to see this woman at home? What made me as if part of her family, a tie not only of professional duty but also of earthy desire? I did it because of literature.

"Her life is now simply inconceivable to him. Until he starts to tell her story."[1] Michael Stein, an internist, writes in a novel called *This Room Is Yours* about a middle-aged high school teacher who takes on the responsibility of overseeing his demented mother's care. He supervises things in the assisted living faculty in Providence, Rhode Island, that he has chosen for her and, in the process of coming to terms with her loss of memory, finds himself recreating her life—writing, if you will, his mother's memoir. That Dr. Stein himself moved his demented mother to live in an assisted living facility close to his own home in Providence is no coincidence. He wrote his mother's story not just to understand it but to inhabit it. Only in the writing does the protagonist and the author behind the protagonist come to occupy what the mother went through and, as a dividend, what the son went through at her hands. What emerges toward the end of the text (it is hard to specify a genre for the work) is a gutsy, scrappy, possessive son unconditionally, exhaustively, and irrationally on the side of his mother, a state of commitment altogether new for this son and this mother. What a gift for the mother, for the son, and for the reader. "A year earlier . . . he would not have thought of crying over her shame and embarrassment or over the work her uncontrollable, unconscious, ingrained behaviors caused. What's happened to him? Has he simply opened himself to her story?"[2]

When Mrs. Nelson and I first met around 1985, we didn't get along. Her care was transferred to me, when I was a very junior doctor, from a physician who had retired. I found her difficult to care for, headstrong, not interested in doing the things I wanted her to do for her health. Here is how I described her in a paper I wrote seven years ago:

Mrs. Ruby Nelson is an 82-year-old obese, diabetic, hypertensive woman with osteoarthritis who has been in my practice for around 15 years. Our early years together were marked by disagreement over silly things: she insisted on brand name medicines, even when generics were just as good, and I bristled at the extra work and cost. She never took seriously the need to address her obesity. Consequently, her diabetes was ill-controlled and her degenerative knee disease disabling. One morning, as she sat on the examining table waiting for me to take her blood pressure (which was invariably alarmingly high and triggered in me anxiety, fear of reprisal, great impatience, and the felt duty to scold), she mentioned that she sang in the church choir. I don't know why, but I asked her to sing me a hymn. This woman, whose body habitus I routinely described as "morbidly obese," was transfigured into a form of stateliness and dignity as she raised her heavy head, clasped her hands, and sang in a deep dark alto about the Lord, on the banks of the river, bringing her home. From then on, I would do anything for her and she for me. A moment of epiphany indeed, those few bars of mournful powerful song transported us into a new geography of respect and value together.

Since then, she has developed cerebrovascular disease, requiring multiple hospitalizations to stave off strokes. She has remained for me, throughout her many weeks in the hospital, a figure of great dignity and spirituality. Despite the firm recommendations of the social workers and visiting nurses [to place her in a nursing home], I backed her deep desire to return to her own apartment, knowing, now, something about the power of her desires. She is now back home, anti-coagulated, her blood pressure effectively controlled, TIAs for the time being absent. She continues to ask me to do her little special favors in the office, and I am always grateful that she asks.[3]

I often find myself writing about my patients. I am able to discover things about them by virtue of writing the two of us into stories. At the beginning, I was a little worried about this tendency. It seemed voyeuristic, or at least unprofessional. If I didn't know something, I would even make it up. Before I knew how writing gives the writer access to unconscious material, I was spooked when the parts I made up turned out to be true. But slowly I came to understand that writing about my patients is just part of how I do my general internal medicine. Sometimes I show my patient what I have written about him or her, and this is invariably therapeutic. Patients have absolutely no idea how much their doctors brood about them. They have no idea that we dream about them and worry endlessly about them and treasure our lives with them. Our patients get into our bones, making us the doctors we are. And so making a patient the hero of a story is the most natural thing for a doctor to do.[4]

I learned a great deal by writing about Mrs. Nelson, becoming curious about and so learning about nonmedical aspects of her life, entering into my deep awe at her faith and courage, finding words and forms with which to represent my dramatic conversion to her side. Finding out Mrs. Nelson was a minister helped me to interpret correctly what I had mistaken in her as imperiousness. Hearing—if only in the songs she sang—of her vision of this life as doomed and the next life as the treasure helped to put into perspective some of her seeming disdain for things of the flesh.

The protagonist in William Maxwell's brilliant novel *So Long, See You Tomorrow* thinks back, in old age, to himself as a ten-year-old boy who lost his mother to the 1918 influenza epidemic and who suffered his grief silently and inconsolably. The novel weaves in a fictionalized account of a real murder that took place in the boy's hometown, in which a man kills his best friend out of jealousy and then kills himself. The speaker recreates or invents memories, feelings, and motivations for the characters who stand for actual people, especially the ten-year-old son of the murderer/suicide. In psychoanalytic treatment many years later, the protagonist relives the nights, after his mother's death, pacing with his father from one room to the next: "From the library into the dining room, where my mother lay in her coffin. Together we stood looking down at her. I meant to say to the fatherly man who was not my father, the elderly Viennese . . , '*I couldn't bear it*,' but what came out of my mouth was 'I can't bear it.'"[5] No matter the decades elapsed, no matter the loves that replaced that earliest one, the man-boy is compelled to recapitulate and repeat his early wounds so as to work them through, not to "find himself" or to "come to terms with his losses," but to make it happen, to make his life happen, and even to make the past happen.

Like Michael Stein's fictionalized autobiography of his mother who has lost her mind, this work is a multigenre work. Indeed, William Maxwell's mother died of influenza in 1918 when the author was ten years old. Like the fictional protagonist, the author grew up in Lincoln, Illinois, and then moved with his remarried father to Chicago. The murder/suicide took place in the author's hometown when he was a boy. It is in the friction between the memoir and the fiction that the point of the work emerges, as if neither fact nor fiction alone is quite enough impetus for the human mind to behold the truth. The speaker of *So Long, See You Tomorrow* writes, "What we, or at any rate what I, refer to confidently as memory—meaning a moment, a scene, a fact that has been subjected to a fixative and thereby rescued from oblivion—is really a form of storytelling that goes on continually in the mind and often changes with the telling. Too many conflicting emotional interests are involved for life ever to be wholly acceptable, and possibly it is the work of the storyteller to rearrange things so that they conform to this end. In any case, in talking about the past we lie with every breath we draw."[6]

It is as if Maxwell can remember accurately—or forgivingly—some aspects of his own real life only by imagining and "getting inside of" the stories of others, well enough, in fact, to tell their stories himself. If Michael Stein can only expose his own childhood and his relationship with his mother by the process of imagining *her* life from the inside, William Maxwell can only expose *his* own boyhood grief and loss by imagining the lives of relative strangers from his hometown, facing horrible tragedies that repeat to some extent his own felt experiences of abandonment and dread. As it turns out, and I think now that this may be Maxwell's point, we may, when we remember, "get inside" a stranger who happens to be ourselves.

In writing about my patient whom I am calling here Mrs. Nelson, I stick to the facts, but I am certainly selective about which facts to include in my story. While not lies, my descriptions of Mrs. Nelson were scenes chosen from an infinite assortment of potentially tellable scenes. Ordinarily, when doctors write about their patients, they choose from among a restricted assortment of tellable scenes—substernal chest pain, abdominal cramps and bloody diarrhea, euphoria alternating with despair. The liberties I took in writing about Mrs. Nelson were not liberties of fiction but liberties of plot. I chose some plots that mattered for me, personally, and, I thought, perhaps for Mrs. Nelson. It is a different kind of *matter* from the internist's ordinary preoccupation.

I continued the story about this patient in a later essay, chapter nine in a book I am now finishing on narrative medicine*:

The patient was able to stay home for many years with phalanxes of visiting nurses, home health attendants, physical therapists, and wound specialists who came to visit her at home. I was on the phone with one or another of her homecare providers maybe twice a week. It was not easy, and I sometimes grew out of patience for being quarterback of this increasingly complex team.

In 2003 and 2004, the patient required multiple hospitalizations for falls, infections, and worsening diabetes. By the fourth or fifth admission in as many months, the nurses and social workers and I all finally relented and transferred Mrs. Nelson to a nursing home. I told her it might be temporary, but within myself I knew she would die in the nursing home.

About three months after her discharge to the nursing home, her niece called me at the office. I assumed, when I heard her voice on my voice mail, that she was calling to tell me her aunt had died, and I felt the guilty pang of having abandoned this patient to whom I had once felt such allegiance. But it was not

* This book is completed and published as *Narrative Medicine: Honoring the Stories of Illness* (New York: Oxford UP, 2006).

a death call. Mrs. Nelson absolutely insisted that the nursing home discharge her back to her apartment. She refused to sign papers that would allow them to keep her in the home. My advice to her niece was to *not* back her aunt's desire to return home. I remembered how very difficult it had been the last time she was home. I felt that letting her go home was just too dangerous—she would fall again and break her hip; she would have a major bleed; she would have another stroke. Finally, I realized, I did not relish resuming the complex and wearing responsibilities of overseeing her homecare from afar.

Her niece thanked me most politely for my advice. But then, a few days later, I found myself within blocks of the patient's nursing home. I could not help myself from paying her a visit. There she was—turban on head, sprawled in bed, gazing mutely at the ceiling, foot dressed where she had had a toe amputated. I called out her name softly and, when she first looked at me somewhat blankly, said my name. She rose. "Dr. Charon. You came to see me." We were silly with joy to be in one another's presence again. I drew a chair up to her bed and listened as she told me, with woe, what life was like for her in the home. I wanted to know specifically how life would be different for her were she to be back home. I asked what she would do in the apartment, who would help her out, how she'd spend her days.

"What would you eat at home that you can't eat here?" I asked her. She gazed into the middle distance and said, with eloquent and precise gestures of her angularly deformed arthritic hands, "I would get a piece of fish this big, and I would fry it up in the skillet, or have the girl to do it for me, and I would make some grits to go along with it." The look on her face of anticipatory pleasure reached my heart and formed my resolve. I introduced myself to the head nurse as Mrs. Nelson's internist of twenty-three years. If, I told her, the staff here thinks she is stable enough to be discharged home, I, as her "community physician," would be happy to resume direction of her care.

I would not have developed this loyalty without having written about the patient, without having spent time in my imagination with her and, by doing so, realizing how I valued the years we had spent as a dyad. I have a screw loose for her, as John Marcher says about May Bartram in Henry James's "The Beast in the Jungle," and the screw loosened in the narrative acts of inventing, imagining, and finding the words to speak for her and about her. These narrative acts showed me what I did not know until I committed them: that this patient stands for something transcendent for myself, something primal for my life as a doctor, and something resolutely spiritual in my life. It is as irrational as it is clinically salient. I have a screw loose for her, and that means I will accept the slightly foolhardy clinical assignment toward fulfilling her deep wishes for her future.[7]

My writing has helped us both. Because I found some forms—some literary forms—in which to capture the otherwise formless perceptions and sensations triggered by Mrs. Nelson's presence, I could mount a vigorous state of attention when with her. Because I found ways to represent her, I paid better attention to her. My state of attention let me widen my gaze to include not only the finger-stick-glucose and the body mass index but the deep dark alto and the tremendous faith. I let this patient speak to me. I let her speak *for* me—as I am doing now—in papers and lectures about narrative medicine.

I let her speak about myself too, of course. Transference and countertransference are not phenomena reserved for psychiatrists and analysts. We internists and other ordinary doctors also practice our medicine with the self. We realize that effective medicine requisitions of the doctor not just the obvious things like intellect and scientific competence and the senses of humor and proportion. It impresses as well one's savage imagination, one's tragic certainty, one's aesthetic capacity, and one's courage to face others' and one's own traumas and losses. An overlooked dividend of clinical practice is that medical practice mobilizes the doctor's authentic self, making it available for his or her own review and recognition. Not only does the doctor get to use the self in the care of patients; he or she gets to meet it, sometimes for the first time.

Novelist Pat Barker knows this about medicine, and so she chose a doctor as her protagonist for her historically based trilogy of novels. In *Regeneration*, Barker represents psychiatrist W. H. R. Rivers at work caring for shell-shocked soldiers at Craiglockhart War Hospital in Edinburgh during World War I. Some of the characters for the novel are drawn from Rivers's case reports, some of which were published in *The Lancet* in the early twentieth century. Rivers's publications in psychiatry, neurology, and anthropology are liberally called upon in depicting the protagonist. And yet the work qualifies as a novel in having imaginatively and originally recreated a whole out of the given parts, much as memory works for Maxwell.

Pat Barker usurps the memory of Rivers, who in turn tries to entice his shell-shocked soldier-patients to remember their unspeakable experiences in the trenches instead of repressing them. "The typical patient, arriving at Craiglockhart, had usually been devoting considerable energy to the task of *forgetting* whatever traumatic events had precipitated his neurosis. . . . Rivers's treatment sometimes consisted simply of encouraging the patient to abandon his hopeless attempt to forget, and advising him instead to spend some part of every day remembering. Neither brooding on the experience, nor trying to pretend it had never happened."[8] The remembering is the basis for the therapy, for the reconstitution of self that must be done prior to recovery. The novel slowly reveals how all of us—shell-shocked or not—need to create ourselves out of the fragments we are given, and that serious and committed listeners can help that process to occur.

All doctors are potentially such serious and committed listeners. My group at Columbia in the Program in Narrative Medicine has of late turned to the work of trauma scholars, oral historians, and chaplains to learn how one bears witness to another's suffering. Traumas of any kind need to be met with recognition, with confirmation that this loss or injury has happened, has altered the self, but that the self, albeit perhaps in a new form, can continue. Pat Barker adds a fresh and urgent dimension to her depiction of how one bears witness to another's suffering: she reveals the mutuality of suffering between doctor and patient and the mutuality of healing. Dr. Rivers, too, is a man who has evidently suffered, although his own suffering is muted in the novel. His care for these damaged and courageous men calls forth a domestic, maternal, attentive presence from him, a presence the men crave. One particularly wounded soldier, Burns, elopes from Craiglockhart, returning late at night after a day of perilous exposure. "All the way back to the hospital Burns had kept asking himself why he was going back. Now waking up to find Rivers sitting by his bed, unaware of being observed, tired and patient, he realized he'd come back for this."⁹

When I taught this novel recently in a seminar to fourth-year medical students, one of my students wrote in a reader-response paper, "Central to the novel was the concept of trauma and how dealing with horrific circumstances affects a person. Repression and denial have a lot to do with it. . . . All of the men at Craiglockhart are damaged from the traumas they have experienced, including the doctors . . . As a future physician and psychiatrist . . . I thought deeply about my own way of dealing with conflict as a man in society and the possible benefits of 'manly' repression. It displays strength in some manner, but I can't think of a good reason why men should continue to close off certain emotional avenues other than to avoid ridicule." The intertwining of the suffering of the doctor and his patients in their efforts to rescue experience from repression—that is, to remember—had reached this student, illuminating anew an aspect of his chosen work destined to hurt him as well as to let him perform his work.

What also slowly becomes evident to the reader of *Regeneration* is how much Dr. Rivers needs his work to live. Although he tends to his patients with maternal devotion, he feeds off them and their traumas so as to live. One patient had said to him, "I don't see you as a *father*, you know. . . . More a sort of . . . *male mother*." This comment speaks the truth to Rivers, who "had often been touched by the way in which young men, some of them not yet twenty, spoke about feeling like fathers to their men. Though when you looked at what they *did*. Worrying about socks, boots, blisters, food, hot drinks. And that perpetually harried expression of theirs. Rivers had only seen that look in one other place: in the public wards of hospitals, on the faces of women who were bringing up large families on very low incomes. . . . It was the look of people who are totally responsible for lives they have no power to save."[10] The soldiers enact their maternality at the extreme expense of war and exposing themselves to death, while Rivers gets to experience his maternality only by virtue of caring for his men in the safety of the war hospital. It is, indeed, an unequal division of suffering, with the patients doing the lion's share of it and the doctor reaping compound interest from their pain.

The lives of doctor and patient, then, are parallel, even though the suffering is not symmetrical. The effort underway in the healing process is to see the suffering, to remember it, to tell it straight so as at least to overhear it oneself, to derive some consolation from its being told. The therapeutic method Rivers chooses to treat his shell-shocked soldiers is appropriate for all of us clinicians who face the catastrophic traumas of war, genocide, and rape as well as the uncatastrophic traumas of dementia, influenza, and asthma. What Rivers does is to join his men, and both doctor and patient derive comfort, perhaps primal comfort, from that unity. If what they suffer from, in the end, is isolation, then the treatment cures the condition, for both patient and doctor. What cures the condition is no longer being alone with it.

As I reread what I have written about Mrs. Nelson over the years, I see it is more about me than about her. You learn more about me and my doctoring from my excerpts than you do about my patient. Literary scholar Walter Benjamin said that storytelling "sinks the thing into the life of the storyteller, in order to bring it out of him again. Thus traces of the storyteller cling to the story the way the handprints of the potter cling to the clay vessel."[11] I know that Mrs. Nelson grew up in the American South, that she came to New York as a young woman to do domestic work for wealthy white families, and that her faith—including her own ministry—has been the North Star of her life. I know about her church, her singing, her extended family. I know she never had children, a choice I know not much about. I know that she has been a caregiver all her life—for her relatives, her neighbors, her congregants, and, more recently, her fellow residents in the nursing home. I know how she values independence and self-governance in this life and how she looks forward, with a complex and concrete belief, to an everlasting life with God upon her death. And yet this is her life as told to me and by me, inflected with my own brand of curiosity, my sense of what matters, my search.

Rereading my account of Mrs. Nelson now propels me to fill these lacunae, to ask about, learn about, bear witness to not only her recent and current traumas of chronic illness but also her youthful traumas—living through Southern racism and then Northern racism, holding in her breast the fire of faith, perhaps a doomed faith whose golden paradise will most likely not be materialized in this life or after it. Writing and then rereading my version of Mrs. Nelson's story prompts me to attend to aspects of her life still in the shadows, to look beyond my own *uses* of her story to see it whole, to bring myself as authentically as I can to her side. If indeed my authentic self is my clinical instrument, my clinical duty is to know myself as well and as honestly as I can so as to see—and therefore be able to treat—my patient whole.

I know that I turn naturally to stories—the reading of them and the writing of them—in my practice as a doctor and as a means to know my own interior. These are the methods we are developing in narrative medicine. I realize that my own acts of writing about patients, reading what I have written, and seeing my patients afresh in the wake of having represented them alters what I do. It alters how I conceive of our lives together. I recognize that my reading and teaching of certain novels nourishes the clinical contact between me and my patients, as I hope it will strengthen the contact possible between my students and their future patients.

But why did I find myself turning to these particular novels? It is an odd assortment, I allow. In the seminar from which this paper emerged, we turned next to W. G. Sebald's novel *Austerlitz* to continue the search. We could have read novels by Paul Auster or Michael Ondaatje as well. We could have read *Moby Dick* or *The Turn of the Screw*. These novels share a method: the interpenetration of fact with fiction, of truth with imagination, perhaps because the truth is only available to the one who has had her eyes opened by the imagination, by the effort to make it make sense, to make it happen. So-called reality, we know, doesn't happen by itself; we make it happen by putting it in a certain way. As my literary "mentor" Henry James wrote, "To put things is very exactly and responsibly and interminably to do them."[12]

So, then, my narrative methods achieve several potentiating goals. By representing my patients in writing and by reading what I write, I prime and sharpen my state of attention—trying, as James says about the novelist, "to be one of those people on whom nothing is lost."[13] I turn to stories—to well-written stories—that help me on my quest to behold others, to represent them, and also to remember and recreate myself, to admit to what all is inside there. As a result of these simultaneous "knowings"—of my patient and of myself—we together emerge as affiliated, as on the same search for recognition and for contact, joined with all humans as they muddle modestly toward goodness and rightness and health. I really think I am becoming a different kind of doctor by virtue of my literary acts. The membranes between me and my patients seem to have become more permeable. I find I am more available to them in many ways. I find that caring for them nourishes me in fresh ways.

You can see how Michael Stein aids me in my search in his modeling a way to open himself to his mother's story and using the challenge of representing the obscure interior world of his demented mother as a goad to attend all the more particularly and lovingly to her manifest life and, as a consequence, to their lives as mother and son. You can see how Pat Barker's portrayal of her shell-shocked soldiers and their grave and generous Dr. Rivers shows the power of affiliation in unearthing painful memory and living by its side and how readers' experiences, as they travel with these men through their cursed roles in world history, can be altered, remade, moved, and changed by painful exposure to strangers' suffering. And William Maxwell gives us names for all that we do in these realms of narrating, recovering, and recreating. We rescue events or thoughts from oblivion, we "fix" them, and so we render even the horror somehow acceptable or at least tellable.

Most health care professionals who work with us in narrative medicine are women. Although most nurses and medical social workers are women, and so participation from these health care professions will favor women, doctors are still more likely to be men than women, and yet those doctors who are attracted to our narrative work are predominantly women doctors. When we offer seminars for medical students in illness narratives—either reading published pathographies or writing one's own illness narratives—those who enroll are by and large women students.[14] This is not an accident. The doctoring of women doctors differs from doctoring of men doctors.[15] Nursing practice honors its sources in mothering, less prickly than medicine in admitting the intensely intimate and familial sources of caring.[16]

Michael Stein's unnamed protagonist is reaching for his mother. He locates the motherly in himself by virtue of recreating her memories from within her past but placing them squarely within *his* imagination. William Maxwell's protagonist is, in his old age, seeking for connection with his mother, who died so young. The loss that he never surmounts is the desertion, by death, by his mother, the only woman in his then ten-year-long life; she who has no surrogate in his father or brother. The effort of Maxwell's elderly protagonist is, analytically, to remake himself into the mother who can now, in projection and imagination and transference, adequately care for him, even now in his eighties. Dr. Rivers goes out of his way to identify his work and his soldiers' caregiving work as maternal. In so doing, both the doctor and his patients bow to the evident, the ordinary, the givens of gender where mothers are the ones with that look in their eyes, "the look of people who are totally responsible for lives they have no power to save." No one, it comes to this, has the power to save anyone's life—one's own, one's children, one's patients, one's dying brood. This might be the peculiarly womanly aspect of beholding others' suffering that all three novelists are after—the savage recognition of the doom of care along with its absolute and irrevocable necessity.

We were five women in the community of presence around Mrs. Nelson's bed, and that was not an accident. Carol Gilligan's pioneering work in listening carefully to adolescent girls to hear the difference gender makes in moral development has led her recently to study love and gendered fate in relational connection.[17] In *The Birth of Pleasure: A New Map of Love*, she opens up a radical discourse examining how girls and boys and women and men learn how to give voice to or to repress knowledge of tragedy, loss, and pleasure, suggesting not only that such voices are from early on gendered but also that love and pleasure are, in part, the dividends of the tragic experienced and loss counted.[18] In the care of the sick, of course, the dimensions of tragedy and loss can never be ignored or eclipsed by technical concerns, although indeed much of mainstream medicine tries hard to do so.

We can perhaps understand deeper aspects of our narrative medicine work by examining particularly the forces of *women together* at work and the ways in which the particularly female voices might influence care. Feminist scholar Hélène Cixous described the singularity of women's voices and texts: "All the feminine texts I've read are very close to the voice, very close to the flesh of language, much more so than masculine texts. . . . There's tactility in the feminine text, there's touch, and this touch passes through the ear."[19] Perhaps the womanliness of our nascent communities of presence in such places as Mrs. Nelson's bedroom, especially because they provide the tactile, personal care of bodies, tells us something about the demands, the sources, and the rewards of caring for the sick.

What we are after here is not only representation but the cultural memory that subtends representation and its resultant interpretation and metabolism into self. My clinical work with Mrs. Nelson over the years has rested, I am suggesting, on the workings of this cultural memory between us, deepened by acts of imagination and kept whole by acts of fidelity. It is the memory that the three novels examined here embody and call forth, suggesting that the work of art is, in part anyway, an avenue toward remembering. "The practice of great art" suggests Toni Morrison, "is memory, it is perception, it is imagination, and it is knowledge. There is no combination more powerful than these four, and there is no void more dangerous to the human project than their loss."[20] When we engage in routine clinical work with authenticity and narrative skill, we find, with great joy, that we can partake in great art.

Recent work in cultural memory by literary scholars, historians, performance scholars, and life writers emphasizes the implications of embodied and performed locations for the individual acts of insight and display that emerge as a result of the remembering. If, as Diana Taylor puts it in *The Archive and the Repertoire: Performing Cultural Memory in the Americas,* "cultural memory is shaped by ethnicity and gender," then our emerging work examining narrative medicine practices of memory will by definition too be shaped by ethnicity and gender.[21] Rather than essentialize illness or practice for the woman patient or caregiver, such inquiry deepens the singularity of each witness or sufferer, contributing Morrison's thoughts on memory, perception, imagination, knowledge to the effort to understand the workings of remembering and its implications in clinical practice.[22]

We can recognize, with the help of these literary frameworks and fictional texts, that our communities of presence matter to ourselves and our patients, that they enact and embody some deep currents within our selves and our culture that yearn toward the genuine and the healing. Such work, perhaps not unlike testimony studies and oral history, gives voice to silenced accounts of suffering and also gives body to instances of care. Perhaps we can see that repression, however "manly" some may find it, stands in the way, first, of the trauma and loss and, second, of the love and the pleasure that come as a result of having seen and faced them. Our communities of presence can include women and also men, whom we overhear here in the voices of Stein and Maxwell and Rivers, to crave the maternality of care. Finally, such communities—of presence, of touch, of joy—will in the end nourish and support those who are ill, those who commit themselves to the care of the ill, and those who, leaving out no one, have always more to be remembered.

NOTES

1. Michael Stein, *This Room Is Yours* (Sag Harbor, NY: Permanent Press, 2004) 17.

2. Stein 126.

3. Rita Charon, "The Seasons of the Patient-Physician Relationship," *Clinics in Geriatric Medicine* 16 (2000): 37–50.

4. There is a growing literature, on the part of patients and caregivers, about writing in clinical settings. See Charles Anderson and Marian MacCurdy, *Writing and Healing: Toward an Informed Practice* (New York: National Council of Teachers of English, 2000); Charles Anderson, ed., "Writing and Healing," special issue of *Literature and Medicine* 19 (2000): 1–132; and Gillie Bolton, *Reflective Practice: Writing and Professional Development* (London: Paul Chapman, 2001) for research and reflection on the methods and outcomes of narrative writing in health care settings.

5. William Maxwell, *So Long, See You Tomorrow* (New York: Vintage/Random House, 1996) 131.

6. Maxwell 27.

7. Rita Charon, *Narrative Medicine: Honoring the Stories of Illness* (New York: Oxford UP, 2006) 195–96.

8. Pat Barker, *Regeneration* (New York: Penguin, 1993) 26.

9. Barker 40.

10. Barker 107.

11. Walter Benjamin, "The Storyteller," *Illuminations,* trans. Harry Zohn (New York: Schocken Books, 1968) 91–2.

12. Henry James, preface to *The Golden Bowl, The Art of the Novel* (Boston, MA: Northeastern UP, 1984) 347.

13. Henry James, "The Art of Fiction," *Selected Literary Criticism,* ed. Morris Shapira (Cambridge: Cambridge UP, 1981) 57.

14. Sayantani DasGupta and Rita Charon, "Personal Illness Narratives: Using Reflective Writing to Teach Empathy," *Academic Medicine* 79 (2004): 351–6.

15. Ellen Singer More and Maureen A. Milligan, eds., *The Empathic Practitioner: Empathy, Gender, and Medicine* (New Brunswick, NJ: Rutgers UP, 1994).

16. Suzanne Gordon, Patricia Benner, and Nel Noddings, eds., *Caregiving: Readings in Knowledge, Practice, Ethics, and Politics* (Philadelphia: U of Pennsylvania P, 1996).

17. Carol Gilligan, *In a Different Voice: Psychological Theory and Women's Development* (Cambridge: Harvard UP, 1982).

18. Carol Gilligan, *The Birth of Pleasure: A New Map of Love* (New York: Vintage Books/Random House, 2003).

19. Hélène Cixous, "Castration or Decapitation?" *Authorship from Plato to the Postmodernists: A Reader,* ed. Sean Burke (Edinburgh: U of Edinburgh P, 1995) 175.

20. Toni Morrison, Gayatri Chakravorty Spivak, and Ngahuia Te Awekotuku, "Guest Column: Roundtable on the Future of the Humanities in a Fragmented World," *PMLA* 120 (2005): 715–23, 717.

21. Diana Taylor, *The Archive and the Repertoire: Performing Cultural Memory in the Americas* (Durham: Duke UP, 2003), 86.

22. See Marianne Hirsch and Valerie Smith, eds., "Gender and Cultural Memory," special issue of *Signs* 28 (2002).

# Contributors

༺૭

REGINA A. ARNOLD was professor of sociology and associate dean of studies at Sarah Lawrence College, specializing in contemporary American sociology with an emphasis on criminology, deviance, and issues of race, class, and gender. She published articles on stigma, female criminality, minority judges, and women in prison and is the author of *7 Garden South,* an unpublished memoir.

JOAN BARANOW is assistant professor of English at Dominican University of California. Her poems have appeared in *Antioch Review, Feminist Studies, Spoon River Poetry Review, U.S. 1 Worksheets, Western Humanities Review, Western Journal of Medicine,* and in the online journal *Feminism and Nonviolence Studies.* Her book of poems, *Living Apart,* was issued by Plain View Press in 1999.

FRAN BARTKOWSKI is associate professor of English at Rutgers University. She is the author of *Feminist Utopias* (University of Nebraska, 1989) and *Travelers, Immigrants, Inmates: Essays in Estrangement* (University of Minnesota, 1995). She is completing work on *Kissing Cousins: A Kinship Bestiary for a New Century.*

LARA BIRK studied the sociology of trauma at Amherst College and is currently working on an interdisciplinary theory of chronic pain in her graduate work at Tufts University, where she also is a program director at the Academic Resource Center.

MARISSA BOIS is a recent graduate of Sarah Lawrence College, where she concentrated on writing and participated in the illness narratives seminars on campus.

KATHY BOUDIN was part of a community effort to cope with the AIDS epidemic in prison during her twenty-two-year incarceration. Articles about her work in prison, focusing on literacy, mothering, higher education, and HIV/AIDS, have appeared in *Harvard Education Review, Women and Therapy, Journal of Nursing, Social Justice,* and in Correctional Association publications. Boudin received the first prize in the PEN Prison Writing Award contest. She is currently completing a doctoral studies program.

SUCHENG CHAN is professor emerita of Asian American studies and global studies at the University of California, Santa Barbara. She is the recipient of two distinguished teaching awards and is the author or editor of fifteen books. Her most widely read publication, "You're Short, Besides!" has been reprinted in more than thirty anthologies.

RITA CHARON is a general internist and literary critic at Columbia University and director of the Program in Narrative Medicine. She is coeditor of the journal *Literature and Medicine*, coeditor of *Stories Matter: The Role of Narrative in Medical Ethics* (Routledge University Press, 2003), and author of *Narrative Medicine: Honoring the Stories of Illness* (Oxford University Press, 2006). An earlier version of her essay was delivered as "The Poetics of House Calls" in the lecture series Literature and Medicine: King's Dialogues between Disciplines, at King's College, London, in March 2005.

FERN W. COHEN is a New York psychoanalyst and psychotherapist in private practice who supervises psychology graduate students, and is the author of a prize-winning essay on a psychoanalytic perspective in ordinary life ("Attachment Is Where You Find It"). Cohen completed analytic training both at NYU's postdoctoral program and at IPTAR, the Institute for Psychoanalytic Training and Research, where she is also a member. Her memoir is titled "From Both Sides of the Couch: Reflections of a Psychoanalyst, Daughter, Tennis Player, and Other Selves" (Booksurge, 2007).

SAYANTANI DASGUPTA is a faculty member in General Pediatrics and the Program in Narrative Medicine at Columbia University. She teaches courses on illness narratives and narrative genetics, as well as a summer workshop called "Writing the Medical Experience" at Sarah Lawrence College. She is the author of *The Demon Slayers and Other Stories: Bengali Folktales* (Interlink, 1995) and *Her Own Medicine: A Woman's Journey from Student to Doctor* (Ballantine, 1999), and she serves on the editorial board of the journal *Literature and Medicine*.

CORTNEY DAVIS is a poet, nurse-practitioner, and author of three poetry collections: *The Body Flute* (Adastra Press, 1994), *Details of Flesh* (Calyx Books, 1997), and *Leopold's Maneuvers* (University of Nebraska Press, 2004). In 2003 she won the Prairie Schooner Book Prize in Poetry. She is also coeditor, with Judy Schaefer, of *Between the Heartbeats: Poetry and Prose by Nurses* (University of Iowa Press, 1995). Davis and Schaefer's second anthology from University of Iowa, *Intensive Care: More Poetry and Prose by Nurses* (2003), was named a 2003 Book of the Year by *American Journal of Nursing*. Her memoir about her work in women's health, *I Knew a Woman* (Random House 2001/Ballantine Books 2002) won the Connecticut Center for the Book nonfiction prize in 2002.

ANGELEE DEODHAR is an eye surgeon, haiku poet, and artist from India, with a keen interest in promoting haiku and its related forms all over the world. Her haiku/haiga has been published internationally in various books, journals, and online publications. She is a member of the Haiku Society of America, the Haiku Society of Canada, the Haiku International Association, and the World Haiku Association.

DIANE DRIEDGER, a writer, poet, painter, and teacher, is the author of *The Last Civil Rights Movement: Disabled Peoples' International* (Hurst and St. Martin's,

1989) and *The Mennonite Madonna* (poems, gynergy, 1999). She has coedited two anthologies: *Imprinting our Image: An International Anthology by Women with Disabilities* (1992) and *Across Borders: Women with Disabilities Working Together* (1996), both published by gynergy books. Driedger is currently a doctoral candidate in the Faculty of Education, University of Manitoba, Canada.

PATRICIA DUNN is a graduate of the Sarah Lawrence College writing program. She is a regular contributor to MuslimWakeUp.com and has written for *Women's enews, Village Voice, The Nation,* and *LA Weekly.* Her fiction most recently appeared in *Global City Review* where she also acted as editor for the international issue.

JAN FELDMAN died in 2002 of an epileptic seizure in her sleep. This narrative, about her diagnosis twenty years earlier, was submitted by her sisters, Myrna Silverman and Sondra Zeidenstein. Feldman was a mother, a psychiatric nurse, sculptor, writer, mountain hiker, windsurfer, and gardener. In addition to having a psychotherapy practice, she facilitated cancer survivor groups, provided counseling to incarcerated adolescents, and taught yoga and exercise therapy to community groups.

MARY FELSTINER is professor of history at San Francisco State University and author of *To Paint Her Life: Charlotte Salomon in the Nazi Era* (HarperCollins, 1994), for which she was awarded the American Historical Association Prize in women's history. Her recent work includes essays, fiction, and a memoir-plus-history called *Out of Joint: A Private and Public Story of Arthritis* (American Lives Series, University of Nebraska Press, 2005).

MAUREEN TOLMAN FLANNERY, author of *Ancestors in the Landscape: Poems of a Rancher's Daughter* (John Gordon Burke, 2004), was nominated for the 2005 Pulitzer Prize. Her other books are *Secret of the Rising Up: Poems of Mexico* (John Gordon Burke, 1998), *Remembered Into Life* (John Gordon Burke, 1998), the anthology *Knowing Stones: Poems of Exotic Places* (John Gordon Burke, 2000), and *A Fine Line* (Fractal Press, 2004), which was produced as musical theater. Her work has appeared in four anthologies and over a hundred literary reviews.

ARTHUR FRANK is a professor of sociology at the University of Calgary in Canada. He is the author of *At the Will of the Body: Reflections on Illness* (Mariner Books, 1992), *The Wounded Storyteller: Body, Illness, and Ethics* (University of Chicago Press, 1995), and, most recently, *The Renewal of Generosity: Illness, Medicine, and How to Live* (University of Chicago, 2004). Among his editorial positions, he is book review editor of the journal *Health* and a contributing editor to the journal *Literature and Medicine.*

SUZANNE E. W. GRAY is a writer who lives in Brooklyn, New York.

AMY HADDAD teaches at the School of Pharmacy and Health Professions and directs the Center for Health Policy and Ethics at Creighton University Medical Center in Omaha. Her poetry and short stories have been published in the *American Journal of Nursing, Reflections, Journal of General Internal Medicine, Journal of Medical Humanities,* and in the anthologies *Between the Heartbeats: Poetry and Prose by Nurses* (University of Iowa Press, 1995), *The Arduous Touch: Women's Voices in Health Care* (Purdue University Press, 1999), and *Intensive Care: More Poetry and Prose by Nurses* (University of Iowa, 2003).

DONNA HENDERSON is a psychotherapist currently pursuing an MFA at the Warren Wilson College Program for Writers. Her poetry has been published in *Calyx, Christian Century, First Things, Writers' Forum, A Room of One's Own, Feminist Broadcast Quarterly,* and *Cutbank.* She has published two poetry chapbooks, one of which was a finalist for the Oregon Book Award in Poetry in 1997.

MAGGIE HOFFMAN is founding codirector of Project DOCC, a program that educates pediatric residents about how families care for children at home with chronic health care needs. Project DOCC is used in more than twenty-six residency programs in the United States and abroad.

MARSHA HURST is the director of the Health Advocacy graduate master's program at Sarah Lawrence College, where she also teaches courses on women's health and the history of health care. Her research interests have focused on women's health advocacy and on the role of narrative in advocacy. She speaks widely about health advocacy, and her research is published in a range of medical, social science, and consumer journals.

CAROL LEVINE directs the Families and Health Care Project at the United Hospital Fund in New York City. She is former editor of the *Hastings Center Report* and managing editor of *IRB: A Review of Human Subjects Research.* In 1993 she was awarded a MacArthur Foundation Fellowship for her work in AIDS policy and ethics. Her most recent books are *Always On Call: When Illness Turns Families into Caregivers* (Vanderbilt Press, 2004) and *The Cultures of Caregiving: Conflict and Common Ground among Families, Health Professionals, and Policy Makers* (Johns Hopkins, 2004).

LYN LIFSHIN, whose *Before It's Light* (Black Sparrow Books, 1999) won the Paterson Poetry Award, has published more than a hundred books of poetry, and her work has appeared in hundreds of journals and anthologies. Her recent books include *The Daughter I Don't Have* (Plan B, 2005), *The Liconie Daughter: My Year with Ruffian* (Texas Review Press, 2005), and *Another Woman Who Looks Like Me* (Black Sparrow Books, 2006).

VENETA MASSON is a nurse, poet, and essayist living in Washington, D.C. She is the author of *Rehab at the Florida Avenue Grill* (Sage Femme Press, 1999), a collection of poems, and *Ninth Street Notebook—Voice of a Nurse in the City* (Sage Femme Press, 2001), essays from her years as a nurse in an inner-city neighborhood.

VICTORIA MAXWELL, BPP (Bi-Polar Princess), is a mental health educator and speaker and directs Crazy for Life Co., a company specializing in keynotes, workshops, and performances on a range of mental health topics. Her one-person show, "Crazy for Life," depicts her real-life story of accepting and overcoming bipolar disorder. It tours worldwide and recently won the Gaia Award for best stage play at the 2005 Moondance International Film Festival.

DAWN MCGUIRE is a neurologist and researcher in AIDS and other neuro-degenerative diseases. As an undergraduate, she won the Academy of American Poets and Morris Croll Poetry prizes from Princeton University. Her first book, *Sleeping in Africa,* was published by the Maine Writers and Publishers Alliance in 1982. She recently won prizes from *Villa Montalvo, The Clackamas Review,* and *The Spoon River Poetry Review.* Her book *Hands On* was published by Creative Arts Book Company in January 2002.

ELISSA MEITES is a medical student at a university in California, where she was reproductive health director for a free clinic and president of Medical Students for Choice.

JOAN MILANO is a psychotherapist and psychoanalyst working in the Mental Health Clinic at White Plains Hospital, New York, and in private practice. Following the death of her son, Daniel, she began specialized work with patients undergoing treatment for cancer. She currently leads a support group for cancer patients at the Dickstein Cancer Center and a bereavement group at Gilda's Club Westchester for family members who have lost loved ones to cancer.

MARJA MORSKIEFT studied theology and pediatrics. She has been chronically ill for sixteen years and works as a teacher and coach in nursery schools. She gives workshops and publishes political columns and essays about living with chronic illness. A selection of her columns was published in "Ik wil alles anders dan anders," *Versiegroep,* Amsterdam, February 2005. Her essay was written in Dutch and translated to English by Hanneke Meulenbroek.

MURIEL MURCH is a nurse whose *Journey in the Middle of the Road* was published in 1995 by Sibyl Publishing. Her work is included in both *Between the Heartbeats: Poetry and Prose by Nurses* (University of Iowa Press, 1995) and *Intensive Care: More Poetry and Prose by Nurses* (University of Iowa Press, 2003). Murch continues to write stories while working as an independent radio producer in Berkeley, California.

JUDITH NADELL is an associate professor of communication at Rowan University in Glassboro, New Jersey, where she has taught for almost twenty years. Author of six textbooks and a two-time cancer survivor, Nadell is a frequent speaker at health-related support groups and medical institutions. In her presentations, she examines a popular but dangerously oversimplified mind-body belief: that the wrong kinds of thoughts and feelings create illness and that it's only by changing these that the ill get well.

ANDREA NICKI, a feminist philosopher, is currently a research associate at the Center for Women's Studies at the University of British Columbia. Two years ago she was a postdoctorate fellow at the Center for Bioethics at the University of Minnesota. There she began a book project titled *Marginalized Moral Voices,* which has been granted a contract by Broadview Press. Her poetry has appeared in Canadian and international publications such as *Rampike, Sophie's Wind,* and *In Our Own Words.* "Adventures of Amelia" is excerpted from a longer poem of the same title.

JENNIE PANCHY is a graduate of Vassar College and a poetry graduate of the Sarah Lawrence College writing program. A secondary-school English teacher for nearly a decade, she lives in northwestern Connecticut.

REBECCA A. POPE is coauthor with Susan J. Leonardi of *The Diva's Mouth: Body, Voice, Prima Donna Politics* (Rutgers, 1996) and *It's Been Marvelous: Ida and Louise Cook's Life of Opera, Romance, and Rescue* (forthcoming). Her published essays range in topic from Wordsworth to opera to AIDS. After many years of teaching literature and medicine at a university in Washington, D.C., she now lives in California, where she has a private practice in Chinese medicine.

SUNITA PURI is a recent graduate of Yale University and attended Oxford University as a Rhodes Scholar in South Asian history. She has worked as a domestic violence counselor for women and published work on domestic violence among South Asian immigrants in the United States and the United Kingdom. She is currently a second-year medical student in the Joint Medical Program between Berkeley and UC San Francisco, where she continues advocacy work with children and adolescents survivors of domestic violence.

BUSHRA REHMAN is the author of *Marianna's Beauty Salon* (Thomson Gale, 2006) and is coeditor, with Daisy Hernandez, of *Colonize This! Young Women of Color on Today's Feminism* (Seal Press, 2002). She has been featured in *NY Newsday,* and her work has appeared in *Curve* magazine, *SAMAR, Bottomfish,* and *Writing the Lines of Our Hands: An Anthology of South Asian-American Poetry* (Creative Arts Press, forthcoming). She performs her work regularly around the country and has traveled with the Asian American Literary Caravan.

JANET REIBSTEIN is a psychologist, writer, and broadcaster who teaches at the University of Exeter (UK), where she runs the training in family therapy. Reibstein is author of *Staying Alive: A Family Memoir* (Bloomsbury, 2003), *The Best Kept Secret: Stories of Enduring Love* (Bloomsbury, 2006), and *Love Life,* a TV series produced in the UK. She is coauthor, with Roger Bamber, of *The Family through Divorce* (HarperCollins, 1997) and, with Martin Richards, of *Sexual Arrangements: Marriage and Affairs* (William Heinemann, 1992).

RACHEL NAOMI REMEN is clinical professor of Family and Community Medicine at UCSF School of Medicine and the founder and director of the Institute for the Study of Health and Illness at Commonweal. She is one of the pioneers of integrative medicine and the founder and director of the Healer's Art curriculum for medical students, which is now being taught in thirty-three medical schools nationwide. She is cofounder and medical director of the Commonweal Cancer Help Program, featured in the 1993 Bill Moyer's PBS series *Healing and the Mind.* Remen is the author of *Kitchen Table Wisdom* (Riverhead, 1997) and *My Grandfather's Blessings* (Riverhead, 2001), which have been published in eighteen languages. She has a fifty-one-year history of Crohn's disease and her work is a synthesis of the perspectives of physician and patient.

ROBYN DESANTIS RINGLER is a nurse, lawyer, and writer in Ballston Lake, New York. A regular contributor to *Nursing Spectrum* and *Multicultural Review,* Ringler is writing a memoir about the ten days she cared for President Ronald Reagan after the assassination attempt in 1981. Her work has been published in newspapers as well as on various Web sites, and she has recorded personal essays for Northeast Public Radio and other nationally syndicated programs. Her "Letter to Al Pacino" appeared in *Women's Letters: America from the Revolutionary War to the Present* (Dial Press, 2005).

XAN L. ROBERTI recently finished her graduate work in poetry at Sarah Lawrence College. She has meandered through many creative genres, including singer-songwriter, drag performer, cabaret dancer, and painter. Her work has appeared or is forthcoming in *Goodfoot: A Poetry Magazine* and *Sophia.* She has taught creative writing to secondary school students at the Fordham Lutheran Youth Ministries, the Sarah Lawrence College High School Writers' Program, and the Baccalaureate School of Global Education in Queens.

GAIL ROSEN is a professional storyteller, certified bereavement facilitator, hospice volunteer, and workshop leader for women's groups, bereavement groups, schools, and special populations. Gail is also the founder of the National Storytelling Network's Special Interest Group, the Healing Story Alliance. Rosen has released two audiotapes, "Darkness and Dawn: One Woman's Mythology of Loss and Healing" and "Listening after the Music Stops: Stories of Loss and Comfort."

LAURIE ROSENBLATT is an assistant professor of psychiatry at Harvard Medical School and has published book chapters on grief and psychosocial and spiritual issues at the end of life, as well as articles on narrative and medicine in *Medical Humanities, Ars Medica,* and *Storytelling, Self, and Society.* Her poetry has appeared in *JAMA, Medical Humanities, Bellevue Literary Review, Academic Medicine, Borderlands: Texas Poetry Review, Ibbetson Street,* and elsewhere.

LAURA ROTHENBERG recorded over two years for NPR. This audio diary was aired when she was twenty-one years old, a year before she died from complications of a lung transplant she required due to cystic fibrosis. Rothenberg was a Brown University student and her memoir *Breathing for a Living* was published by Hyperion in 2004.

KATE A. SCANNELL is a physician with the Kaiser Permanente Medical Group in Oakland, California, where she practices geriatrics and internal medicine and serves as the director of the clinical ethics department. She has published extensively in both lay and professional venues, and she authored *Death of the Good Doctor:*

*Lessons from the Heart of the AIDS Epidemic* (Cleis, 1999). She writes about contemporary sociopolitical and ethical issues in her syndicated op-ed column that appears regularly in the *Oakland Tribune* and other newspapers.

LYNNE SHARON SCHWARTZ is a writer whose most recent novel is *The Writing on the Wall* (Counterpoint Press, 2005). Her eighteen books include the novels *Rough Strife* (Playboy Press, 1980), *Disturbances in the Field* (HarperCollins, 1983), *Leaving Brooklyn* (Minerva, 1990), the memoir *Ruined by Reading* (Beacon Press, 1996), the poetry collection *In Solitary* (Sheep Meadow Press, 2002), and several collections of short stories, essays, and translations from Italian. A nominee for a National Book Award and PEN/Faulkner Award, she has taught at writing programs throughout the United States and abroad.

C. SEBASTIAN wrote this as a medical student.

CHERYL HARRIS SHARMAN is a writer specializing in health, women, and multiethnic communities. Her work has appeared in the *Pan-American Health Organization's Perspectives in Health* magazine, the *San Francisco Chronicle,* the *Miami Herald,* the *American Book Review,* and elsewhere. This piece stems from five years of ethnographic fieldwork in East Harlem, New York, where she lives part of the year. She is also working on a novel set in Costa Rica, where she resides the remainder of each year.

PATRICIA B. STANLEY is a recent graduate of the program in Health Advocacy at Sarah Lawrence College. She is a faculty member in the program in narrative medicine at Columbia University.

NANCY STOLLER is a sociologist and professor of community studies at the University of California–Santa Cruz. She is the author of *Forced Labor: Maternity Care in the United States* (Pergamon, 1975) and *Lessons from the Damned: Queers, Whores, and Junkies Respond to AIDS* (Routledge, 1997). Her current book project is titled *Life and Death in American Prisons: A Twenty-Five-Year Trajectory.*

LAURIE STROBLAS has had poetry published in numerous journals and anthologies, and she served as editorial coordinator for *Hungry As We Are,* a poetry anthology. She has been poet-in-residence at Children's National Medical Center in Washington, D.C., from which a Safe Kids Campaign anthology of poems was published, and at Georgetown University Hospital's pediatrics unit. She founded the District Lines Poetry Project, which brings poems of the community to "Metro Muse," poem posters placed in the Washington, D.C.-area subways and buses and on station platforms.

EDITH WYPLER SWIRE was a professional violist and teacher with an advanced music degree from Sarah Lawrence College. When a shoulder injury precluded further performance and teaching, she enrolled in the Health Advocacy Graduate Program at Sarah Lawrence. She wrote "The Bag," based on personal experience, to fulfill a class assignment in a course on illness narratives.

MARCY PERLMAN TARDIO is a midwife in New York City. She reopened her homebirth practice in 2004, five years after being diagnosed with Wegener's Granulomatosis, an autoimmune disease, and two years after receiving a kidney transplant from her son. This piece is taken from a memoir she is writing on receiving her son's kidney.

JASMINA TEŠANOVIĆ, born in Belgrade, is a full-time freelance writer. She is extensively published in fiction and nonfiction, including *The Invisible Book* (KOV, Vrsac, Yugoslavia, 1992), *In Exile* (Publisher 94, Belgrade, Serbia, 1994), *A Women's Book* (Publisher 94, Belgrade, Serbia, 1996), *The Mermaids* (Publisher 94, Belgrade, Serbia, 1997), which received the Borislav Pekic award, *The Suitcase: Refugee Voices from Bosnia and Croatia* (UC Berkeley, 1997) with J. Mertus, and *Diary of a Political Idiot* (*Granta*, Cleis Press, 2000), which has been translated into twelve languages. She has made several films and is an activist of Women in Black, Serbia, and founder of feminist Publisher 94. "All Patients are Political Women" is an excerpt from a larger unpublished work titled *My Matrimony*.

ANNE WEBSTER has written full time since 1995, when illness ended a twenty-five-year nursing career. Her poems have appeared in many journals, including *Southern Poetry Review, The New York Quarterly, Mediphors,* and *13th Moon.* Her work has been anthologized in *Ethnic American Woman, O! Georgia,* and *Intensive Care: More Poetry and Prose by Nurses* (University of Iowa Press, 2003), and an essay was short-listed in a recent Faulkner Words and music writing competition. She is currently completing *Captive,* a memoir about her experience of being both a nurse and a patient. Her book of poems, *Body Parts,* is forthcoming by Zona Rosa Books.

ANNE WENZEL has an advanced degree in science writing from Johns Hopkins University and an MFA in creative nonfiction writing from Sarah Lawrence College. Originally from Mobile, Alabama, she now resides in New Rochelle, New York.

PENNY WOLFSON is a faculty member in creative writing at Sarah Lawrence College. She won a National Magazine Award for an essay that appeared in *The Atlantic Monthly* in 2001; her memoir, *Moonrise,* was based on that article and was published by St. Martin's in 2003. Her work has appeared in the *New York Times,* the *Washington Post, Exceptional Parent, Good Housekeeping, Chelsea, Iris: A Journal of Women,* and *Kaleidoscope: International Journal of Art and Disability.* She has been anthologized in both *Best American Essays* (2002) and *Best American Magazine Writing* (2002). Her essay was adapted from a talk given at the University of Virginia Medical School in April 2004.

# Permissions and Acknowledgments

Joan Baranow: "Watching the Laparoscopy," originally published in *Western Humanities Review* 49.4 (1995), reprinted with permission of the author; "Follicles," originally published in *Feminist Studies* 23.2 (Summer 1997), reprinted with permission of *Feminist Studies Inc.* and the author.

Cortney Davis: "Anorexia," originally published in the *Women's Review of Books* 14.7 (April 1997), reprinted with permission of the author; "It Is August 24th," originally published in *Calyx: A Journal of Art and Literature by Women* 20.1 (Summer 2001), reprinted with permission of the author.

Angelee Deodhar: "Storm Warning," previously published in *frogpond* 20:2 (1997), and "Eight Hours," previously published in *frogpond* 20.3 (Dec. 1997), reprinted with permission of the author.

Diane Driedger: "Give my Regrets," from the chapbook *The Mennonite Madonna* (Canadian Scholars' Press Inc./Women's Press, 1999), reprinted with permission of Canadian Scholars' Press Inc./Women's Press and the author.

Patricia Dunn: "Pure and Predictable," originally published in *Women's eNews* (11 Feb. 2004) with the title "My Name Means Pure, Says Egyptian Mother-in-Law"), reprinted with permission of *Women's eNews* <www.womenseNews.org>.

Mary Lowenthal Felstiner: "Casing My Joints: A Private and Public Story of Arthritis" (now titled "Casing the Joints: A Story of Arthritis"), originally published in *Feminist Studies* 26.2 (Summer 2002), reprinted with permission of *Feminist Studies Inc.*

Katrina Haslip's "Forward" (reprinted in full within the essay "Stories from the Inside" by Kathy Boudin), originally published in *Breaking the Walls of Silence: AIDS and Women in a New York State Maximum-Security Prison* (1998), reprinted with permission of the Overlook Press, New York.

Donna Henderson: "Vigils, III," originally published in a limited edition self-published chapbook, reprinted with permission of the author.

Carol Levine: "Night Shift," originally published in *Ms.* magazine, (Aug./Sept. 2000), reprinted with permission of *Ms.* magazine and the author.

Veneta Masson: "Pathology Report," originally published in the *Annals of Internal Medicine* 117 (1992), reprinted with permission of *Annals of Internal Medicine* and the author.

Rachel Naomi Remen: "A Front Row Seat," from *Kitchen Table Wisdom*, reprinted with permission of Riverhead Books, an imprint of Penguin Group (USA) Inc.

Laura Rothenberg: "My So-Called Lungs" is the audio diary of Laura Rothenberg. The story was produced by Joe Richman and Radio Diaries, and originally broadcast on National Public Radio. To hear Laura's diary and for more information visit: www.radiodiaries.org

Kate A. Scannell: "Leave of Absence," originally published in the *Annals of Internal Medicine* 132 (2000), reprinted by permission of *Annals of Internal Medicine* and the author.

Lynne Sharon Schwartz: "So You're Going to Have a New Body," from the book *The Melting Pot and Other Subversive Stories* (Harper and Row, 1987), reprinted with permission of the author.

Patricia B. Stanley: "The Patient's Voice: A Cry in Solitude or a Call for Community" (revised and now titled "The Female Voice in Illness: An Antidote to Alienation, a Call for Connection"), originally published in *Literature and Medicine* 23.2 (Fall 2004), reprinted with permission of the Johns Hopkins University Press.

Anne Webster: "Doppelgänger," originally published in *Intensive Care: More Poetry and Prose by Nurses* (University of Iowa Press, 2003), reprinted with permission of University of Iowa Press and the author.

# Index

やの

*Literature and Medicine Series*

Editors Carol Donley and Martin Kohn are cofounders of the Center for Literature, Medicine, and Biomedical Humanities at Hiram College. Since 1990 the Center has brought humanities and the health care professions together in mutually enriching interactions, including interdisciplinary courses, summer symposia, and the Literature and Medicine book series from The Kent State University Press.

The first three anthologies in the series grew out of courses in the Biomedical Humanities Program at Hiram. Then the series expanded to include original writing and edited collections by physicians, nurses, humanities scholars, and artists. The books in the series are designed to serve as resouces and texts for health care education as well as for the general public.